RENAL AND UROLOGIC DISORDERS

ISSUES IN DIALYSIS

RENAL AND UROLOGIC DISORDERS

Additional books in this series can be found on Nova's website
under the Series tab.

Additional E-books in this series can be found on Nova's website
under the E-book tab.

Renal and Urologic Disorders

Issues in Dialysis

Stephen Z. Fadem
Editor

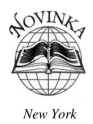

New York

Copyright © 2013 by Nova Science Publishers, Inc.

All rights reserved. No part of this book may be reproduced, stored in a retrieval system or transmitted in any form or by any means: electronic, electrostatic, magnetic, tape, mechanical photocopying, recording or otherwise without the written permission of the Publisher.

For permission to use material from this book please contact us:
Telephone 631-231-7269; Fax 631-231-8175
Web Site: http://www.novapublishers.com

NOTICE TO THE READER

The Publisher has taken reasonable care in the preparation of this book, but makes no expressed or implied warranty of any kind and assumes no responsibility for any errors or omissions. No liability is assumed for incidental or consequential damages in connection with or arising out of information contained in this book. The Publisher shall not be liable for any special, consequential, or exemplary damages resulting, in whole or in part, from the readers' use of, or reliance upon, this material. Any parts of this book based on government reports are so indicated and copyright is claimed for those parts to the extent applicable to compilations of such works.

Independent verification should be sought for any data, advice or recommendations contained in this book. In addition, no responsibility is assumed by the publisher for any injury and/or damage to persons or property arising from any methods, products, instructions, ideas or otherwise contained in this publication.

This publication is designed to provide accurate and authoritative information with regard to the subject matter covered herein. It is sold with the clear understanding that the Publisher is not engaged in rendering legal or any other professional services. If legal or any other expert assistance is required, the services of a competent person should be sought. FROM A DECLARATION OF PARTICIPANTS JOINTLY ADOPTED BY A COMMITTEE OF THE AMERICAN BAR ASSOCIATION AND A COMMITTEE OF PUBLISHERS.

Additional color graphics may be available in the e-book version of this book.

Library of Congress Cataloging-in-Publication Data

Issues in dialysis / editor, Stephen Z. Fadem.
    p. ; cm.
  Includes bibliographical references and index.
  ISBN: 978-1-62417-576-3 (softcover)
  I. Fadem, Stephen Z.
  [DNLM: 1. Renal Dialysis. WJ 378]

  617.461059--dc23

2011040286

Published by Nova Science Publishers, Inc. † New York

Contents

About the Contributors		vii
Acknowledgements		xv
Introduction		xvii
	Tom F. Parker, III	
Chapter I	Milestones in Dialysis	1
	Stephen Z. Fadem	
Chapter II	The Course of Therapy: Changing the Paradigm	35
	Thomas A. Golper and Martin J. Schreiber, Jr.	
Chapter III	Accept This Kidney or Continue Dialysis?	
	A Strategic Approach to Donor Options	49
	Amy L. Friedman	
Chapter IV	Dialysis at Home, the Seattle Experience	65
	Christopher R. Blagg	
Chapter V	How do Clinical Outcomes of Automated Peritoneal	
	Dialysis Compare with those of Continuous	
	Ambulatory Peritoneal Dialysis?	85
	Sunil V. Badve, Carmel M. Hawley and David W. Johnson	
Chapter VI	Intensified Hemodialysis Programs	
	for Children and Adolescents	103
	Julia Thumfart and Dominik Müller	
Chapter VII	The Wearable Artificial Kidney: A Paradigm Change	
	in the Treatment of ESRD	113
	Victor Gura	
Chapter VIII	Is Dialysis Ever an Inappropriate Therapy?	123
	Susan Higley Bray	

Chapter IX	The Pre-Eminent Role for Control of Extra-Cellular Volume in Dialysis Therapy *Richard J. Glassock*	**135**
Chapter X	Mechanisms Causing Muscle Wasting in Kidney Disease and Other Catabolic Conditions *William E. Mitch*	**149**
Chapter XI	The Dysregulated Immune System of Patients on Dialysis *Alexander Grabner, Hermann Pavenstädt, Detlef Lang and Stefan Reuter*	**167**
Chapter XII	Is Serum Albumin a Useful Marker of Nutritional Status in Chronic Kidney Disease? *Allon N. Friedman*	**193**
Chapter XIII	The Chronic Kidney Disease-Mineral Bone Disorder (CKD-MBD) and Vascular Calcification *Keith A. Hruska, Yifu Fan and Toshifumi Sugatani*	**207**
Chapter XIV	Update on Anemia and Kidney Disease *K. M. Goli, A. Pinkhasov, D. L. Landry, Y. Chait, J. Horowitz, C. V. Hollot, R. P. Shrestha and M. J. Germain*	**221**
Chapter XV	Accumulation of Toxic Metals and Trace Elements in Chronic Dialysis Patients *Tzung-Hai Yen, Dan-Tzu Lin-Tan and Ja-Liang Lin*	**251**
Chapter XVI	Adequacy of Dialysis *James Tattersall*	**265**
Chapter XVII	The AV Fistula *Fahad A. Syed and Eric K. Peden*	**295**
Chapter XVIII	Cardiac Surgery in the End-Stage Renal Disease Population: General Considerations, Risk Factors and Clinical Outcomes *Javier E. Anaya-Ayal, Mark G. Davies and Michael J. Reardon*	**309**
Chapter XIX	Assessing Health-Related Quality of Life with the KDQOL-36 *Dori Schatell*	**321**
Chapter XX	Integrated Renal Disease Care *Franklin W. Maddux*	**331**
Index		**341**

About the Contributors

Javier E. Anaya-Ayala, M.D.
Research Fellow, Department of Cardiovascular Surgery
Methodist DeBakey Heart & Vascular Center
The Methodist Hospital, Houston, TX USA
Cardiac Surgery in the End Stage Renal Disease Population: General Considerations, Risk Factors and Clinical Outcomes

Sunil V. Badve, MBBS, M.D., DNB, FRACP
Senior Lecturer, Staff Nephrologist
Department of Nephrology, Princess Alexandra Hospital
School of Medicine, University of Queensland, Brisbane, Australia
How do Clinical Outcomes of Automated Peritoneal Dialysis Compare with those of Continuous Ambulatory Peritoneal Dialysis?

Chris Blagg, M.D.
Professor Emeritus of Medicine, University of Washington Executive Director Emeritus
Northwest Kidney Centers, Seattle, Washington USA
Dialysis at Home - The Seattle Experience

Susan Higley Bray, M.D., MBE, FACP
Clinical Associate Professor of Medicine
Drexel University College of Medicine
Philadelphia, Pennsylvania USA
Is Dialysis Ever An Inappropriate Therapy?

Yossi Chait, PhD
Professor in the Department of Mechanical and Industrial Engineering
University of Massachusetts, Amherst, Massachusetts USA
Update on Anemia and Kidney Disease

Mark G. Davies, M.D., Ph.D., M.B.A.

Professor of Surgery, Weill Medical College of Cornell University
Vice Chairman of Department of Cardiovascular Surgery
Methodist DeBakey Heart & Vascular Center
The Methodist Hospital, Houston, Texas USA
Cardiac Surgery in the End Stage Renal Disease Population: General Considerations, Risk Factors and Clinical Outcomes

Stephen Z. Fadem, M.D., FACP, FASN

Clinical Professor of Medicine, Division of Nephrology
Baylor College of Medicine
Medical Director, Houston Kidney Center/DaVita Integrated Service Network
Chief Medical Officer, Kidney Associates, Houston, Texas USA
Milestones in Dialysis

Yifu Fang, M.D., M.Sc.

Senior Research Technician
Department of Pediatrics
Washington University School of Medicine
St. Louis, Missouri USA
The Chronic Kidney Disease-Mineral Bone Disorder (CKD-MBD) and Vascular Calcification

Allon Friedman, M.D.

Assistant Professor of Medicine, Division of Nephrology
Indiana University School of Medicine
Indianapolis, Indiana USA
Is Serum Albumin a Useful Marker of Nutritional Status in Chronic Kidney Disease?

Amy L. Friedman, M.D., FACS

Director of Transplantation and Professor of Surgery
SUNY Upstate Medical University, Syracuse, New York
Medical Director, Finger Lakes Donor Recovery Network, Rochester, New York USA
Accept this Kidney or Continue Dialysis? A Strategic Approach to Donor Options

Michael J Germain, M.D.

Professor of Medicine Tufts University School of Medicine
Springfield, Massachusetts USA
Update on Anemia and Kidney Disease

Richard J. Glassock, M.D., MACP

Emeritus Professor
David Geffen School of Medicine at UCLA
Los Angeles, California USA
The Pre-eminent Role for Control of Extra-cellular Volume in Dialysis Therapy

Kiran M Goli, M.D.
Clinical Instructor, Tufts University School of Medicine
Baystate Medical Center/Tufts University School of Medicine
Springfield, Massachusetts USA
Update on Anemia and Kidney Disease

Thomas A. Golper, M.D., FACP, FASN
Professor of Medicine
Division of Nephrology and Hypertension
Vanderbilt University Medical Center
Nashville, Tennessee USA
The Course of Therapy – Changing the Paradigm

Alexander Grabner, M.D.
Physician, Nephrology
Department of General Internal Medicine and Nephrology
University Hospital Münster, Münster, Germany
The Dysregulated Immune System of Patients on Dialysis

Victor Gura, M.D.
Clinical Associate Professor
David Geffen School of Medicine at UCLA
Los Angeles, California USA
The Wearable Artificial Kidney – A Paradigm Change in the Treatment of ESRD

Carmel M. Hawley, MBBS, FRACP, MMedSci
Associate Professor of Medicine, Senior Staff Nephrologist
Department of Nephrology, Princess Alexandra Hospital
School of Medicine, University of Queensland, Brisbane, Australia
*How do Clinical Outcomes of Automated Peritoneal Dialysis Compare with those of
    Continuous Ambulatory Peritoneal Dialysis?*

Christopher V. Hollot, PhD
Professor in the Department of Electrical and Computer Engineering
University of Massachusetts, Amherst, Massachusetts USA
Update on Anemia and Kidney Disease

Joseph Horowitz, PhD
Professor Emeritus in the Department of Mathematics and Statistics
University of Massachusetts, Amherst, Massachusetts USA
Update on Anemia and Kidney Disease

Keith A. Hruska, M.D.
Professor of Pediatrics, Medicine and Cell Biology
Director, Pediatric Nephrology Division
Washington University School of Medicine
St. Louis, Missouri USA
The Chronic Kidney Disease-Mineral Bone Disorder (CKD-MBD) and Vascular Calcification

David W. Johnson, MBBS (Hons), FRACP, PhD, PSM
Professor of Medicine and Population Health, Director of Nephrology
School of Medicine, University of Queensland, Brisbane, Australia
Department of Nephrology, Princess Alexandra Hospital, Brisbane, Australia
Director, Metro South and Ipswich Nephrology & Transplant Services (MINTS)
Chair, Queensland Statewide Renal Clinical Network
Co-Director, Centre for Kidney Disease Research
How do Clinical Outcomes of Automated Peritoneal Dialysis Compare with those of Continuous Ambulatory Peritoneal Dialysis?

Daniel L. Landry D.O.
Assistant Professor of Medicine, Tufts School of Medicine
Western New England Renal & Transplant Associates
Springfield, Massachusetts USA
Update on Anemia and Kidney Disease

Detlef Lang, M.D.
Assistant Professor, Nephrology
Department of General Internal Medicine and Nephrology
University Hospital Münster, Münster, Germany
The Dysregulated Immune System of Patients on Dialysis

Ja-Liang Lin, M.D.
Professor of Nephrology and Clinical Toxicology
Chang Gung Memorial Hospital; Chang Gung University and School of Medicine
Taipei, Taiwan Republic of China
Accumulation of Toxic Metals and Trace Elements in Chronic Dialysis Patients

Dan-Tzu Lin-Tan, R.N.
Chang Gung Memorial Hospital; Chang Gung University and School of Medicine
Taipei, Taiwan Republic of China
Accumulation of Toxic Metals and Trace Elements in Chronic Dialysis Patients

Franklin W. Maddux, M.D., FACP
Senior Vice President & Chief Medical Information Officer
Fresenius Medical Care Waltham, Massachusetts USA
Integrated Renal Disease Care

William E. Mitch, M.D.
Gordon A. Cain Chair in Nephrology and Director, Division of Nephrology
Baylor College of Medicine
Houston, Texas USA
Mechanisms causing Muscle Wasting in Kidney Disease and other catabolic conditions

Dominik Müller, M.D.
Consultant,
Department of Pediatric Nephrology
Charité
Berlin, Germany
Intensified Hemodialysis Programs for Children and Adolescents

Tom F. Parker, III, M.D.
Clinical Professor, University of Texas Southwestern Medical School
Consultant, Baylor University Medical Center
Chief Medical Officer, Renal Ventures Management
Dallas, TX
Introduction

Hermann Pavenstädt, M.D.
Professor, Nephrology
Department of General Internal Medicine and Nephrology
University Hospital Münster, Münster, Germany
The Dysregulated Immune System of Patients on Dialysis

Eric K. Peden, M.D.
Chief of Vascular Surgery
Assistant Professor of Cardiovascular Surgery
Weill Medical College of Cornell University
The Methodist Hospital. Houston, Texas USA
The AV Fistula

Arkadiy Pinkhasov M.D.
Clinical Instructor, Tufts University School of Medicine
Baystate Medical Center/Tufts University School of Medicine
Springfield, Massachusetts USA
Update on Anemia and Kidney Disease

Michael J. Reardon, M.D.
Professor of Surgery, Weill Medical College of Cornell University
Senior Attending Surgeon of Department of Cardiovascular Surgery
Methodist DeBakey Heart & Vascular Center
The Methodist Hospital. Houston, Texas USA
Cardiac Surgery in the End Stage Renal Disease Population: General Considerations, Risk Factors and Clinical Outcomes

Stefan Reuter, M.D.
Assistant Professor, Nephrology
Department of General Internal Medicine and Nephrology
University Hospital Münster, Münster, Germany
The Dysregulated Immune System of Patients on Dialysis

Fahad A. Syed, M.D.
CV Surgery Research Fellow
The Methodist Hospital, Houston, Texas USA
The AV Fistula

Dorian Schatell, M.S.
Executive Director, Medical Education Institute, Inc.
Madison, Wisconsin USA
Assessing Quality of Life with the KDQOL-36

Martin J. Schreiber, Jr., M.D.
Vice Chair, Glickman Urological and Kidney Institute
Chairman, Department of Nephrology and Hypertension
Cleveland Clinic, Cleveland, Ohio USA
The Course of Therapy – Changing the Paradigm

Rajiv P. Shrestha MS
Doctoral student in the Department of Mechanical and Industrial Engineering
University of Massachusetts, Amherst, Massachusetts USA
Update on Anemia and Kidney Disease

Toshifumi Sugatani, D.D.S., Ph.D.
Research Instructor,
Department of Pediatrics
Washington University School of Medicine
St. Louis, Missouri USA
*The Chronic Kidney Disease-Mineral Bone Disorder (CKD-MBD) and Vascular
    Calcification*

James Tattersall, MBBS, M.D., MRCP
Staff Grade Nephrologist
Department of Renal Medicine, Leeds Teaching Hospitals
Leeds, United Kingdom
Medical Director and software developer
Mediqal Health Informatics Limited, Stevenage, United Kingdom
Adequacy of Dialysis

Julia Thumfart, M.D.
Consultant
Department of Pediatric Nephrology
Charité
Berlin, Germany
Intensified Hemodialysis Programs for Children and Adolescents

Tzung-Hai Yen, M.D., PhD.
Associate Professor of Nephrology
Chang Gung Memorial Hospital; Chang Gung University and School of Medicine
Taipei, Taiwan Republic of China
Accumulation of Toxic Metals and Trace Elements in Chronic Dialysis Patients

Acknowledgments

This book stands as a combination of major efforts by several authors, each with a level of expertise, dedication and experience to discuss an area of topical concern in depth. To these authors, not only for their personal contributions, but also for reviewing the other chapters, I am grateful. I would especially like to thank Tom Parker, Richard Glassock and Chris Blagg for their superb guidance and the suggestions they offered.

I would also like to acknowledge other reviewers, namely Allen Nissenson and Fred Finkelstein for their insights and perspectives. The partners at Kidney Associates, Ruth Wintz, Han Dang, Dana Mitchell, Joey Buquing, Emil Abdulhayoglu and Wasae Tabibi, and our physician assistant, Cassie Brown greatly helped to make this book practical and meaningful for nephrologists and clinicians.

The assistance of Ronica Bandel, Charlotte Hicks, and Rany Heng has been invaluable in producing this book. Also, the team at Nova Science Publishers, particularly Carra Feagaiga, Nick Longo, Alexandra Columbus and Donna Dennis have been extremely supportive in shepherding me through this process and helping make this book possible.

Finally, I would like to thank my wife, Joyce for her encouragement and support, and as well as for proofreading text and offering valuable suggestions. She and my family have demonstrated extraordinary patience and understanding in letting me devote a disproportionate fraction of my time to the preparation of this book.

Introduction

Tom F. Parker, III

Baylor University Medical Center, Dallas, Texas US
University of Texas Southwestern School of Medicine, Dallas, Texas US
Renal Ventures Management. Lakewood, Colorado, US

The prospect for survival from "end-stage" renal disease (ESRD) was dramatically addressed in a conference held in Dallas, TX in 1989. For the first time, the nephrology community faced the unacceptable outcomes, at that time, for patients undergoing dialytic renal replacement therapy. Since, despite vast improvements in technology, introduction of exciting pharmaceuticals, the development of clinical performance guidelines (CPGs) and clinical performance measures (CPMs), close oversight by governmental regulators, development of widespread protocols by multi-national companies and expert panels and ongoing concern expressed on the 10th and 20th anniversaries of that hallmark meeting, the outcomes that really count have only shown minimal improvement.

Of course we have improved the quantification of dialysis, anemia and metabolic bone disease control and access to care; entities such as aluminum toxicity and uremic neuropathy have virtually disappeared. Vast improvements in water preparation have decreased exposure to pyrogens and other inorganic toxins. Yet, hospitalizations remain essentially unchanged (2 per patient per year) in spite of many procedures now performed on an outpatient basis. Hospital days remain at about 2 weeks per year, mortality is still above 20% and the costs per patient and for the overall ESRD program are enormous (over $40,000,000,000 per year.) This is neither acceptable nor sustainable.

Yet, this is one of those moments in time when there is a convergence of forces, where science and necessity are merging to allow (force) outcomes to vastly improve. There is a marvelous passage in the book *Solar* by Ian Mc Ewan, "Sometimes in a grave situation, even a crisis, we understand, sometimes too late, that it is not in other people or in the system or in the nature of things that the problem lays, but in ourselves, our own follies and unexamined assumptions. And second, there are moments when the acquisition of new information forces us to make a fundamental reinterpretation of our situation." Mr. McEwan goes on to note, and I paraphrase: The Stone Age didn't end because of shortage of stones. The Stone Age ended because we had new information. [1]

And so it is. We now have the information to transform outcomes, paying very close attention to those entities that cause the greatest harm to our patient. Absolutely we must continue to pay attention to those traditional CPMs. After all, this is what continuous quality improvement is all about. Fix one thing and another will emerge needing to be fixed. But while we pay attention to these, we now know there are very large problems and we have the solutions.

We know that we must save the left ventricle at all costs and that the current model in which the majority of dialysis is delivered even worsens it. Our patients die of volume overload and the associated damage to the left ventricle and resulting fibrosis. Chapter 9 by Richard Glassock points out how to fix this. This one entity is responsible for about 40% of all deaths.

We know that the second cause of death is infection and that the source of that infection, in most cases, is the catheter. We recognize this to be an iatrogenic issue and we know how to fix it.

We know that huge numbers of patients die in the first year of care, especially in the first 120 days. Yes, many of those patients should not have initiated dialysis in the first place - palliative care having been more appropriate, as discussed in Chapter 8, by Susan Bray. But for the remainder, we know how to fix that.

We know that our patients are inflamed, but we know how to ameliorate that in part. And we know that that will lead to better nutrition. Chapters 10 through 12 address this.

We know these things and many others.

Given this, why indeed must change occur? Because it's the right thing to do. And, looming on the horizon are models of care that will not tolerate the current rate of hospitalizations, the lack of rehabilitation, the exorbitant costs. We have to apply the science to meet the personal needs of our patients and the social needs of our community.

Stephen Fadem has chosen authors to address these issues crisply and with the understanding that change must occur. Included in this textbook is the prospect of emerging modalities associated with bio-membranes, nano-technology breakthroughs, changes in the acquisition process of organs for transplantation, longer and more frequent treatments.

Perhaps it was best said by Albert Einstein: "(Our) world is (what it is), not because of those who do bad things, but because of those who look on and do nothing." Do not do nothing.

References

[1] Mc Ewan I. Solar. London: Random House Group Ltd; 2010.

In: Issues in Dialysis
Editor: Stephen Z. Fadem

ISBN: 978-1-62417-576-3
© 2013 Nova Science Publishers, Inc.

Chapter I

Milestones in Dialysis

Stephen Z. Fadem[*]
Nephrology Division, Baylor College of Medicine, Houston, Texas, US
Kidney Associates, Houston, Texas, US
Houston Kidney Center Integrated Service Network, Houston, Texas, US

Abstract

Dialysis has reached many milestones in its nearly 200 year course. It started with observations by Richard Bright and Thomas Graham that described the underlying causes and potential therapy for chronic kidney disease. Yet, treatment had to wait around 100 years until advancements in membrane technology and coagulation would make it practical. Willem Kolff is credited with inventing the dialysis machine in 1943. Until the discovery of practical access methods, it could only be regarded as a therapy for acute kidney injury or a stopgap for patients awaiting a kidney transplant. Belding Scribner deserves credit for developing a practical way to provide chronic dialysis therapy. As need and demand quickly outgrew capacity, home dialysis became a viable option. The engineering triumph of the single pass system dialysis machine lent itself well to the home machine, but became the prototype for center therapy as well. The development of a commercial infrastructure made dialysis easily accessible throughout the USA, and was followed by the only Medicare legislation ever passed to solely insure therapy for a specific disease. Advances, such as more efficient dialyzers followed the development of hollow fiber technology. Peritoneal dialysis has shown great promise, but it is still underutilized. Economic challenges led to the first wave of payment reform, the composite rate in 1983, but threatened dialysis quality. The new era of restrictive funding saw the development of Kt/V - a marker for adequacy, the USRDS - a national registry, and the NKF K/DOQI Guidelines. A major advance, the genetic engineering of human erythropoietin, improved the quality of life, but added greatly to the cost burden. Legislation was passed to bundle the costs of this therapy and other ancillary services with the composite rate around the same time as the conditions for coverage were updated to provide structure for the regulatory oversight of quality. The discovery of the

---

[*] Correspondence to: Stephen Z. Fadem, M.D., Kidney Associates, 6624 Fannin, Suite 1400, Houston, Texas 77030. Telephone 713-795-5511. Email: fadem@bcm.edu.

mechanisms causing vascular calcification and cardiac disease is ongoing. As the population of dialysis patients ages, guidelines developed by the Renal Physician's Association are proving necessary to help clinicians assess prognosis and the appropriateness of care. The challenges of providing quality, covering the vast need for service and meeting economic demands has created the many issues that form the topics of this chapter, as well as this book.

Table 1. Milestones in Dialysis

MILESTONES IN DIALYSIS

Milestone 1: Dialysis discovered by Thomas Graham (1861)
Milestone 2: Heparin (1916)
Milestone 3: Cellophane for dialysis (1937)
Milestone 4: The first practical dialysis machine (1943)
Milestone 5: Kidney transplantation (1954)
Milestone 6: Developing The Arteriovenous Access (1960)
Milestone 7: Home Dialysis (1960s)
Milestone 8: Hollow Fibers And Membrane Technology (1960s)
Milestone 9: Infrastructure For Dialysis Development – National Medical Care (1960s)
Milestone 10: Social Security Amendment Of 1973 (1973)
Milestone 11: Peritoneal Dialysis (1978)
Milestone 12: Omnibus Budget Reconciliation Act (OBRA) (1981)
Milestone 13: Kt/V (1985)
Milestone 14: USRDS – OBRA 1986
Milestone 15: Erythropoiesis Stimulating Agents (ESAs) (1989)
Milestone 16: The National Kidney Foundation K-DOQI Guidelines
Milestone 17: Chronic Kidney Disease - Mineral Bone Disorders (CKD-MBD) (2005)
Milestone 18: Conditions For Coverage (2008)
Milestone 19: Medicare Improvements For Patients And Providers Act (MIPPA) (2008)
Milestone 20: RPA Guidelines - Appropriate Dialysis (2010)

Introduction

The history of the management of renal failure has been an amazing journey that spans nearly two hundred years. While appreciation of this journey may be nostalgic for those who have grown up with the availability of dialysis, it is much more in that it lends great insights that make our profession more lucid to those entering it. Our journey is defined by a landscape, upon which is set distinctive milestones marking major advancements. Throughout the nearly seventy year history of dialysis, and fifty years of chronic dialysis therapy for end-stage renal disease, economics intermingled with technology and need for care have played key roles. As we enter a new era of enduring cost-cutting pressures, these early experiences will seem to some like déjà vu. Through the discussion of these milestones one can gain insights that will aid in understanding the issues presented in this book.

The milestones (Table 1) intersperse discovery, development, implementation, and ethics. There is always the interplay between cost and technology. Initially, these milestones take us from insight and discovery to the practical application of therapies. Later milestones mark overcoming ethical hurdles and the development of corporate and legislative infrastructures. As the therapy matures, milestones mark meeting economic challenges and developing data registries. They denote the introduction of novel therapies and advances. We end by introducing a reasonable solution to the major ethical challenge facing us – providing appropriate care.

Milestone 1 – Thomas Graham Discovers Dialysis (1861)

In the 1820s and 1830s, the English physician, Richard Bright of Guy's Hospital in London, did pioneering work on the etiology of "dropsy" or edema, and identified that in some forms it is associated with "albumen" in the urine. Bright's Disease is an old term for glomerulonephritis, and memorializes Bright as the father of nephrology. Equally as important, Bright, along with George Owen Rees recognized the retention of urea in kidney disease. [1] He also noted that some patients with nephritis had left ventricular hypertrophy. [2] By 1839, it was becoming established that kidney disease was associated by the retention of urea, a nitrogenous substance known to be present in urine. [3] Almost parallel with the observations of Bright, Thomas Graham of Glasgow discovered that colloids could be separated from crystalloids using a "semipermeable membrane" or "dialyzer." He demonstrated that urea and sodium chloride could pass through a membrane, were both elements of urine, and could be separated from blood. [4,5]

In 1861, Graham coined the term "dialysis." Yet, despite knowledge of this concept, successful treatment for uremia was not available for nearly 100 years. The disappointment is understandable in that early membrane experiments were performed with tissues from animal internal organs, and while in vitro, peritoneal membranes could effectively separate blood from electrolytes and urea, and could prove the concept well, decay and putrefaction prevented their practical application in a clinical device. [3] Thus, the application of this early principle would have to await the emergence of suitable synthetic or chemically altered substances. An alternative therapy, restricting dietary protein intake was also tried. The low protein diet was probably introduced in the late 1800s by Mariano Semmola [6] and culminated in a popular, but relatively unsuccessful form of therapy, the Giovannetti diet, introduced in 1964. [7] By then, advances in therapy that were to an impact on shaping the landscape that defines the clinical practice of kidney disease were on their way.

Milestone 2: Heparin (1916)

In 1913, John Jacob Abel of Johns Hopkins University attempted to direct blood outside the body through collodion membranes. [8] Abel's anticoagulant was prepared from leeches, and known as hirudin, but was too toxic to be practical for human use. In 1924, George Haas also tried to perform dialysis in humans using collodion membranes, and was the first to use heparin as an anticoagulant.

The sulfated glycosaminoglycan, heparin, was first isolated from the canine liver in 1916, hence its name – (hepar is Greek for liver). Its odyssey in revolutionizing health care as we know it today can be the subject of another treatise. This strongly negatively charged molecule occurs naturally in vertebrates and some non-vertebrates. It is a misnomer that it should be called heparin, however, in that the yield is much higher from lung and intestines. Its isolation was first accomplished by a second year medical student, Jay McLean, in the laboratories of William Henry Howell at Johns Hopkins University. Howell was searching for thromboplastins at the time, and sent his student to look for natural anticoagulants. Howell was initially surprised that the liver "phoshatid" was an anticoagulant, and not a procoagulant as he had anticipated. In 1928, it was shown that heparin was not a phosphorus-containing lipid, but a highly sulfated glycosaminoglycan. Efforts at purification were delayed for several years because the original publications reported its primary production was the liver, not the intestine. Luckily, its therapeutic value was being explored during the period when techniques for its production were being developed. Leonard Roundtree, who had by now relocated at the Mayo Clinic, but had previously worked with John Jacob Abel at Johns Hopkins, was interested in the role of the anticoagulant in therapy of pulmonary embolism. Despites its experimental use, heparin was not commercially practical for clinical use until 1937; [9] its introduction paralleling the practical use of cellophane as a dialyzer membrane that year. Charles Best, who was renowned for discovering insulin, played a role in developing methods for standardization and purification of heparin, and confirmed that it should be isolated from the intestines and lung, and not liver. [9]

Milestone 3: Cellophane for Dialysis (1937)

Collodion is made by reacting nitric acid with cellulose in cotton or wood, creating the highly explosive component of dynamite, guncotton, or nitrocellulose. When dissolved in ether and ethyl alcohol, the product dries as a thin film. This film, though flammable, was used in early photography and the early film industry. " Abel probably chose collodion because Adolf Fick had used it for in vitro dialysis in 1855, and it was used to impregnate filter paper in 1907. Abel's experiments with collodion were in animals. However, his efforts, as well as those of his team, Benjamin Turner and Leonard Roundtree were noteworthy in demonstrating that endogenous substances could be removed by dialysis. The dialyzer they developed became a very early prototype for future devices. The story of their "vividiffusion" experiments on dogs was published in *The Times* of London on August 11, 1913. It was in this article that the term "artificial kidney" was first used, and was followed by an article published January 18, 1914 in The *New York Times*, entitled "Machine Purifies Blood and Restores it to the Body." [8] Despite its promise as a blood purification membrane, the stability of collodion was poor. The product was fragile and unstable; it had to be prepared immediately before use. Hence, collodion film was not practical for commercial application and advancement in membrane stability was essential for dialysis to become a reality.

Cellophane was just being developed at the time of Abel's work, and had been patented the year before by Jacques E. Brandenberger. It was used primarily to wrap Whitman candy in the well-known and still popular Whitman Sampler. It was not waterproof, ironically, unless sprayed with nitrocellulose. Nitrocellulose and its by products were always of interest to E.I. du Pont de Nemours and Company (DuPont), a major manufacturer of gunpowder and dynamite. In 1924, DuPont opened a US plant to inexpensively manufacture cellophane, although the process was not perfected until 1927. After 1927, it no longer needed to be imported from Europe, and quickly found its way into commercial packaging. In 1925, Edmund O. Freund of Chicago discovered regenerated cellulose tubing was more suitable than purified animal intestines for sausage casing. In 1927, he founded The Visking Company, and introduced cellophane tubing to the sausage packing industry. The term "visking tubing" remains in use for dialysis membranes made of regenerated cellulose or cellophane. The term Cellophane^{TM} was registered as a trademark of DuPont. As its price fell and its popularity rose, it became the logical choice as a potential dialysis membrane substitute for collodion. Perhaps, this should seem less a coincidence in that heparin forms a suitable anticoagulant on the surface of medical materials such as glass and plastics. In 1937, William Thalheimer [10] demonstrated that dialysis worked well with the cellophane sausage casing he acquired from the Visking Company. His major interest was in blood transfusion and exchange transfusion, and even considered exchange transfusion with heparinized blood as a potential treatment for uremia in dogs. His construction of an artificial kidney of cellophane that would work for 3 to 5 hours in dogs to remove urea was a vital contribution to the field of dialysis. [9]

Milestone 4: The First Practical Dialysis Machine (1943)

The first practical dialysis machine, developed by Willem "Pim" Kolff (Figure 1) of the Netherlands between 1939 and 1943, consisted of a rotating drum wrapped with 20 meters of cellophane sausage casing. The dimensions of this membrane were calculated by Kolff to be sufficient to remove an adequate amount of urea. During the time of its development, the Nazis invaded the Netherlands, necessitating Kolff to also contribute his creativity and skill to the war effort. He has been credited with setting up the first blood bank in Europe, and has always claimed his experiences of handling blood outside the body gave him added confidence when working with the artificial kidney. [3] In 1943 the first person, a 29-year-old homemaker with malignant hypertension was treated with 12 courses for kidney failure with this prototype, but ultimately died. Kolff did not achieve success until 1945. [11]

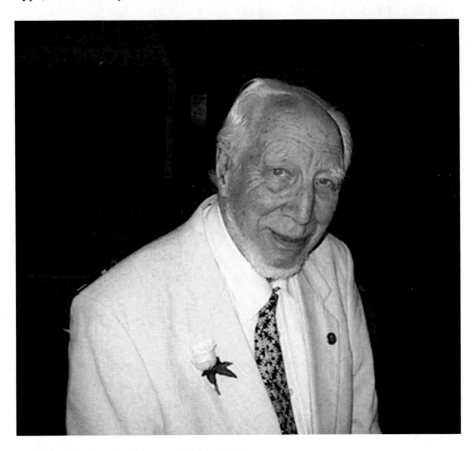

Figure 1. Willem Kolff. (Photo by Stephen Z. Fadem, MD.)

This machine used glucose to increase the osmotic gradient across the membrane, creating a risk that serum glucose could rise. Later research would culminate in more ideal dialysates. Kolff's device became popular in the USA. In 1947, Isadore Snapper of Mt. Sinai Hospital in New York, a legendary physician in his own right, invited Willem Kolff to visit and to set up a dialysis program. George Thorn, the Hersey Professor of Medicine at Peter Bent Brigham Hospital visited Mt. Sinai Hospital to witness the Kolff machine, and invited him to "The Brigham" to help develop a second-generation machine. Many of the duties related to dialysis management were assigned to his resident, John Merrill (Figure 2). The result was the Kolff-Brigham Kidney, built of stainless steel by Edmund Olson and Carl Walter (Figure 3). This machine was considered a "deluxe toy" by many skeptics, among who were some of the most prominent leaders in medicine of the time. Both John Peters and Louis Welt, representing the height of early scientific investigation in this infant specialty, questioned the utility of dialysis. Despite skepticism, the device was ultimately shipped to various centers around the world. Early hemodialysis was proven successful in treating acute kidney injury during the Korean War, and was well along its way as the main therapy for acute kidney injury. John Merrill went on to help shape and develop the new specialty of nephrology, not only serving as a pioneer in dialysis and transplantation, but also in training future physicians who would not only apply this new, innovative technology, but also assure its widespread adoption. [12] Merrill's dream was initially that in addition to acute care, dialysis would be useful as a stopgap measure for a revolutionary procedure developed at his hospital, transplantation.

Milestone 5: Kidney Transplantation (1954)

The next advance was the development of kidney transplantation, and the discovery of the role the immune system would play in its success or failure. This milestone took place in 1954 with the successful transplant of a kidney in an identical twin by Joseph Murray and his team at The Peter Bent Brigham Hospital in Boston. [13] This helped substantiate the notion it was immune system rejection causing previous kidneys to fail. To tackle these immune system challenges, the team performed a series of transplants using various combinations of irradiation and corticosteroids. It was the development of tissue typing, and by 1962 the introduction of immunosuppressive medications, that made kidney transplantation a more reliable option. [14] The next milestone of the Brigham team was to successfully perform a cadaveric kidney transplant, which they did in 1963. Transplantation opened the door to an entirely new field of medicine.

Milestone 6: Developing the Arteriovenous Access (1960)

Although viable for acute therapy, the landscape in the 1950s was not at all conducive for chronic therapy. The major challenge to the care of the end stage renal disease patient was access to the circulation. Were it not for the emergence of a variety of "plastic" polymers after World War II, dialysis as we know it today would not be possible. These advances in synthetic materials mirror several of the milestones that mark our dialysis story. Repeated dialysis treatments would require that the conduit between the dialysis system and the patient's circulation be nonreactive with body tissues, resist clotting, and easy to connect with existing equipment. In 1960, Belding Scribner, a professor at the University of Washington in Seattle worked with Wayne Quinton, an instrument maker, to develop a U-shaped shunt devised of a slippery fluorinated ethylene plastic that was becoming widely used in industry – and the kitchen – as a non-stick coating. This DuPont plastic, now well known as Teflon®, was at that time being primarily used as an insulator for pacemaker wires. Teflon was deemed ideal by Scribner because it would not react with tissues. Surprisingly, its non-stick properties made it useful by preventing clotting. The first patient, a machinist, Clyde Shields was initiated on dialysis March 9, 1960 with this prototype. His ultimate survival heralded the beginning of a new era in the management of kidney failure. This shunt only lasted four months before it had to be replaced. [15] Shields lived for 11 more years. Later, Wayne Quinton used a more flexible plastic – a silicone elastomer trademarked Silastic,® which when combined with Teflon tips in the body of the "Scribner Shunt" greatly extended its life. [16] The shunt achieved wide use well into the late 1970s.

In 1961, Stanley Shaldon, who started his career as a hepatologist at the Royal Free Infirmary in London, was placed in charge of the hospital's dialysis machine by his professor, Sheila Sherlock. Although initial patients were connected via the "Scribner Shunt," Shaldon was successful in pioneering the use of silicone-Teflon femoral catheter. Economic necessity, like advancing technology will prove to be a recurring theme shaping the practical application of dialysis. As his hospital would only purchase three twin-coil dialyzers per month, he developed a protocol to reuse dialyzers. [17]

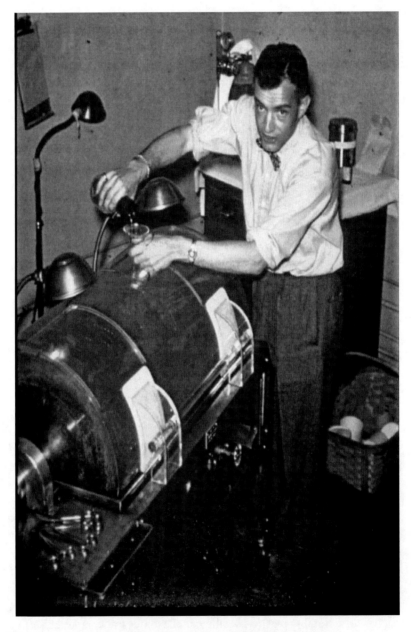

Figure 2. John P. Merrill preparing the dialysate bath for the Kolff-Brigham Kidney. (Photo by Eli A. Friedman, MD.)

The arteriovenous communication known as a traumatic arteriovenous fistula can occur as the result of healing military wounds. James Cimino, who had previously worked as a phlebotomist, observed that soldiers returning from the Korean War with traumatic fistulae were very easy to cannulate. Working with Kenneth Appel and Michael Brescia, the Brecia-Cimino fistula was developed at the Bronx Veterans Administration Hospital in 1962 and refined by 1966. [18,19] It is still the preferred means of dialysis today, replacing earlier access initiatives, also pioneered by Wayne Quinton. It is preferred over the synthetic arteriovenous graft as the therapy of choice due to its native endurance and decreased propensity to clot, stenose or become infected. In 1969, Wilbert H. Gore, patented his work on tetraflouroethylene polymers as a sealant. Later, along with Rowena Taylor and Robert Gore, his son, he discovered the process for making these polymers porous and "breathable," yet water resistant. As the story goes, they attempted to stretch the polymer as far as they could, but instead of fracturing, it returned to its former shape more porous and with unique properties. They patented their product, GORE-TEX. (USPTO 3,953,966), and initially promoted it as ideal for electrical insulation, and as a pipe-sealant. GORE-TEX is widely used in sportswear and raingear, but is also highly suitable for implantable devices. In 1981, Gore developed a cardiovascular patch using GORE-TEX and since then, this material enjoyed wide use as the material of choice for the arteriovenous graft. Its popularity has recently dwindled because it does not last as long as a well-placed AV fistula, but is still one of the mainstays of dialysis in cases where the fistula is not suitable. [20] In 2006 Flixene, a third generation porous polytetrafluroethylene laminate [21] was approved by the FDA. It may prove superior to GORE-TEX for implantable vascular grafts as it is claimed that it can be cannulated within 24 to 72 hours. [22]

Milestone 7: Home Dialysis (1960s)

The first proportioning machine was from the University of Washington Hospital, and was devised to mix concentrate with water centrally and proportion it to each machine. Albert "Les" Babb, Professor of Chemical and Nuclear Engineering at the University of Washington, developed the proportioning technology that was used. The in-center machine along with its proportioning system was known as "The Monster." The capacity to of the small center to provide dialysis services was exceeded soon after opening, and the need for home dialysis equipment arose out of necessity – and emotion.

A16-year-old girl, Caroline Helm, (see picture in Chapter 4) was never eligible for review by a selection committee in Seattle as she was under the required age of 18. This led to the development by Babb of a single-patient proportioning system with monitors and safety devices. So the story goes, the young girl was the daughter of an acquaintance of Babb. The original "Mini-1" was built for her by Dr. Babb's staff, and was a miniature version of the Monster. The Milton Roy Company got the contract from the University of Washington to build the "Mini-2" in 1964. It used a Kiil Dialyzer, and was designed exclusively for home dialysis; it even had wood veneer so that it would match furniture in the house. Milton-Roy ultimately joint-ventured with Extracorporeal and was acquired by Johnson & Johnson, but then sold to Delmed in 1984. This negative pressure machine evolved into Baxter-Travenol SPS machines that culminated in the Baxter Arena dialysis machine. [23-26]

The design and concept behind the dialysis machines used today in dialysis centers was based upon original machines intended for home use. Recently, interest in home dialysis has been reborn, not only out of economic necessity, but because of patient preference. New models for personal dialysis machines were designed initially by Aksys Ltd. and more recently by NxStage Medical, Inc.

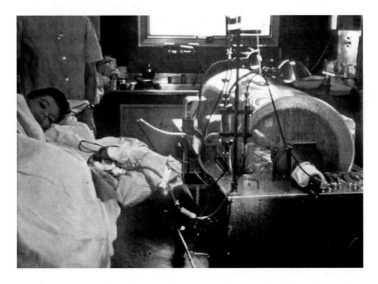

Figure 3. The Brigham Dialysis Unit in Use (note the gauze at the coupling).
(Photo by Eli A. Friedman, MD.)

In 1963, a 30 year old draftsman in London, who after becoming uremic, was referred to the Royal Free Hospital, where he was treated with a low sodium diet and hospital-based daily self-dialysis. He improved and was discharged on twice weekly 12 hour dialysis, totally dialyzing himself using reusable coil dialyzers. He was maintained on a 22 mEq sodium diet, which was not unusual in 1963. The patient was able to return to work, and the following year fathered another child. [27] His success underscored the value of dialysis, and the feasibility of self-care. In 1964, the Royal Free Hospital started their home dialysis program and in 1965, Shaldon reported unattended overnight self-care dialysis using the pump-free Kiil dialyzer and the Scribner Shunt. [16]

The home dialysis experience was most successful in Seattle, as well as in London. [28,29] In Chapter 4 of this book, Chris Blagg provides a first-hand account of some of the historical events, which were mentioned above.

Milestone 8: Hollow Fibers (1960s) and Membrane Technology

Equally, significant advancements in plastics technology enabled both reverse osmosis, widely used to generate pure water, and the dialyzer. The story of dialyzers is fascinating, and has been recounted in a historical perspective by Zbylut Twardowski, one of the premier pioneers in dialysis technology. [3]

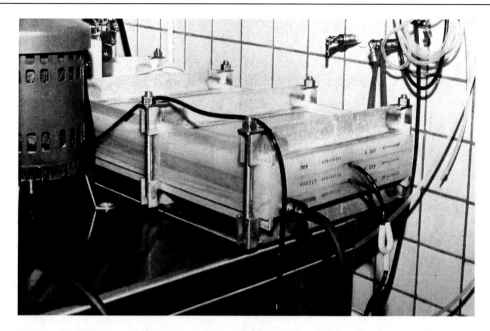

Figure 4. The Kiil Dialyzer as modified by Belding Scribner. (Photo courtesy Chris Blagg, MD, University of Washington, Seattle.)

In addition to the contributions of Kolff, Nils Alwall had been working on dialysis in Lund, Sweden since the 1940s. His efforts were independent and parallel to those of Kolff insofar as he also developed an artificial kidney and an early prototype dialyzer. With his dialyzer, cellophane was wrapped around a coil over which was placed a support. Thus, the Alwall method, which introduced ultrafiltration, was more successful in treating fluid overload than the Kolff rotating drum dialyzer. [16]

Leonard Skeggs and Jack Leonard of Case Western Reserve University in Cleveland, Ohio collaborated to develop a more portable, compact dialyzer. By 1948, they were able to modify the earlier prototypes by wrapping cellulose between parallel plates. The parallel plate dialyzer was the first to use negative pressure, and was an advance in that it enabled a more successful control of volume. This dialyzer was used by Scribner in 1960 when he dialyzed Clyde Shields.

Skeggs, who worked in a hospital laboratory, then moved on to develop the SMA-12 autoanalyzer, which he sold to the Technicon Corporation. This device was revolutionary in that it automated the analysis of blood chemistries. Ironically, advancements in nephrology could have never been possible were it not for this concomitant contribution to laboratory science. The autoanalyzer technique was ultimately applied by Skeggs to flame photometry, a technique already in use by John Peters of Yale in the 1940s for the measurement of sodium and potassium. This made the measurement of electrolytes practical for the members of the new specialty. [30]

In 1950, Kolff moved to Cleveland where he developed a prototype kidney by coiling cellophane around orange juice cans. By using two lengths of cellophane, he was able to prevent a pressure drop across the dialyzer. Hence, the name "twin coil kidney" was used to describe the first disposable dialyzer. The dialyzer was produced by Travenol and became commercially available in 1956. Cellulose is derived from cotton fibers, and regenerated from solution. Cellulosics were developed in 1862, and original products were cellulose acetate, celluloid and rayon. Cellophane was developed in the early 1900s and the more porous cuprophane in 1937. These became popular as polymers used in early-day dialyzers. Due to their poor ability to clear beta microglobulins, and thus contributing to acquired amyloidosis, they are hardly used in modern practice, and have since been replaced by more biocompatible materials.

The Skeggs-Leonard flat plate dialyzer consisted of a multiple layers, and was thus difficult to assemble. It was modified by a Norwegian urologist, Frederic Kiil, who used cuprophane, instead of cellophane, and replacing the rubber pads with those of plastic. This consisted of five boards interspersed with four layers of cuprophane. Scribner learned of it in 1961, and started using it in Seattle for all dialysis patients, adapting it for home use when his program started in 1964. It was well suited for home use because no blood pump was needed. [31] He modified the design of the Kiil dialyzer, converting it from a four-layer to a two-layer device by removing two of the boards. Scribner commissioned local machinists at Western Gear Corporation to mill the boards, and used this dialyzer for over 10 years. (Figure 4) Later cuprophane was used in coil dialyzers.

In the early 1960s, Twardowski concluded that the ideal dialyzer would require high efficiency and not rupture easily when obtaining a high transmembrane pressure, and thus should be made of capillary tubing as opposed to plates or coils. He secured a patent for this in 1965 in Poland, but not elsewhere. The hollow fiber had been developed in the 1940s, although commercialization was not possible until the mid-1960s when the Dow Chemical Company started to manufacture fibers for reverse osmosis. Richard Stewart, at the University of Michigan, recognized its potential in dialysis, and in collaboration with Joseph Cerny and Henry Mahon pursued the idea for a hollow fiber dialyzer. In a further collaboration with Ben Lipps and John Sargent of Dow Chemical Company, the Western Division Research Laboratories, Marquette University School of Medicine and the Wood Veteran's Administration Hospital, a hollow fiber dialyzer was developed. A joint venture with the Cordis Company formed Cordis-Dow. [32] As concerns with biocompatibility grew, other plastics were tried. By 1981, it was estimated that there were 23 companies manufacturing 100 different dialyzers, mainly cuprophane and cellulose acetate. [3]

Union Carbide introduced polysulfones in 1965, and they figured prominently in both the space and electronics industries. Fresenius collaborated and supported using them for manufacturing hollow fiber membranes, as their high permeability made them ideal for clearing beta microglobulins. Polysulfones were popular because they demonstrated a suitable biocompatibility profile. Although they have been modified since originally introduced, polysulfone membranes remain the major component of the current Fresenius line of dialyzers. [33] Currently, newer modifications of polysulfone, such as polyarylethersulfone are in use by Gambro. These new membranes are engineered to provide highly efficient, stable, and biocompatible dialysis treatments.

Reverse Osmosis

The concept of osmosis was first observed by Abbe Nottet, a French cleric, in 1748. It is well known now that a difference in solute concentrations across a semipermeable membrane creates a pressure, the osmotic pressure, which drives solutions to the compartment with the highest concentration. While the quantitative relationships of osmotic pressure were studied in 1887 by Jacobus Henricus van't Hoff, it was only in the twentieth century that pressure was recognized as the driving force in the movement of fluids across a membrane. While conventional osmotic pressures will move fluids from the compartment with a lower to that with the higher concentration, this osmotic pressure can be overcome. By increasing the pressure on the other side of the membrane, fluid is driven backward to the side of the lower concentration. Thus, overcoming the natural osmotic pressure of a system forces water from the highly concentrated to a less concentrated compartment. By applying several passes, one can achieve a very pure sample of a fluid.

In the late 1940s and 1950s, reverse osmosis was attempted, [34] but its evolution to a commercially practical method of purifying water depended upon the advancement in thin-film membrane technology. Spiral wound polyamide membranes have been available and in use since 1977, and are available through many manufacturers. These membranes generally do not tolerate chlorine, and while this presents a vexing dilemma for community water purification systems, is quite convenient for dialysis facilities that routinely remove chlorine before processing with reverse osmosis. Currently, RO is the major source of pure water for dialysis facilities.

Milestone 9: Infrastructure for Dialysis Development – National Medical Care

Initially, hemodialysis was adopted and developed by academic centers of excellence. In 1962, Merrill started his own dialysis program at the Brigham, having been inspired by Belding Scribner's program in Seattle. Merrill recruited fellows to purchase and boil the cellophane, wrap the dialyzers and mix the chemicals. Three of the fellows, Edward "Ted" Hager, Eugene "Gene" Schupak and Constantine "Gus" Hampers have become famous as founders of the largest dialysis company in the world. Their story is well recounted in Tim McFeely's *The Price of Access*. [35]

By 1965, the Peter Bent Brigham Hospital's six stations were the only source of dialysis for the growing numbers of patients in the New England area who required it. As word of its availability spread, patients sought their care, and were not turned away, even though many lacked insurance coverage. Soon dialysis services consumed a disproportionate share of the hospital's resources, and became a financial burden to the hospital. As the major academic institution adjacent to Harvard Medical School, the provision of routine chronic services was not aligned with being a model, innovative research center. By 1966, the hospital's dialysis center was at capacity, and the Brigham, along with the Massachusetts Department of Public Health offered support to Hager and Hampers to establish a program in Boston's Normandy House, an extended care facility. Their outpatient center was able to provide dialysis services at a fraction of the cost of the hospital, and soon their model was replicated. Their new company, National Medical Care (NMC), began to grow. They next set up a center on Babcock Street, and planned to replicate the project around the country. By 1971, the company, along with Biomedical Applications in Queens, managed by Schupak, was successfully capitalized. Centers were opened in Bethesda, Maryland; Philadelphia, Pennsylvania; Dallas, Texas; Miami, Florida; Torrance, California; Pittsburgh, Pennsylvania; Beverly Hills, California; San Francisco, California; Portland, Maine; Tampa, Florida and other cities. During this period, dialysis was largely funded through insurance and for some, Medicaid, as this preceded the passage of legislation creating a Medicare coverage benefit.

Over the years that followed, particularly given that end stage renal disease (ESRD) patients now qualified for Medicare benefits, the company grew, and became a major US corporation. In 1984, it was purchased by W.R. Grace, and later sold to Fresenius. In its wake, NMC developed an infrastructure for cost effective, accessible and efficient dialysis care. [35]

Milestone 10: Social Security Amendment of 1973 (1973)

Selection Committees

As word of Scribner's success grew, it became apparent in Seattle that the hospital per se would be short lived as an ongoing site for dialysis. The original dialysis program in Seattle was funded by the National Institute of Health, but it was soon discovered that other funding would be necessary, and the center would have to be moved out of the hospital. Scribner thus initiated a program through the King County Medical Society, a three-station non-profit outpatient center. It was the first outpatient dialysis center in the world, and was located in the newly remodeled basement of the nursing residence of Swedish Hospital. [15] In the summer of 1961, in light of the reality that there would be too many possible applicants, two committees were established to help select patients for dialysis. The first, a medical committee composed of nephrologists and internists, applied very strict medical criteria. Those who were successfully screened were then reviewed by a second committee, the Admissions and Policy Committee, an anonymous group of people representing the community. These committees accepted the first four patients, one in September and three in December of 1961, and they started dialysis therapy at the University Hospital, transferring to the Seattle Artificial Kidney Center when it opened in January 1962.

The Seattle Artificial Kidney Center ultimately became the world-renown Northwest Kidney Centers. [15] Soon the center was at capacity, and a serious ethical conundrum was born. It was estimated that 10,000 persons were in need of dialysis in the USA, and strict criteria were established to determine who would be deemed eligible. Some who were considered "unfit" for therapy because they were too young - under 18 or too old - greater than 45, had co-morbid conditions (except hypertension) or no rehabilitation potential were never even considered. The Admissions and Policy committee was comprised of six community leaders and a non-nephrologist physician. It only considered patients who met stringent criteria for review. Of the thirty candidates referred in Seattle in 1962, thirteen were reviewed by the medical panel and found medically unsuitable. The remaining seventeen were reviewed by the Admissions and Policy Committee. Only ten could be selected for the three-station program; the other seven died. Aside from a grant from the Hartford Foundation, there were insufficient funds, as well as space to accommodate more than the ten patients. Criteria among those medically fit included net worth, marital status, nature of occupation, extent of education, number of children and church attendance.

In November 1962, Life Magazine ran a feature story by Shana Alexander, "They Decide Who Lives, Who Dies," which achieved national attention. [36] This story stimulated the development of the discipline of bioethics. Gradually, the Seattle program expanded, but not at a rate to meet capacity. On November 18, 1965, Edwin Newman of NBC Broadcasting Company ran an hour-long television documentary about the Seattle selection committee, entitled "Who Shall Live." Produced by Lucy Jarvis, this stirred further debate about the ethical issues surrounding dialysis. [37] As dialysis spread as a viable treatment option, controversy over the balance of scarcity vs. rationing continued. In some areas IQ tests and personality tests were administered to determine who would qualify for treatment. In Los Angeles, candidates were selected by lottery. Circumstances such as this sparked the controversies that ultimately led to the passage of legislation to cover dialysis. [38]

Legislation Passes

Although pressure was placed on Congress in 1963, it would be a decade before dialysis would be widely available. However, in 1963 and 1964 the Veterans Administration and the Public Health Service both announced plans to build dialysis centers. In 1965, the Budget Bureau established a committee headed by Carl Gottchalk to study its feasibility, its cost and to make recommendations. Although dialysis legislation was delayed, an act was passed to provide coverage to Americans over 65 years old.

During this era, dialysis was becoming more widely accepted. In 1968, National Medical Care was incorporated (see above). As in Seattle, the renal staff at the Peter Bent Brigham Hospital in Boston was also unable to receive continued funding through the hospital. The physicians set up a small program – the Babcock Unit - in a neighboring hospital, and using outside financing developed a corporation to manage dialysis therapy. Centers spread throughout the country, staffed by young physicians trained at the major academic centers pioneering dialysis.

In 1966 a young college student, Andrew Peter Lundin, III developed renal failure, and underwent home training at the University of Washington in Seattle. He completed his premedical education at Stanford University and wished to attend medical school. In Brooklyn, Eli Friedman was beginning a program that would serve as a nidus for the development of patient-centered health care. Dr. Friedman took a chance on the young applicant, and Lundin became the first dialysis patient to graduate from medical school in the USA. Lundin had a distinguished career as a nephrologist, and as a community leader. [39][1]

The young man Friedman accepted, in collaboration with fellow dialysis patients in Brooklyn and Queens formed a patient group, The National Association of Patients on Hemodialysis. This group would later become The American Association of Kidney Patients, but in the interim served to persuade Congress to enact legislation covering dialysis costs. The prediction to Congress that there would never be more than 35,000 persons on dialysis,

---

[1] The first dialysis patient to ever graduate medical school was Robin Eady, who graduated in the 1960s from Guy's Hospital (the same hospital where Richard Bright attended). The story goes that when his parents contacted Scribner, he was initially turned away because he was not a local resident, however, Scribner agreed to accept him and train him as a dialysis technician for the dialysis facility to soon open in Edmonton, Alberta. After Alberta, he returned to medical in England. He is alive today, (August 10, 2011) and a retired distinguished Professor of Dermatology at the University of London (Chris Blagg – personal communication)

and that the program would never cost more than 250 million dollars became the nidus legislation to make all ESRD patients eligible for health coverage. Congress was also told that most people who underwent home dialysis return to work. It was likewise presumed kidney transplantation would enable patients to regain employment, qualifying them for private insurance benefits and immunosuppressive therapy coverage. [40]

The combined efforts of scientists, physicians such as George Schreiner, his neighbor, Charles Plante, the lobbyist for the National Kidney Foundation, and the public brought increasing pressure on Congress. In November 1971, Bill Litchfield, an engineer from Houston, Samuel Orenstein and Lundin joined Shep Glazer in the Ways and Means Committee Room. Schreiner nervously provided the machine for Glazer, who had traveled from Queens to Washington. Glazer dialyzed briefly before Wilbur Mills and his committee while Schreiner's fellow anxiously stood by (personal communication). [41]

In a unique experiment, Medicare amended their coverage policy to include a single disease, rather than basing eligibility upon age. In this act, they also extended coverage for disability. Tragically for some, they fell short of continuing long-term eligibility for the expensive and necessary immunosuppressive agents required to maintain a kidney transplant. In October1972, when Congress enacted legislation that amended The Social Security Act, there were 10,000 persons on dialysis, of whom 40% were on home therapy. [42]

Milestone 11: Peritoneal Dialysis (1978)

While home hemodialysis was established long before, chronic peritoneal dialysis did not become successful as a home therapy until 1978. This procedure was first attempted on guinea pigs and rabbits in 1923 by Georg Ganter, [43] who was able to note removal of non-protein nitrogen along with improvement in the animal's uremic symptoms. He also made unsuccessful attempts to try his new procedure on patients. Throughout the late 1940s [44] and throughout the 1950s it became a preferred technique for the treatment of acute renal failure. [45] Catheters in use during this period were stiff. Without a permanent access, it would not be practical as a therapeutic regimen for chronic care. A flexible catheter was first developed by Arthur Grollman in 1952, and in 1959, Paul Doolan developed a polyethylene catheter for chronic use. When Fred Boen moved from Holland to Seattle in 1961 he initiated an intermittent outpatient peritoneal dialysis program.

Russell Palmer was an internist stationed in the Netherlands during World War 2. He visited with Kolff, and received a blueprint for the dialysis machine. Palmer introduced hemodialysis and later peritoneal dialysis into Vancouver, Canada. In 1964, home peritoneal dialysis programs were initiated in Seattle as well as in Vancouver, Canada. Seattle had begun a small outpatient peritoneal dialysis program twice weekly in 1962. [15] Here, the physician went to the patient's home, cannulating the peritoneal space using a trocar. After each treatment the catheter was removed. [15] It was not until 1968, when Henry Tenckhoff modified an earlier prototype of Palmer's and Wayne Quinton's Silastic implantable peritoneal catheter that chronic peritoneal dialysis could become practical. [46-48] Intermittent peritoneal dialysis showed great promise. Tenckhoff modified Palmer's catheter by adding two Dacron cuffs into which tissue grew to anchor the catheter and close the sinus tract around the catheter to minimize infection. One cuff was below the skin and the other immediately outside the peritoneal cavity. [15] Further advancements by Jack Moncrieff and Robert Popovich in Austin, Texas led to chronic ambulatory peritoneal dialysis (CAPD). This therapy was based upon calculations of the contact time of dialysate with the peritoneal membrane – "the dwell time." The concept called for fluid to constantly remain in the peritoneal space. In 1978, Dimitrios Oreopoulos developed dialysis containers made of plastic bags instead of glass bottles. This revolutionized the practical application of peritoneal dialysis therapy. Others who contributed greatly to the development of peritoneal dialysis were Zbylut Twardowski and Karl Knolph. [49] The Home Choice™ peritoneal dialysis system was developed for Baxter International by renowned inventor, Dean Kamen, automating the dialysis procedure. This made it easier for patients to undergo convenient nightly, peritoneal dialysis. Peritoneal dialysis is more economical to provide than hemodialysis, and it shares similar outcomes with respect to mortality. It enables patients to have a more flexible schedule. Hence, it is ideal for patients who continue to work. It is very popular in cities such as Hong Kong, and gaining popularity in the USA due to economic restrictions created by recent changes in reimbursement.

This book extensively discusses issues related to peritoneal dialysis, in particular the role it plays in a key new paradigm for ESRD management (See Chapter 2 by Tom Golper). Chapter 5, by Sunil Badve, Carmel Hawley and David Johnson, critically and comprehensively compares automated peritoneal dialysis and chronic ambulatory peritoneal dialysis, and is quite timely for this era of economic challenge.

Milestone 12: Omnibus Budget Reconciliation Act (OBRA) (1981)

During the first ten years of the Medicare ESRD Program, dialysis availability greatly expanded. No longer were patients restricted by age or comorbidities. In 1974, based upon data from the Health Care Financing Administration (HCFA) the prevalence of dialysis was 15,993. In 1983, it was 86,354. That same year, the incidence rose from 21,927 to 25,155. Total Medicare expenditures for all dialysis patients in 1974 were 229 million, but by 1983, it had jumped to 1.898 billion dollars. This 729% change, when corrected for inflation, still represented a 331% change. During this time, Medicare payment policy was to reimburse outpatient dialysis services based upon reasonable charges. Reimbursement was set at $138.00 per treatment, but home dialyses for patients were paid separately. [50] The original ESRD legislation underfunded home dialysis, and despite efforts to correct reimbursement in 1983, there were serious challenge to the growth of this modality.

Efforts to curb costs were apparent, as Congressional hearings were held as early as 1976, and in 1977 and 1978. The passage of PL 95-292 in 1978 enabled the establishment of prospective payment rate for dialysis providers. A Notice of Proposed Rulemaking was not issued until 1980, but was rejected by the Reagan administration. The passage of OBRA 1981 successfully mandated the establishment of a prospective payment system, and a Notice of Rulemaking issued the following year. A composite rate was established in a Final Rule effective August 1, 1983. This consolidated dialysis reimbursement to an average rate between $127 and $131 per treatment depending upon a geographic wage adjustment. In 1986, HCFA proposed to calculate the dialysis rates based on the median cost per treatment for all dialysis facilities in the entire sampled patient population, arguing this would be a more accurate reflection than by median per facility. This resulted in a proposal to cut the dialysis rate by an additional $6.00. After it was argued that this was in response to pressure from the Office of Management and Budget to reduce the ESRD program by $100 million dollars, HCFA reconsidered; the amount was only cut by 2 dollars in 1986. Between 1986 and 1991, the composite rate continued to fall regularly, and by 1991 was $124 per treatment. HCFA used the argument that dialysis rates were initially set too high, as was evidenced by the growth and profitability of companies like NMC. What was not considered, however, was when Medicare was the primary and sole payer and only covered 80% of the rate. Given that primary insurance payments from other patients were higher, there resulted a compensatory shift of costs from Medicare to private health insurers. The Institute of Medicine issued a report in 1990, highlighting several issues: while dialysis reimbursement rates were lowered, facilities remained financially solvent by obtaining lower supply costs, reducing treatment times, reusing dialyzers and decreasing staff to patient ratios. Concerns were raised that the quality of core medical services was threatened. HCFA countered the IOM argument by revealing the cost reports from 1985 and 1987. They demonstrated that in 1985, despite a variation between facilities, payment for treatment exceeded unaudited costs by 8 dollars. HCFA was criticized for not adjusting dialysis prices for inflation, but argued back that price drops in dialyzers offset inflation-rated raises in salaries. It was argued that as long as dialysis facilities were expanding capacity, they must have been making a profit. They also argued that vertical integration of large chains would allow them to offset negative costs from profits in other aspects of their business, such as manufacturing. Likewise, they argued that professional fees could offset any procedure losses in physician-owned facilities. Concerns by regulators were that facility profits were at the expense of quality because their quality was not monitored systematically. [41]

This price change, in retrospect, had quite a sobering effect upon dialysis care. NMC was already looking for a buyer before the establishment of a composite rate. By 1984, W.R. Grace had agreed and the deal closed on December 20, 1984. [35] More than ever, the strain between providing services for those in need conflicted with the availability of discretionary resources; and this would challenge the quality of care provided. Many providers contend that reimbursement rate declines force compromises in care, and adversely affect patient outcomes. The Institute of Medicine Report of 1990 suggested that quality had deteriorated, but that this was not conclusive. They expressed concerns that as real payments decreased, units would survive by reducing services to patients, even to the point of reducing standards. The IOM recommended that the composite rate not be reduced, but that the rate be updated yearly, rebased only when an ESRD quality assessment program was in place, and that payment policy be reviewed on a regular basis. [50]

Milestone 13: Kt/V(1985) [51]

The optimal time for acute dialysis treatment was initially determined in Leeds, England. [15,52,53] Optimal dialysis time for chronic renal failure was increased from once to three times a week over the course of three years in Seattle, based upon clinical observation, and the amelioration of symptoms. It balanced clinical well-being with cost factors, and was more practical than alternate day dialysis. In 1965, analog simulations showed more frequent dialysis improved removal of solutes that moved slowly from the intracellular to the extracellular space. [29,15] Yet, a true mathematical relationship between urea equilibrium had yet to be established until 1985. Such a relationship, the single pool Kt/V (spKt/V), defined equilibrium kinetics of solute clearance in dialysis procedures, and was a major advance in kidney health care. The spKt/V formula states that the logarithmic expression of urea reduction equals the urea clearance of the dialyzer multiplied by the contact time of dialysis divided by the volume of distribution of urea. Measuring the Kt/V immediately post dialysis is not accurate because different compartments or pools in the body each have urea transfer characteristics. Thus, the urea measured immediately post treatment from the extracellular pool does not reflect an equilibrated state, and it takes around 30 to 60 minutes for it to shift back from the intracellular and interstitial compartments. It is not practical for patients and staff to wait for this to occur. Calibration for the time that it takes urea to return to equilibrium between these other compartments was taken into consideration by later modifications of the formula, hence the more accurate eKt/V used in the HEMO Study. [54-58] Initially, the therapeutic goal was to maintain the spKt/V at a value that would balance out the protein catabolic rate, i.e., maintain sufficient dialysis to remove wastes products generated through the combination of food breakdown and muscle turnover. The National Cooperative Dialysis Study (NCDS) first reported that increased urea clearance during dialysis was associated with better patient outcomes. [59,60] Based on these data, Gotch and Sargent later predicted that a single pool spKt/V lower than 0.8 was associated with worse clinical outcomes. [51]

The application of dialysis as a service was being shaped and molded by the confluence of industrial advancement and the necessities determined by the economics of providing for the needs of a growing population of patients with ESRD. The consequence of this, amidst new budgetary and economic constraints of 1983, was a shift to shorter, but more efficient dialysis. The institution of reuse was also gaining in popularity as a cost-saving measure.

However, as the cottage industry of dialysis care advanced, a reality check was needed, particularly in light of data gleaned from the USRDS in contrast with the registries of other nations. While initially acceptable, it became obvious by the end of the 1980s that inadequate dialysis dosing in the United States was accounting for inferior patient outcomes compared to other nations. [61,62] This was noted in a key stakeholder meeting in Dallas in 1989. The 1989 Dallas Conference on Morbidity and Mortality in Dialysis will be remembered as a turning point in nephrology; [63] it resulted in a multicenter study initiated by Dallas Nephrology Associates to capture key observational data: As they increased the Kt/V from 1.18 to 1.46 between 1989 and 1992, their mortality fell from 21.8 to 19.5%, which was better than that of the rest of the USA. Similar observations were noted at NMC, which between 1990 and 1992 increased its urea reduction ratio from 57.1 to 62.5%, and achieved a standard mortality rate of .77 when referenced to the rest of the USA. [64]

As these were not randomized trials, the debate continued as to what was optimal dialysis, and whether or not increasing the Kt/V could extend patient life. A large, multi-center, randomized, controlled trial, the HEMO study was published in 2002. [65] It failed to demonstrate an improvement in mortality in the group with the higher eKt/V. To the surprise of many, it was not shown that an eKt/V greater than the original NKF Dialysis Outcome Quality Initiative (DOQI) recommendation improved mortality. [66,67] The HEMO study showed the survival advantage of a higher Kt/V for women over men. As this was based upon an ad hoc analysis, it was not considered strictly evidence-based. It is unknown, though strongly suggested that men and women have different body characteristics that might determine a more selective determination of their dose, [68-71] and further studies are needed to demonstrate this.

MIPPA 2008 (see below) calls for a "pay for performance" quality incentive program (QIP) that withholds 2% of each treatment reimbursement, and rewards it back if minimal criteria are met. Among these criteria are a minimum URR of .65, and this translates to accepting a spKt/V of less than 1.2.

While the Kt/V was valuable in establishing a measure of adequacy, it is being challenged as less valid for identifying issues that might make a more substantial contribution to outcomes. This challenge gains significance given the historical perspectives discussed above, and the consequences sustained by combining a strict payment reform and adequacy metrics that validate underperformance. [120] Randomized controlled trials are confirming earlier notions that more frequent dialysis is associated with better the composite outcome of left ventricular mass and death. Chapter 16 by James Tattersall continues this debate regarding dialysis adequacy, and elegantly highlights many of the mathematical principles of dialysis kinetics. Dialysis adequacy, as quantified by the transfer of urea, does not take into account the transfer of middle molecules. Richard Glassock (Chapter 9) discusses the issues relating to assessing volume in dialysis. In retrospect, the major lesson to future nephrologists might be to never rely upon a sheer number without considering its clinical context.

Milestone 14: USRDS– Omnibus Budget Reconciliation Act (OBRA) (1986)

For the first four years after the ESRD program was established, it was administered by the Bureau of Health Insurance and the Public Health Service Bureau of Quality Assurance. This resulted in a lack of coordination in data management. In 1977, the Health Care Financing Administration (HCFA) was established. Public Law 95-292 of 1978 created a specific program for ESRD information management – the ESRD Program Management and Medical Information System, which was fully implemented by 1980. It established several medical data source documents, calling for national uniform bill (Form UB-82), a medical evidence report (Form 2728) and an ESRD death notification form (Form 2746). In addition, it provided for forms to report health cost information (Form 2552) and to record the facility survey (Form 2744).

After much discussion with stakeholders, Congress passed OBRA 1986, establishing an "ESRD registry." In 1988, the registry, USRDS, was established, and the contract was awarded to the University of Michigan. The USRDS contract is currently managed by the University of Minnesota. Its current goals, as defined on the USRDS web site, [72] are to characterize the ESRD population, describe the prevalence and incidence of ESRD along with mortality trends and disease rates, to investigate demographic, treatment and morbidity relationships, identify areas for special studies and support research, and to provide data sets and samples of national data to support research by special studies centers.

Milestone 15: Erythropoiesis Stimulating Agents (ESAs) (1989)

One of the great advances in technology came when scientists were able to clone the gene that produced erythropoietin and genetically engineer immortal Chinese hamster ovary cells to produce it. Previous efforts such as managing anemia included attempts to stimulate red blood cell production with anabolic steroids such as nandrolone. These were met with limited success. In some instances, blood transfusions were the only option to manage anemia. The anemia management story has been fraught with challenges. It is discussed in depth by Michael Germain and colleagues in Chapter 14 of this book.

Since 1974, it was known that dialysis was associated with accelerated cardiac disease. Seventy-four percent of patients presented with abnormal cardiac function, and anemia, along with hypertension and accelerated atherosclerosis was considered a causative factor. When Palfrey studied 434 dialysis patients for 41 months during a period between 1982 and 1991, he and his group demonstrated that 31% had congestive heart failure at the onset of disease and another 25% developed it. Those with heart failure had a survival time of 36 months as compared with 62 months for the rest. Anemia was identified as one of the risk factors. [73] During this period, the mean hemoglobin was 8.5 gm/dL±1.5. After adjusting for age, diabetes, blood pressure, serum albumin and ischemic heart disease, each 1 gram decrease in hemoglobin was associated with worsening left ventricular hypertrophy and worsening mortality. [74]

Recombinant human erythropoietin (rHuEPO) was welcomed by nephrology in the late 1980s. The phase III clinical trials for this product were conducted by Joseph Eschbach, and targeted a hematocrit between 33 to 38%. In the multicenter trial, 333 hemodialysis patients with a hematocrit of less than 30% at initiation showed that with a rise in hematocrit, there was the elimination of blood transfusions, improvement in quality of life and control of iron overload. [75] These results were submitted to the FDA, which approved epoetin alfa in June 1989 at a target of 30 to 33%. In1994, they widened their target to 30 to 36%. These initial trials demonstrated that at the start of the study, the baseline hematocrit was 23.7, and was maintained at the second (six month) evaluation at 34.2% and at the tenth month, 33.9%. The Karnofsky Score [76] demonstrated that the patients who were able to carry out normal activity rose from only 19.8% to 37.3% in 6 months, and was maintained at 35.5% at ten months (p <= 0.01 compared with baseline). Activity levels using the Nottingham Health Profile also significantly improved. Activity levels and energy levels paralleled these scores. Since then, many studies demonstrated the relation between quality of life and anemia management with ESAs. [77-92]

In 1993, the mean hematocrit was 30.2%, still with 43% of patients having hematocrits below this value. [72] The National Anemia Cooperative Project was established in 1994, and set the target for hematocrit at 30%. When the National Kidney Foundation Dialysis Outcome Quality Initiative (DOQI) [93] was released in the autumn of 1997, the average hematocrit was already up to 32.4%. [72] The KDOQI Guidelines raised the targets to between 33 and 36%, and the Clinical Performance Measurements established by HCFA were based upon these guidelines. [94]

In 1998, the Normal Hematocrit Study was published. It is the only hard evidence against normalizing the hematocrit using ESA. In this study of dialysis patients with cardiac disease,

618 were assigned to receive ESA to maintain a target of 42% and the remaining 615 to maintain a target of 30%. Although the study never reached statistical significance, it was terminated when the higher hematocrit target group had a higher mortality. This group also required more intravenous iron, and had poorer adequacy outcomes. Nevertheless, it was recommended that dialysis patients not be targeted to a normal hematocrit. [95]

Despite this study, the next eight years realized a steady rise in the average hematocrit of dialysis patients, and by 2007, the mean hemoglobin was 12 gm/dL. The Clinical Performance Measures (CPM) project also demonstrated that the ratio of ESA/hemoglobin levels also rose during the years of 1998-2004, indicating an increase in epo hyporesponsiveness. [94] Epo hyporesponsiveness will be discussed in Chapter 14.

In 2000, the updated KDOQI guideline target was 11-12 gm/dL. The Normal Hematocrit Study was challenged by observational data such as a study in 2002 by Collins, whose team reported that the risk of death was not different in groups who had higher (36 to 39%) vs. lower (33 to <36%) hematocrits. The higher hematocrit arm also had a lower hospitalization rate, hence lower costs. [96] Randomized clinical trials to determine the benefits of ESAs were thus initiated.

Two such trials, the CREATE Study in Europe and the CHOIR Study in the USA were reported in November 2006, [97,98] and failed to demonstrate an advantage to targeting high hemoglobin levels. In both trials, study subjects were targeted to higher or baseline hemoglobin levels. In 2006, the NKF KDOQI anemia guideline specified a target > 11 gm/dL, and caution when maintaining a hemoglobin > 13gm/dL.

Those patients with a higher hemoglobin target did worse in the CHOIR Trial, resulting in an FDA advisory and a Congressional Hearing the following month. An FDA Black Box warning initially advised the use of ESAs solely to prevent drug transfusions, but was revised to allow a target hemoglobin of 10 to 12 gm. Early in 2007, the NKF revised the KDOQI guideline to specify a hemoglobin target between 11 and 12 gm/dL, and advised that levels should not exceed 13 gm/dL. In 2009, the TREAT trial was published. [99] This was a randomized controlled trial comparing a placebo arm with an arm targeted to achieve a hemoglobin of 13 gm/dL. Although results were similar, the higher target group had slightly worse outcomes. In January 2011, the Centers for Medicare & Medicaid Services (CMS) convened a Medicare Evidence Development & Coverage Advisory Committee (MEDCAC) hearing, but did not change its coverage decision. On June 24, 2011 the FDA modified its labeling recommendation and removed the target hemoglobin levels of 10 to 12 gm/dL, substituting language that non-dialysis patients should receive treatment with ESAs only when the hemoglobin level is below 10 gm/dL, and that the dose should be reduced or interrupted when the level reaches 10 gm/dL. For dialysis patients, it was suggested that the dose be reduced or interrupted if the hemoglobin rises above 11 gm/dL. [100]

As part of the Medicare Improvements for Patients and Providers Act of 2008 (MIPPA 2008), and the establishment of a prospective payment system, Medicare was authorized to implement a quality incentive payment program (QIP) that would withhold up to 2% of the reimbursement to facilities for dialysis treatments if specified performance measures were not met. The three finalized measures published for the initial year of the ESRD QIP were the percentage of Medicare patients with an average hemoglobin of less than10.0 gm/dL, the percentage with an average hemoglobin of greater than 12.0 gm/dL and the percentage with an average urea reduction ratio of less than 65%. This is historically significant in that it is the first time a pay for performance program has been fully implemented in an ESRD reimbursement program. However, in direct response to the change in FDA labeling recommendations, CMS retired the measure of patients with a hemoglobin less than 10 gm/dL, equally weighting the other two.

There is no doubt that the development of a synthetic form of rHuEPO has had a positive impact upon the lives of patients with ESRD. There is therefore room for an argument that this milestone's benefit to kidney patients could be blunted. This is based upon the historical observation that the quality of patient care falls when economic pressures increase, particularly in a capitated system. There is a risk that not having a minimal standard for hemoglobin could lead to increased blood transfusions, hospitalization rates and worsening in the quality of life for dialysis patients.

Milestone 16: The K-DOQI Guidelines

In 1950, the National Nephrosis Foundation was started by Ada and Harry Debold. In 1958, the name was changed to the National Kidney Disease Foundation and in 1964 to the National Kidney Foundation. The Foundation has been instrumental in providing a variety of resources to the kidney community. In March 1995, the NKF launched an ambitious program, the Dialysis Outcome Quality Initiative (DOQI) under the leadership of Garabed Eknoyan. This was an effort to develop evidence-based clinical practice guidelines to aid providers in the care of patients. Multidisciplinary workgroups were established to methodologically review published literature on hemodialysis, peritoneal dialysis, anemia and vascular access. [60,61] These guidelines then underwent expert and public review, and were published 1997. An Internet version was also established under the direction of Stephen Fadem. The MDRD Study Equation for glomerular filtration rate was released around the same time, and would have a crucial impact on future guidelines.

These guidelines were widely disseminated and have become well accepted by the community. The NKF continued to publish other guidelines, first in nutrition, and later in bone disease, hypertension [101] and lipid management. [102]

By 2002, the guidelines had been extended to chronic kidney disease, extending beyond ESRD and greatly expanding their range of involvement. They consolidated and simplified terminology, suggesting that "chronic kidney disease" replace "early renal insufficiency" and "preESRD." By eliminating vagueness, and in establishing a lexicon and classification system for kidney disease, communication and collaboration across specialties could be greatly improved. [103] This system would be based upon the calculated GFR presented in 1997, initially available as a web tool, but then integrated into standard laboratory testing. DOQI became KDOQI – Kidney Disease Outcomes Quality Initiative. The CKD guidelines have helped to integrate care better between primary care physicians and specialists, and increase understanding of CKD. [104] The guidelines have been updated regularly.

An international iteration of clinical guidelines, Kidney Disease: Improving Global Outcomes (KDIGO) (http://www.kdigo.org) developed guidelines for hepatitis C, chronic kidney disease related mineral and bone disorders (CKD-MBD), care of the kidney transplant recipient and acute kidney injury. In progress are KDIGO guidelines for glomerulonephritis, hypertension, chronic kidney disease and anemia.

Milestone 17: Chronic Kidney Disease – Mineral Bone Disorders (CKD-MBD) (2005)

As part of the KDIGO initiative, a consensus conference was held to redefine and classify renal osteodystrophy. [105] The serum phosphorus has in the past two decades emerged as an independent risk factor for mortality in kidney disease. In addition, the association between the severity of vascular calcification and mortality has been established. The relationship between calcium and phosphorus elevation, mortality rate and extraskeletal vascular calcification and their contribution to morbidity established the need for a classification to encompass all the diverse manifestations of this disease process. [106] The disorder was defined as a triad of laboratory abnormalities, bone abnormalities and vascular calcification. The morbidities were identified as cardiovascular disease, fractures and mortality. [105] This has opened a field of discovery that enabled us to visualize the relationship between skeletal and vascular mineralization, and is discussed by Keith Hruska in Chapter 13. Under this milestone should also go advances in our understanding of the relationship between volume overload and the mechanisms of cardiac disease, discussed by Richard Glassock in Chapter 9, and the role of inflammation and nutrition also discussed in this book.

Milestone 18: Conditions for Coverage

Conditions for Coverage for dialysis facilities were established in 1976. [107] These included specifications for the fulfillment of services, furnishing of data and information, compliance with laws and regulations, governance, a care plan, patient rights, medical records, the physical environment, medical director responsibilities, staff responsibilities and minimal service requirements. It also established that a social worker and dietitian are required to see patients regularly, and that state surveys be performed under contract by HCFA. The statute also required that each ESRD network have a medical review board and paved the way for the formation of ESRD Networks in 1977. These conditions for coverage remained in effect for over 30 years.

By 2005, a new set of regulations for Medicare coverage of dialysis services were completed and went to final review after extensive public comment. After revision and approval by the necessary components of HHS, they were released in active form on April 8, 2008. [108] The conditions became effective on October 14, 2008.

These conditions, and their attendant interpretive guidelines and tools, created a uniform survey environment with the expressed effort to eliminate variations in quality between dialysis facilities. They dealt mainly with general compliance and patient safety, with special attention to infection control, the water and dialysate systems, reuse and the physical environment, and updated infection and water quality control guidelines. They required cardiac defibrillators in dialysis facilities, better fire safety and disaster management standards, and created a requirement for dialysis technician certification.

They also dealt with specifics of patient care, including improved patient rights, responsibility, grievance and involuntary discharge provisions. They provided structure for improved patient assessments at chair side and during interdisciplinary team conferences. The program provided for a patient assessment at least once yearly for stable patients, but once monthly for patients considered unstable. The patient plan of care was to be completed and dated by inter-disciplinary team members with 30 days of initiating treatment, and adjusted as frequently as monthly if achieved outcomes were not being met.

Additionally, the new conditions specified medical director responsibilities, and explicitly gave more authority to medical directors, providing for a tight structure in which to assess, trend and improve a series of quality measures. This Quality Assessment and Performance Improvement program (QAPI) required that dialysis centers achieve measurable improvement in health outcomes and the reduction of medical errors by measuring, analyzing and tracking quality indicators. This would become an essential tool to assure quality after the enactment and implementation of legislation to achieve payment reform by bundling separately billable ancillary services with the composite rate.

Milestone 19: Medicare Improvements for Patients and Providers Act (MIPPA) (2008)

The Omnibus Budget Reconciliation Act of 1981, Public Law 97-35 established the prospective payment system and required that payments be made using a single composite weighted formula. However, substantial expenditures were excluded from this rate, particularly erythropoiesis stimulating agents and vitamin D analogues. By 2008, these services comprised around 40% of the total spending for outpatient chronic dialysis. Previously, the Medicare Payment Advisory Commission (MedPac) and the Government Accountability Office (GAO) reviewed the Medicare payment system and suggested a bundled prospective payment methodology that would combine the composite rate with separately billable services under a single payment. The passage of MIPPA 2008 offered compromising legislation to dialysis stakeholders. First, it tied an adjustment to the composite rate to inflation. This was something stakeholders had asked Congress to enact, as it would enable costs to maintain pace with salary changes, and this is critical in a service-based operation. It also legislated that payment reform based upon MedPac and GAO recommendations be enacted starting January 1, 2011. The Final Rule was published after much debate with respect to the possibility of including phosphate binding agents and calcimimetics. [109] Although facilities had four years to transition into the reformed payment system, the majority of facilities began at the starting date. The expanded bundle of services also included dialysis-related laboratory studies as well as the oral equivalents to injectable medications (vitamin D analogs). In 2014, it will include phosphate binder therapy as well as calcimimetics.

Like the composite rate in 1983, the prospective payment reform creates an environment where cost reduction strategies compete with efforts to provide quality service. On a global level, market consolidation is occurring. Protocols that stress comparative effectiveness will prevail when outcomes achieved through less costly alternatives are comparable. Changes in the dialysis prescription, ESA dosing regimens and CKD-MBD management strategies are underway, and underline the need for effective quality assessment at all levels. As the Dallas Meeting of 1989, [110] the IOM report of 1990 [50] and the NIH Consensus report of 1993

[61] demonstrated, the quality of US dialysis care worsened in response to the institution of the composite rate in 1983. Might we expect this to happen again if we are not vigilant?

MIPPA 2008 also directed Medicare to establish payment methodology for six education sessions to be provided by office-based nephrology teams to patients who had Stage 4 CKD. [111] Herein lie multiple opportunities for cost savings coupled with quality improvement through a relatively simple and economical task of better patient preparedness. The USRDS [112] demonstrates that the initial hospitalization period associated with starting dialysis is three times more costly than the rest of the time Medicare patients (over 67 years old) receive care, and 6 times higher for those not yet receiving Medicare. It also reflects that only around 25% of incident patients receive care from a nephrologist before initiating treatment. Of patients who never saw the nephrologist prior to dialysis initiation, over 80% start dialysis with a central venous catheter (CVC) in place. When patients have been educated in advanced by a nephrologist, the CVC incidence rate drops, but is still alarmingly high. Patients with catheters are four times as likely to have an infectious complication. [113] Better CKD education will also help patient satisfaction. A survey study of 977 patients undertaken by the American Association of Kidney Patients (AAKP) showed patient satisfaction was lowest for in-center hemodialysis (4.1) higher for peritoneal (5.2), and home hemodialysis (5.5) and highest for patients receiving a kidney transplant (6.1) (P < 0.05). Approximately 31% felt treatment options were not presented fairly. [114]

There is some support that cost savings may be effected through the institution of a Medical Home program or an Accountable Care Organization (ACO). The success of large health delivery centers and the objective of better achieving integrated care between primary care teams, nephrology teams and other disciplines forms the basis for that interest. Units going at risk for an entire spectrum of care have a better opportunity to form strategies to allocate resources more efficiently. Federal regulation calls for the creation of ACOs. [115] They represent the potential to create incentives that are performance, rather than cost-based. Integrated health care is discussed in Chapter 20.

Health care costs are highest when patients initiate dialysis with multiple coexisting disease processes. This also creates a need for extra resources for dialysis staff, particularly if these patients have a central venous catheter (CVC). The prognosis for patients with multiple comorbidities is poor. [116] In a recent study, Kaplan-Meier Diagrams demonstrate patients over 75 years of age initiating dialysis with multiple comorbidities do no better than those who select conservative, non-dialysis care. [117] The Renal Physicians Association has developed tools to enable physicians to estimate the prognosis for the incident dialysis patient, and to assist the patient and family to select a palliative alternative when it is apparent that dialysis will not result in a favorable outcome.

Milestone 20: RPA Guidelines (2010)

Since 1961, there has been a dramatic shift from restricting access to care. Often, dialysis therapy is offered beyond the point where patients may benefit. Currently, the median age of incidence dialysis patients is 64.2 years old. [112] There are recognized circumstances where dialysis does not favorably improve survival or quality of life, in particular when coexisting profound dementia, severe peripheral vascular disease, advanced liver disease or metastatic disease are present. [118] The Renal Physicians Association under the leadership of Alvin "Woody" Moss and his team created a stepwise system for determining whether patients who are potentially not good candidates for dialysis can be evaluated and assessed. In circumstances where care is not going to make a difference in the quality of life, and if the patient or designate and family agree, alternate collaborative services can be offered. In 2010, the Renal Physicians Association published a series of updated guidelines and tools to help physicians develop a decision–making process with patients and prepare them for palliative care when appropriate. [119] This has been excellently discussed by Susan Bray in Chapter 8.

Conclusion

This chapter has reviewed several milestones in the history of dialysis as it progressed from a concept to a mature therapeutic application. The renal community has seen advancements in technology and therapy interplay with the need to meet the demands of patients with ESRD and the struggles to reconcile the economic difficulties that were created. However, the challenges that lie ahead are not what we have done, but what we have yet to do. Tom Parker, in the Introduction, points out challenges we face, and have the potential to fix. This chapter provides the historical perspective, and lays the groundwork for the reader to further delve into the topical issues that face the renal community. These issues are discussed in depth in the subsequent chapters of this book, and form the basis of the milestones yet to come.

References

[1] Rosenfeld L. George Owen Rees (1813-1889): an early clinical biochemist. Clin Chem. 1985 June 1;31(6):1068-70.

[2] Nickles SL, Fackler G. Bright's Disease. Culbertson J, editor. Cincinnati: Cincinnati Lancet Press; 1886.

[3] Twardowski ZJ. History of hemodialyzers' designs. Hemodial Int. 2008;12(2):173-210.

[4] Graham T. Elements of Chemistry. Including the applications of the sciences in the arts. 1st American ed. Philadelphia: Lea & Blanchard; 1843.

[5] Mahler J, editor. Replacement of Renal Function by Dialysis A Textbook of Dialysis. Norwell: Kluwer Academic Press; 1989.

[6] De Santo NG, Bisaccia C, De Santo RM, Perna AF, Manzo M, Di Stazio E, et al. Mariano Semmola (1831-1895): the effect of low protein diet in primary albuminuria. J Nephrol. 2006 May-Jun 19;Suppl 10:S48-57.

[7] Giovannetti S, Maggiore Q. A Low-Nitrogen Diet with Proteins of High Biological Value for Severe Chronic Uraemia. Lancet. 1964 May 9;1(7341):1000-3.

[8] Eknoyan G. The wonderful apparatus of John Jacob Abel called the "artificial kidney". Semin Dial. 2009;22(3):287-96.

[9] Cameron JS. Practical haemodialysis began with cellophane and heparin: the crucial role of William Thalhimer (1884 - 1961). Nephrol Dial Transplant. 2000 July 1;15(7):1086-91.

[10] Thalhimer W. A Method for Concentrating Serum in Cellophane Bags and Simultaneously Removing Salts and Other Constituents. Proc Soc Exp Biol Med. 1939 May 1;41(1):230-2.

[11] Kolff WJ. 50th anniversary ASAIO speech. ASAIO J. 2004 Nov-Dec;50(6):xxii-xxiii.

[12] Epstein M. John P. Merrill: The Father of Nephrology as a Specialty. Clin J Am Soc Nephrol. 2009 January;4(1):2-8.

[13] Guild WR, Harrison JH, Merrill JP, Murray J. Successful homotransplantation of the kidney in an identical twin. Trans Am Clin Climatol Assoc. 1955;67:167-73.

[14] Murray JE, Tilney NL, Wilson RE. Renal transplantation: a twenty-five year experience. Ann Sur. 1976;184(5):565-73.

[15] Blagg C. Personal Communication. 2011.

[16] Shaldon S. 40 Years of Dialysis. Nephron Information Center; 2001.

[17] Shaldon S, Silva H, Pomeroy J, Rae AI, Rosen SM. Percutaneous femoral venous catheterization and reusable dialysers in the treatment of acute renal failure. Trans Am Soc Artif Intern Organs. 1964;10:133-5.

[18] Brescia MJ, Cimino JE, Appel K, Hurwich BJ. Chronic hemodialysis using venipuncture and a surgically created arteriovenous fistula. N Engl J Med. 1966 Nov 17;275(20):1089-92.

[19] Cimino JE, Brescia MJ. Simple venipuncture for hemodialysis. N Engl J Med. 1962 Sep 20;267:608-9.

[20] Giacchino JL, Geis WP, Buckingham JM, Vertuno LL, Bansal VK. Vascular access: long-term results, new techniques. Arch Surg. 1979 Apr;114(4):403-9.

[21] Martakos P, Karwoski T, Herweck SA, inventors; Atrium Medical, assignee. Methods of making controlled porosity expanded polytetrafluoroethyleneproducts and fabrication. United States; 1999.

[22] Schild AF, Schuman ES, Noicely K, Kaufman J, Gillaspie E, Fuller J, et al. Early cannulation prosthetic graft (FlixeneTM) for arteriovenous access. J Vasc Access. 2011 Feb 10.

[23] Blagg CR. Belding Hibbard Scribner--better known as Scrib. Clinical journal of the American Society of Nephrology: Clin J Am Soc Nephrol. 2010 Dec;5(12):2146-9.

[24] Blagg CR. The early history of dialysis for chronic renal failure in the United States: a view from Seattle. Am J Kidney Dis. 2007 Mar;49(3):482-96.

[25] Blagg CR. Belding Hibbard Scribner, the individual: a brief biography. J Nephrol. 2006 May-Jun;19 Suppl 10:S127-31.

[26] Rabindranath Kannaiyan S, Adams J, Ali Tariq Z, MacLeod AM, Vale L, Cody JD, et al. Continuous ambulatory peritoneal dialysis versus automated peritoneal dialysis for end-stage renal disease - Cochrane Database of Systematic Reviews. Chichester, UK: John Wiley & Sons, Ltd; 2007.

[27] Shaldon S, Rae AI, Rosen SM, Silva H, Oakley J. Refrigerated femoral venous-venous haemodialysis with coil preservation for rehabilitation of terminal uraemic patients. Br Med J. 1963 Jun 29;1(5347):1716-7.

[28] Blagg CR. The early years of chronic dialysis: The Seattle contribution. Am J Nephrol. 1999;19(2):350-4.

[29] Scribner BH, Cole JJ, Ahmad S, Blagg CR. Why thrice weekly dialysis? Hemodial Int. 2004 Apr 1;8(2):188-92.

[30] Peitzman SJ. The flame photometer as engine of nephrology: a biography. Am J Kidney Dis. 2010 Aug;56(2):379-86.

[31] Kiil F. Development of a parallel-flow artificial kidney in plastics. Acta Chir Scand Suppl. 1960;Suppl 253:142-50.

[32] Mclain EA, inventor DOW Chemical CO, assignee. Wound hollow fiber permeability apparatus and process of making the same. United States; 1969.

[33] Streicher E, Schneider H. The development of a polysulfone membrane. A new perspective in dialysis? Contrib Nephrol. 1985;46:1-13.

[34] Glater J. The early history of reverse osmosis membrane development. Desalination. 1998;117(1-3):297-309.

[35] McFeely T. The Price of Access. Nashua: MDL Press; 2001.

[36] Alexander S. They Decide Who Lives, Who Dies. Life Magazine. 1962 November 9:102-25.

[37] Jarvis L, Newman E. Who shall live? National Broadcasting Company. 1965 November 18.

[38] Satel S. The God Committee. American Enterprise Institute for Public Policy Research [serial on the Internet; cited 23 Nov 2011]. 2008:Available from: http://www.aei.org/article/28156.

[39] A. Friedman E, Bommer Jr. Peter Lundin (1944 - 2001) the physician/patient role model. Nephrol Dial Transplant. 2001 November 1;16(11):2272.

[40] Rettig RA. Special Treatment, The Story of Medicare's ESRD Entitlement. N Engl J Med. 2011;364(7):596-8.

[41] Schreiner GE. Personal Communication. 2002.

[42] Plante CL. 1971 Medicare amendment: Reflections on the passage of the end-stage renal disease Medicare program. Am J Kidney Dis. 2000;35(4, Supplement 1):S45-S8.

[43] Teschner M, Heidland A, Klassen A, Sebekova K, Bahner U. Georg Ganter--a pioneer of peritoneal dialysis and his tragic academic demise at the hand of the Nazi regime. J Nephrol. 2004 May-Jun;17(3):457-60.

[44] Odel HM, Ferris DO, Power MH. Peritoneal lavage as an effective means of extrarenal excretion; a clinical appraisal. Am J Med. 1950 Jul;9(1):63-77.

[45] Maxwell MH, Rockney RE, Kleeman CR, Twiss MR. Peritoneal dialysis. 1. Technique and applications. JAMA. 1959 Jun 20;170(8):917-24.

[46] Tenckhoff H, Schechter H. A bacteriologically safe peritoneal access device. Trans Am Soc Artif Intern Organs. 1968;14:181-7.

[47] Tenckhoff H, Shilipetar G, Van Paasschen WH, Swanson E. A home peritoneal dialysate delivery system. Trans Am Soc Artif Intern Organs. 1969;15:103-7.

[48] Tenckhoff H, Curtis FK. Experience with maintenance peritoneal dialysis in the home. Trans Am Soc Artif Intern Organs. 1970;16:90-5.

[49] Twardowski ZJ. History of peritoneal access development. Int J Artif Organs. 2006 Jan;29(1):2-40.

[50] Rettig RA, Levinsky NG. Kidney Failure and the Federal Government. National Academies Press; 1991.

[51] Gotch FA, Sargent JA. A mechanistic analysis of the National Cooperative Dialysis Study (NCDS). Kidney Int. 1985 Sep;28(3):526-34.

[52] Turney JH, Blagg CR, Pickstone JV. Early Dialysis in Britain: Leeds and Beyond. Am J Kidney Dis. 2011 Jan 14.

[53] Parsons FM, Hobson SM, Blagg CR, Mc CB. Optimum time for dialysis in acute reversible renal failure. Description and value of an improved dialyser with large surface area. Lancet. 1961 Jan 21;1(7169):129-34.

[54] Pflederer BR, Torrey C, Priester-Coary A, Lau AH, Daugirdas JT. Estimating equilibrated Kt/V from an intradialytic sample: effects of access and cardiopulmonary recirculations. Kidney Int. 1995 Sep;48(3):832-7.

[55] Daugirdas JT. Simplified equations for monitoring Kt/V, PCRn, eKt/V, and ePCRn. Adv Ren Replace Ther. 1995 Oct;2(4):295-304.

[56] Priester-Coary A, Daugirdas JT. A Recommended Technique for Obtaining the Post-Dialysis BUN. Semin Dial. 1997 Jan-Feb;10(1):23-5.

[57] Depner T, Beck G, Daugirdas J, Kusek J, Eknoyan G. Lessons from the Hemodialysis (HEMO) Study: an improved measure of the actual hemodialysis dose. Am J Kidney Dis. 1999 Jan;33(1):142-9.

[58] Depner TA, Greene T, Gotch FA, Daugirdas JT, Keshaviah PR, Star RA. Imprecision of the hemodialysis dose when measured directly from urea removal. Hemodialysis Study Group. Kidney Int. 1999 Feb;55(2):635-47.

[59] Lowrie EG, Laird NM, Parker TF, Sargent JA. Effect of the hemodialysis prescription of patient morbidity: report from the National Cooperative Dialysis Study. N Engl J Med. 1981 Nov 12;305(20):1176-81.

[60] The National Cooperative Dialysis Study. Kidney Int Suppl. 1983 Apr(13):S1-122.

[61] Morbidity and mortality of dialysis. NIH Consensus Statement Online. 1993 1993. p. 1-33.

[62] Hull AR. Impact of reimbursement regulations on patient management. Am J Kidney Dis. 1992 Jul;20(1 Suppl 1):8-11.

[63] Hull AR. The 1989 Dallas Conference on Morbidity and Mortality in Dialysis: What Did We Learn? Clin J Am Soc Nephrol. 2009 December 1, 2009;4(Supplement 1):S2-S4.

[64] Parker TF, 3rd, Husni L, Huang W, Lew N, Lowrie EG. Survival of hemodialysis patients in the United States is improved with a greater quantity of dialysis. Am J Kidney Dis. 1994 May;23(5):670-80.

[65] Eknoyan G, Beck GJ, Cheung AK, Daugirdas JT, Greene T, Kusek JW, et al. Effect of dialysis dose and membrane flux in maintenance hemodialysis. N Engl J Med. 2002;347(25):2010-9.

[66] NKF-DOQI clinical practice guidelines for hemodialysis adequacy. National Kidney Foundation. Am J Kidney Dis. 1997 Sep;30(3 Suppl 2):S15-66.

[67] Cheung AK, Yan G, Greene T, Daugirdas JT, Dwyer JT, Levin NW, et al. Seasonal variations in clinical and laboratory variables among chronic hemodialysis patients. J Am Soc Nephrol. 2002 Sep;13(9):2345-52.

[68] Daugirdas JT, Greene T, Depner TA, Leypoldt J, Gotch F, Schulman G, et al. Factors that affect postdialysis rebound in serum urea concentration, including the rate of dialysis: results from the HEMO Study. J Am Soc Nephrol. 2004 Jan;15(1):194-203.

[69] Daugirdas JT, Greene T, Chertow GM, Depner TA. Can rescaling dose of dialysis to body surface area in the HEMO study explain the different responses to dose in women versus men? Clin J Am Soc Nephrol. 2010 Sep;5(9):1628-36.

[70] Daugirdas JT, Hanna MG, Becker-Cohen R, Langman CB. Dose of dialysis based on body surface area is markedly less in younger children than in older adolescents. Clinical journal of the American Society of Nephrology: Clin J Am Soc Nephrol. 2010 May;5(5):821-7.

[71] Daugirdas JT. Is there a minimal amount of time a patient should be dialyzed regardless of measured KT/V? Semin Dial. 2011 Jul 31;24(4):423-5.

[72] USRDS. [cited 2011 Aug 4]. Available from: http://www.usrds.org.

[73] Harnett JD, Foley RN, Kent GM, Barre PE, Murray D, Parfrey PS. Congestive heart failure in dialysis patients: prevalence, incidence, prognosis and risk factors. Kidney Int. 1995 Mar;47(3):884-90.

[74] Foley RN, Parfrey PS, Harnett JD, Kent GM, Murray DC, Barre PE. The impact of anemia on cardiomyopathy, morbidity, and and mortality in end-stage renal disease. Am J Kidney Dis. 1996 Jul;28(1):53-61.

[75] Eschbach JW, Downing MR, Egrie JC, Browne JK, Adamson JW. USA multicenter clinical trial with recombinant human erythropoietin (Amgen). Results in hemodialysis patients. Contrib Nephrol. 1989;76:160-5; discussion 212-8.

[76] Karnofsky Score. [cited 2011 Aug 4]. Available from: http://touchcalc.com/calculators/karnofsky.

[77] Tong EM, Nissenson AR. Erythropoietin and anemia. Semin Nephrol. 2001 Mar;21(2):190-203.

[78] Beusterien KM, Nissenson AR, Port FK, Kelly M, Steinwald B, Ware JE, Jr. The effects of recombinant human erythropoietin on functional health and well-being in chronic dialysis patients. J Am Soc Nephrol. 1996 May;7(5):763-73.

[79] Moreno F, Aracil FJ, Perez R, Valderrabano F. Controlled study on the improvement of quality of life in elderly hemodialysis patients after correcting end-stage renal disease-related anemia with erythropoietin. Am J Kidney Dis. 1996 Apr;27(4):548-56.

[80] Levin NW, Lazarus JM, Nissenson AR. National Cooperative rHu Erythropoietin Study in patients with chronic renal failure--an interim report. The National Cooperative rHu Erythropoietin Study Group. Am J Kidney Dis. 1993 Aug;22(2 Suppl 1):3-12.

[81] Nissenson AR. National cooperative rHu erythropoietin study in patients with chronic renal failure: a phase IV multicenter study. Report of National Cooperative rHu Erythropoietin Study Group. Am J Kidney Dis. 1991 Oct;18(4 Suppl 1):24-33.

[82] Nissenson AR, Nimer SD, Wolcott DL. Recombinant human erythropoietin and renal anemia: molecular biology, clinical efficacy, and nervous system effects. Ann Intern Med. 1991 Mar 1;114(5):402-16.

[83] Wolcott DL, Marsh JT, La Rue A, Carr C, Nissenson AR. Recombinant human erythropoietin treatment may improve quality of life and cognitive function in chronic hemodialysis patients. Am J Kidney Dis. 1989 Dec;14(6):478-85.

[84] Nissenson AR. Recombinant human erythropoietin: impact on brain and cognitive function, exercise tolerance, sexual potency, and quality of life. Semin Nephrol. 1989 Mar;9(1 Suppl 2):25-31.

[85] Keown PA, Churchill DN, Poulin-Costello M, Lei L, Gantotti S, Agodoa I, et al. Dialysis patients treated with Epoetin alfa show improved anemia symptoms: A new analysis of the Canadian Erythropoietin Study Group trial. Hemodial Int. 2010 Apr;14(2):168-73.

[86] Mujais SK, Story K, Brouillette J, Takano T, Soroka S, Franek C, et al. Health-related quality of life in CKD Patients: correlates and evolution over time. Clin J Am Soc Nephrol. 2009 Aug;4(8):1293-301.

[87] Riano-Galan I, Malaga S, Rajmil L, Ariceta G, Navarro M, Loris C, et al. Quality of life of adolescents with end-stage renal disease and kidney transplant. Pediatr Nephrol. 2009 Aug;24(8):1561-8.

[88] Leaf DE, Goldfarb DS. Interpretation and review of health-related quality of life data in CKD patients receiving treatment for anemia. Kidney Int. 2009 Jan;75(1):15-24.

[89] Weisbord SD, Kimmel PL. Health-related quality of life in the era of erythropoietin. Hemodial Int. 2008 Jan;12(1):6-15.

[90] Rebollo P, Baltar JM, Campistol JM, Ortega T, Ortega F. Quality of life of patients with chronic renal allograft rejection and anemia. J Nephrol. 2004 Jul-Aug;17(4):531-6.

[91] Vazquez I, Valderrabano F, Fort I, Jofre R, Lopez-Gomez JM, Moreno F, et al. Differences in health-related quality of life between male and female hemodialysis patients. Nefrologia. 2004;24(2):167-78.

[92] Perlman RL, Kiser M, Finkelstein F, Eisele G, Roys E, Liu L, et al. The longitudinal chronic kidney disease study: a prospective cohort study of predialysis renal failure. Semin Dial. 2003 Nov-Dec;16(6):418-23.

[93] NKF-DOQI clinical practice guidelines for the treatment of anemia of chronic renal failure. National Kidney Foundation-Dialysis Outcomes Quality Initiative. Am J Kidney Dis. 1997 Oct;30(4 Suppl 3):S192-240.

[94] Wish JB. Past, Present, and Future of Chronic Kidney Disease Anemia Management in the United States. Adv Chronic Kidney Dis. 2009;16(2):101-8.

[95] Besarab A, Bolton WK, Browne JK, Egrie JC, Nissenson AR, Okamoto DM, et al. The effects of normal as compared with low hematocrit values in patients with cardiac disease who are receiving hemodialysis and epoetin. N Engl J Med. 1998 Aug 27;339(9):584-90.

[96] Collins AJ. Influence of target hemoglobin in dialysis patients on morbidity and mortality. Kidney Int Suppl. 2002 May(80):44-8.

[97] Drueke TB, Locatelli F, Clyne N, Eckardt KU, Macdougall IC, Tsakiris D, et al. Normalization of hemoglobin level in patients with chronic kidney disease and anemia. N Engl J Med. 2006 Nov 16;355(20):2071-84.

[98] Singh AK, Szczech L, Tang KL, Barnhart H, Sapp S, Wolfson M, et al. Correction of anemia with epoetin alfa in chronic kidney disease. N Engl J Med. 2006 Nov 16;355(20):2085-98.

[99] Pfeffer MA, Burdmann EA, Chen C-Y, Cooper ME, de Zeeuw D, Eckardt K-U, et al. A Trial of Darbepoetin Alfa in Type 2 Diabetes and Chronic Kidney Disease. N Engl J Med. 2009;361(21):2019-32.

[100] FDA Drug Safety Communication: Modified dosing recommendations to improve the safe use of Erythropoiesis-Stimulating Agents (ESAs) in chronic kidney disease. Food and Drug Administration; 2011 [updated 24 Jun 2011; cited 24 Jun 2011]. Available from: http://www.fda.gov/Drugs/DrugSafety/ucm259639.htm.

[101] K/DOQI clinical practice guidelines on hypertension and antihypertensive agents in chronic kidney disease. Am J Kidney Dis. 2004 2004/05//;43(5 Suppl 1):1-290.

[102] Eknoyan G, Levin NW, Steinberg EP. The dialysis outcomes quality initiative: History, impact, and prospects. Am J Kidney Dis. 2000;35(4):S69-S75.

[103] K/DOQI clinical practice guidelines for chronic kidney disease: evaluation, classification, and stratification. Am J Kidney Dis. 2002 Feb;39(2 Suppl 1):S1-266.

[104] Eknoyan G. Meeting the challenges of the new K/DOQI guidelines. Am J Kidney Dis. 2003 Jun;41(5 Suppl):3-10.

[105] Moe SM, Drüeke T, Lameire N, Eknoyan G. Chronic Kidney Disease-Mineral-Bone Disorder: A New Paradigm. Adv Chronic Kidney Dis. 2007;14(1):3-12.

[106] Fadem SZ, Moe SM. Management of Chronic Kidney Disease Mineral-Bone Disorder. Adv Chronic Kidney Dis. 2007 01;14(1):44-53.

[107] Social Security Administration Conditions for Coverage for End-Stage Renal Disease Facilities; Final Rule. 42 CFR Federal Register. 1976 June 3;41:22503-22.

[108] Medicare and Medicaid programs; conditions for coverage for end-stage renal disease facilities. Final rule. Federal Register. 2008 Apr 15;73(73):20369-484.

[109] Medicare program; end-stage renal disease prospective payment system. Final rule. Federal Register. 2010 Aug 12;75(155):49029-214.

[110] Hull AR. The 1989 morbidity and mortality meeting: how far have we come? Am J Kidney Dis. 1998 Dec;32(6 Suppl 4):S6-8.

[111] Centers for Medicare & Medicaid Services. Kidney Disease Education Services. Federal Register. 42 CFR(410.48) [cited 2011 Oct 10]. Available from: http://edocket.access.gpo.gov/cfr_2010/octqtr/pdf/42cfr410.48.pdf.

[112] U.S. Renal Data System, USRDS. 2010 Annual Data Report. 2010.

[113] Collins AJ, Foley RN, Gilbertson DT, Chen S-C. The State of Chronic Kidney Disease, ESRD, and Morbidity and Mortality in the First Year of Dialysis. Clin J Am Soc Nephrol. 2009;4(Supplement 1):S5-S11.

[114] Fadem SZ, Walker DR, Abbott G, Friedman AL, Goldman R, Sexton S, et al. Satisfaction with renal replacement therapy and education: the american association of kidney patients survey. Clin J Am Soc Nephrol. 2011 Mar;6(3):605-12.

[115] Centers for Medicare & Medicaid Services. Medicare Shared Savings Program: Accountable Care Organizations. 42 CFR Part 425. Federal Register. 2011 August 6;76(67):19528.

[116] Conway B, Webster A, Ramsay G, Morgan N, Neary J, Whitworth C, et al. Predicting mortality and uptake of renal replacement therapy in patients with stage 4 chronic kidney disease. Nephrol Dial Transplant. 2009 Jun;24(6):1930-7.

[117] Murtagh FE, Marsh JE, Donohoe P, Ekbal NJ, Sheerin NS, Harris FE. Dialysis or not? A comparative survival study of patients over 75 years with chronic kidney disease stage 5. Nephrol Dial Transplant. 2007 Jul;22(7):1955-62.

[118] Charlson Co-morbidity Index. [cited 7 Aug 2011]. Available from: http://touchcalc.com/cci.

[119] Renal Physicians Association. Shared Decision Making in the Appropriate Initiation of and Withdrawal From Dialysis. 2nd Ed. Rockville, MD: RPA; 2010.

[120] Chertow GM, Levin NW, Beck GJ, Depner TA, Eggers PW, Gassman JJ, et al. In-center hemodialysis six times per week versus three times per week. N Engl J Med. 2010 Dec 9;363(24):2287-300.

In: Issues in Dialysis
Editor: Stephen Z. Fadem

ISBN: 978-1-62417-576-3
© 2013 Nova Science Publishers, Inc.

Chapter II

The Course of Therapy:
Changing the Paradigm

Thomas A. Golper[*]
Division of Nephrology and Hypertension
Vanderbilt University Medical Center, Nashville, Tennessee, US

Martin J. Schreiber, Jr.
Glickman Urological and Kidney Institute, Cleveland, Ohio, US
Department of Nephrology and Hypertension
Cleveland Clinic, Cleveland, Ohio, US

Abstract

We believe that the best outcomes for a patient facing end-stage kidney disease are achieved through an individualized approach. To accomplish this one has to recognize that an entire team may be needed, acting in concert. This includes the patient and immediate family, more distant family, friends, clergy, co-workers, nephrologist, and other health providers. The team assists in an integrated care approach which takes into account the individual characteristics that may favor one direction of care over another. This includes creating an environment where knowledge contributes to decisions in a logical order, such as (1) the decision to undertake kidney replacement therapy vs. conservative care; (2) then if kidney replacement therapy is elected, a decision on type (transplantation vs. dialysis); (3) then if dialysis is elected, in-center vs. home; (4) then, if home dialysis is chosen, hemodialysis vs. peritoneal; (5) then lastly, if home dialysis is selected, the type of home hemodialysis or home peritoneal dialysis. Awareness of the advantages and disadvantages for that patient must be part of the physician's influence and recommendations. The attitude of patients and their influential advisors then comes into play. The overarching strategy is the health care team's awareness of these attitudes

---

[*] Corresponding author address: Thomas A. Golper, MD; S-3303 Medical Center North, Vanderbilt University Medical Center, 21st Avenue South, Nashville, TN 37232. Fax 615 322 8653; Phone 615 343 2220; thomas.golper@vanderbilt.edu

in formulating and executing an individualized end-stage kidney disease life plan. Roadblocks to effective communication abound. We confront some of these recognizing our professional obligations and failings and suggest ways to build this strategy into everyday practice. Forthright discussions, education, empowerment and shared decision making within an environment reflecting a team approach will result in greater satisfaction for all participants.

Introduction

Tremendous strides have been made in delaying the progression of chronic kidney disease (CKD). Awareness of specific pathologic processes has led to targeted therapy, but general interventions have been applied as well including control of blood pressure, hyperglycemia and metabolic acidosis. In addition, the process of kidney scarring has been slowed by renin-angiotensin-aldosterone system blockade. The medical community's awareness of kidney disease has increased in part due to the staging of kidney disease (I-VI) based on an eGFR calculation, and, as a result, patients are referred earlier to nephrologists. Not all of these positive changes have had as much penetration into the general population as we want, but all in all, pretty remarkable progress has been made. Because of the progress in slowing the progressive nature of kidney failure, nephrologists and their collaborative care teams now have time to educate their patients about what to expect and how to develop a plan for successfully living with kidney failure and adjust to renal replacement therapies.

This chapter will discuss the approach to this situation. One strategy will not fit all occasions. Many variables come into play from finances to aging. Therefore, both general and specific tactics will be discussed when appropriate. Assemblage of the team participating in patient education is the starting point.

The Team

Often the physician who refers the patient with progressive kidney disease to the nephrologist is only peripherally involved in the kidney care. However, the relationship of that physician to his/her patient may be a valuable attribute in influencing the patient's outlook, attitude and decisions. As such the nephrologist and kidney team should complement and not replace the primary care physician. Understanding the importance of this primary care physician- patient relationship may have significant benefits. Thus, one key team member must be the primary care physician or the specific referring physician. Occasionally the latter may be subspecialists such as cardiologists or endocrinologists.

After the referring physician, the nephrologist is usually the next provider to meet the patient. That relationship must have a solid foundation in mutual trust and respect, which takes time to nurture and mature. Our experience has been that this relationship must have substance prior to referring the patient to an educational specialist, as we discuss later. The nephrologist will essentially assess the current medical situation and simultaneously perform diagnostic and therapeutic maneuvers. As the patient's kidney function deteriorates it is critically important for the nephrologist to constantly inform the patient as to what will occur and what to do about it. This is the important foundation for the relationship that must be built such that when the difficult decisions are necessary, they will be made in the context of trust and confidence.

As the nephrologist's relationship to the patient matures, there then is an expansion of that relationship to the patient's family. Kidney disease extends beyond the patient to touch family, friends, and co-workers so that the patient needs to understand that this is not just his or her disease. As such, we believe that a key to successful care is having a "sponsor" who is an important patient advocate, information synthesizer, and liaison mediator. The sponsor can be a family member or friend who would accompany the patient to the office visit and be part of the information process, reinforcing what the patient is being told along the way. As will be discussed below, progressive kidney failure involves every aspect of a patient's life, so family cannot be excluded as plans evolve. As the physician-family relationships develop, the nephrologist will bring in his/her provider team members. That could include associate physicians but also office nurses, technicians, phlebotomists, social workers, dialysis nurses, clinical nurse specialists, nurse practitioners, physician assistants or education specialists from dialysis provider organizations or lay organizations.

On many occasions we have utilized kidney failure patients on various therapies to discuss their experiences with treatment and how they live a quality life despite having kidney failure. This is a feature of our larger group classes. To ignore this potential team approach is to miss dramatic opportunities. If the nephrologist's office does not have such resources readily available in house, then local or regional lay organizations may be the best available resource. Internet resources abound and should be exploited.

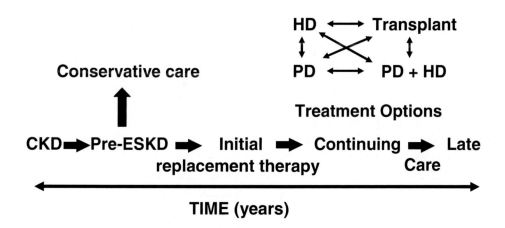

Figure 1. Integrated care across the chronic kidney disease continuum including conservative care, forms of kidney replacement therapies, and acknowledging that transitions points will occur.

We personally utilize every resource mentioned above. Our large group practices have ready access to a hospital/clinic dietician and a dialysis dietician, nurse practitioners in our clinics and dialysis units, and a treatment option program specialist. Furthermore, our clinic hospital phlebotomy and intravenous line teams are aware of the importance to protect future hemodialysis access sites encouraging socially acceptable wrist bands reminding all medical personnel to avoid needle harm to the future fistula arm.

The specific use of the different components of the team is individually addressed, but a standard approach is certainly a reasonable starting point. For example, we have structured two formal classes attended by up to 6 patients, each accompanied by up to three family members (24 total attendees). One class is on kidney function, kidney failure and diet. The second class is on modality options for kidney replacement therapy. Then individual sessions are arranged as needed. The individual sessions could be with the nurse practitioner, the dietician, social worker or educational specialist. We are aware of Medicare payments for some of these services under certain conditions, but have not necessarily designed the educational program around such payments. Throughout these sessions, communication with the nephrologist is mandatory. The nephrologist should discuss any detected or reported concerns promptly to avoid any misunderstandings that may lead later to poor or inappropriate decisions. Keeping the referring or primary care physician in this loop is also important, as well as involving any other consulting specialists who might make a recommendation with potentially adverse outcomes (e.g. pre transplant elective coronary arteriography that changes residual kidney function).

Another advantage of a team approach is the differing perspectives the patient and family will experience by interacting with varied members all projecting a consistent emphasis on patient involvement and choices. Reinforcement of ideas leads to confidence, but also differences of opinions may lead ultimately to a better understanding. The strengths and attributes of the team must be understood by the nephrologist team leader. Within the continuum of kidney disease using all the tools at one's disposal is crucial.

Integrated Care

Figure 1 outlines the breadth of therapies within the concept of the Integrated Care approach to progressive kidney disease. Patients with progressive CKD will either elect kidney replacement therapy to prolong life or to live and then die without it. If replacement therapy is elected there are numerous options to be discussed below. However, it is important to recognize that virtually all options will be utilized in a patient's lifetime and that some level of expertise in all options must be an attribute of the providing nephrologist. For example, education about transplantation should come from the general nephrology care provider just as should education about conservative (non kidney replacement therapy) care, in-center dialysis or home dialysis. That does not preclude input from subspecialists in these areas, but the nephrologist ship captain must be with the patient at the hub of the wheel. We return to this concept of integrated care again below.

The Influence of Attitudes of Patients

For most patients progressive kidney disease leading to end-stage kidney disease (ESKD) can be anticipated. The nephrologist knows this but may not always inform the patient. Even when the patient does know, they are reluctant to really grasp the significance. The "sponsor" who remains with the patient during visits and education sessions can assist in patient comprehension of what the individual hears and is being told. And yet a number of patients want to go it alone, and procrastination of the clinical discussions occurs with many patients sliding unprepared into a default renal replacement option. The consequence of "choice" delays is often insufficient time to discuss management alternatives with other important health care providers such as the primary care physician and other consultants. Even more devastating is the failure to allocate time for discussions with his/her family and others with life-influencing relationships (e.g. employers, co-workers). So the attitude of the patient and his/her inner circle is critical to the development of a rational strategy as ESKD approaches.

Morton and associates have organized helpful perspective about the attitudes of patients and care providers in this setting. [1] The first theme focuses on a patient understanding that CKD is life threatening. As such it offers the opportunity for the patient to re-evaluate and establish new priorities for his/her life. This is done within the context that CKD care is a burden to the patient and those around the patient. Uncertainty as to the timing of events (e.g. access creation, initiating dialysis, transplantation, death) leaves the patient and family in a stressful state of limbo. Should wills be revised, assets liquidated, houses sold and long term care facilities sought? Doing nothing is clearly easier. Maintaining the status quo is almost always preferable to change. Change is risk.

A second theme is choice. Patients may feel or perceive a lack of choice and therefore fail to make a choice and find themselves on a default therapy in a crisis setting, i.e. in-center hemodialysis. Of course education helps overcome this but physical, social or physiological conditions may clearly limit choice. Should these external situations limit choice, letting the patient express frustration and sadness can be therapeutic. Certainly acknowledgement of these emotions is helpful especially in strengthening the relationship between the patient and care providers. A failed hemodialysis fistula, a live donor transplant canceled due to a donor problem, an inability to dialyze in a certain location or at a certain preferred time are all examples of situations where patient choice might be denied. These are losses. It is appropriate to mourn losses to advance to the next stage in one's life. The care provider team has to be prepared to participate and perhaps lead in this evolution of patient attitude. Structuring a Life Plan for each patient is critical to putting all this information and key decision points into an orderly life sensitive approach, best for extending quality survival despite having kidney failure (see below).

Gaining knowledge is critical. So education must be emphasized early, frequently and repeatedly. Maturity and experience help, but is not always an available luxury. Peer influence in education about kidney disease is under-appreciated. Peers in this context include family, friends, co-workers and to some extent we health care providers. Here again timing is important. Procrastination costs us the aid of peer influence simply because the peers do not have adequate time to form their own thoughts and transmit them to patients. It is never too early to educate our patients and families. Doing it consistently and when no medical crises dominate the visit are helpful. Intercurrent illness can require physician time and therapeutic intervention and clearly distracts all parties away from the lower priority issues such as ESKD education. The loss of cognitive skills, employment, external support, general health, and kidney health are all more predictable than not. We must therefore act accordingly and in anticipation.

Following the acquisition of knowledge is the weighing of alternatives. This is where confronting mortality, overcoming the frustration of lack of choice, and knowledge all come together as decisions are made. Patients desire to maintain their current lifestyle but this is shaped by the opinions of family and friends. Outcomes of a treatment often are considered less important than the effect of that treatment on lifestyle. Patients want to uphold their responsibilities and maintain their personal interests. A preference for home dialysis may be based around privacy, freedom and flexibility, attributes often far more influential than the expected duration of one's life. Preference for in-center hemodialysis may be influenced by the importance to that patient for a planned schedule, regular social contact, and a previous experience or knowledge of the therapy.

Table 1. Some Reasons for Choosing a Modality (modified from Morton et al. [1])

Peritoneal Dialysis	Hemodialysis
Self sufficiency	Prefer care from others
Privacy	Prefer a planned schedule
Flexibility	Free days without dialysis
Less travel	Previous experience
Less admissions to hospital	Desire to swim
More spare time	Convenience
Fear of needles	
Arm appearance	
Fear of cross infection	
Vessel preservation for the future	

The Nephrologist's Approach to the Patient

With this insight into the patient's attitudes and with the help of the education team, a nephrologist competent in managing all the different ESKD replacement modalities must help direct the patient's decision making. One often effective approach is to impart knowledge step by step over many visits, building on each previous visit's experience. The success of this transfer of information to the patient is best achieved if the patient has the "sponsor" involved along the way. Therefore, one must start early and not get trapped into having to discuss the difficult or complex issues when there is no time, for example, during medical emergencies.

Once it is clear that the kidney disease is progressive and the team has embarked on therapies to slow its progression, probe for the patient's intentions. What are his/her priorities in their overall life plan? The priorities may be combinations of feeling better, to get a transplant, to experience an upcoming family milestone, to live as long as possible! Is quality or quantity (length) of life more important? The answers are not mutually exclusive but the discussions are crucial to understanding intent. Do not be reluctant to ask patients how long they intend to live. While "as long as possible" is the most common answer, it is by no means the only answer. Again, insight is achieved, and this knowledge is important in trying to help patients make treatment decisions.

Point out to patients that conservative therapy, i.e. no kidney replacement therapy, is an alternative. When a patient replies that this is not an alternative for them, ask why it is not. Some of the worst experiences in ESKD management have been in patients who appear to be dialyzing because someone other than themselves wanted it. This sad situation is unnecessary and can be avoided with early discussion along the lines described above.

Conservative care is no more of a death sentence than is dialysis or transplantation. Its discussion should not be as a last option. On the contrary, it is the first option (see figure 2) because if kidney replacement therapy is selected, than all energy must be directed to that selection, not a passive effort. That may partially explain why some patients come to dialysis with such little motivation to do well. Conservative therapy may not have a poorer outcome then kidney replacement therapy. Murtagh et al. have demonstrated that when co-morbid conditions are present, CKD stage 5 patients that choose conservative therapy live as long as those who choose dialysis. [2] We also know that more often than not, patients do not make decisions based on the effectiveness of therapy such as dialysis. Far more often decisions are based on personal values, beliefs and feelings towards life, suffering, and death. Also highly important and frequently not recognized is the expected difficulty of fitting dialysis into one's life. [3] It is in this context that the very first decision that the patient weighs is on the kidney replacement therapy vs. conservative therapy choice (Figure 2).

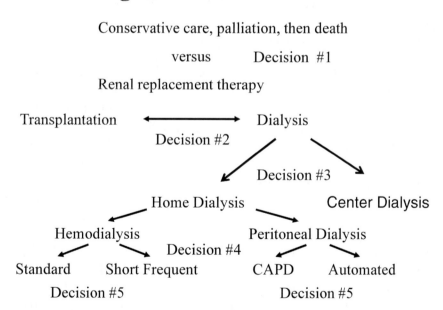

Figure 2. The decisions that must occur in planning ESKD treatment options.

If kidney replacement therapy is the decision, then all energy must be directed to making that decision into the correct decision. For many patients the very next decision is the possibility of transplantation. In our programs formal transplant evaluation cannot begin until the estimated glomerular filtration rate is ≤ 20 ml/min. So even if transplant is opted, begin discussions about dialytic alternatives as a backup. Even with the best of luck, only 5% of our patients experience a pre-emptive transplant. There is little controversy that this is the best approach but because it is often not feasible, move to dialysis discussions, even as a back-up plan, to get the patient's mind-set into that possibility.

The dialysis discussions start with the option of dialyzing in the home vs. in the dialysis center. As we age we all want to remain independent (nursing home vs. independent living) and the same goal should be emphasized in selecting renal replacement therapy. On some occasions a patient's first reaction is that naturally they would do it at home. The more frequent reaction is that they should do it at a dialysis center because they don't know how to do it themselves, feel that they do not have the ability and that someone else can do it better. This reaction should be an immediate launching point about education and about self-care. Make it clear that you as their responsible physician would not allow them to perform self-dialysis with inadequate education. This line of reasoning rapidly moves to having the patient and family meet the home dialysis training staff. Once this decision occurs with visits to the home dialysis unit we quickly dispel the motion that patients would be sent home under-trained. This concern is a variation on the fear of abandonment. Recognition and acknowledgement of this is very important in many medical disciplines. For a patient to understand that they are clearly not alone is quite empowering and an enormous relief. This applies to conservative care and in-center dialysis as well as home dialysis. All members of the health care team must be sensitive to this fear of abandonment.

We confess that we strongly encourage home dialysis. Fifty percent of TG's incident dialysis patients begin at home. As patients deliberate home vs. in-center listen and address their concerns. Sometimes we are asked what we would do. One might specifically respond to that question with "do you mean if I were facing dialysis or if I were you as you face dialysis"? We tell patients who ask the former what we would do and why, and then encourage them to ask that same question of others on the health care team. The "why" is very important because it stimulates thinking. We are particularly pleased if the patient receives specific differing reasons why a health care provider would perform a certain form of dialysis. If the question is what I would do if I were the patient, the response is far more nuanced because each case is so different. But this question leads to more questions, with subsequent answers or at least explanations. In those circumstances where we feel the breadth of options and reasons have been discussed, we will render an opinion as to what we would do if we were the patient. This entire process is a pleasure to experience and builds rapport and trust between patient and physician.

It is after the decision has been made to pursue home dialysis that the options of peritoneal vs. hemodialysis arise. Our programs have no options for in-center peritoneal dialysis, so PD is only performed at home. Figure 2 describes the decision of PD vs. HD as the fourth decision. Most of the literature on dialysis option decision making pits PD vs. HD, when the approach should be home dialysis vs. in-center dialysis. Once home dialysis is preferred, PD and HD options should be discussed and reasons why patients might prefer home HD to home PD are listed in Table 2. A more detailed study of this process is underway at our institutions.

Table 2. Some Reasons for Selecting Home HD vs. PD

Training time needed (1 to 8 weeks)
Cosmetics of the dialysis access
Actual treatment schedule
Portability
Fear of needles
Perceived complexity
Space
Need or availability of a helper

There are a few absolute contradictions to PD including a dysfunctional peritoneal membrane (congenital or acquired by previous surgery) or the absence of a home-like environment. Observational studies inform us statistically as to who is most likely to be on PD vs. HD (Table 3). [4,5] Nephrologists generally suggest that more patients could be on home dialysis than the fraction that actually performs home dialysis. Systematic barriers to home dialysis have been recognized but are not easily overcome (Table 4). [6] So the involvement of the nephrologist in the fourth decision is critical. This cannot be left to chance or to the under-informed. Prudent decisions require education and ample data exist that pre-dialysis education programs improve outcomes and home dialysis incident rates. [7-9]

The final decision is after PD or HD at home is selected and the patient drills down more precisely on the type of home HD or PD that is performed. Even at this very sophisticated decision point many of the previously selected life style decisions come into play. More experience with home nocturnal HD and daily home HD will provide more options. Hybrid modalities will evolve. Remote monitoring, blood leak detection devices, wearable artificial kidneys and other innovations all become game changers as technology advances. Thus the fifth decisions will not be addressed here, but these are exciting times in this field.

Overarching Strategies

A helpful strategy is that of devising a Life Plan for living well with end-stage kidney disease. The steps in developing a Life Plan are listed in Table 5. It becomes the roadmap to extend quality life years by anticipating risk, considering options, and structures decisions for the long term. Anticipating risks eliminates making decisions in a crisis. Complications arise from poor planning (delayed arteriovenous access creation leading to HD initiation with a catheter) and this occurs when one focuses on today's needs rather than planning on how to get to tomorrow. Insisting on some form of plan essentially prompts patient buy-in to participate fully. A properly designed and executed ESKD Life Plan can result in decades of life expectancy. Education and preparation focus has to de-emphasize modality option decisions and emphasize complete Life Plan decisions. Decision # 4 cannot precede decision # 1 (Figure 2). By focusing on the Life Plan, one would leverage all modalities over a lifetime and use each and every therapy if indicated or needed. It would emphasize the right therapy at the right time. Depending on age, disease burden, social situation and life goals, the order of which therapy one selects may vary. This therapy selection approach exists in other chronic diseases such as hypertension, diabetes, COPD, etc. wherein a certain therapy is prescribed and works for a while. But later another therapy is substituted in an attempt to optimize disease control. So in kidney failure for best results we recommend strategic sequencing of therapies. During the Life Plan development exercise no therapy should be demeaned or disparaged. One or another may be preferred, may be more logical for that situation but no therapy should be criticized. All therapies may be needed and to have depended on a therapy later that was criticized earlier is to undermine confidence in going forward.

Table 3. Patients more likely to be on PD vs. HD (modified from references 4 and 5)

Older males
Younger females
Caucasian
Married or not living alone
Physically Independent
Seen by nephrologist earlier and more frequently
More assertive or autonomous
Employed
Living a further distance from dialysis unit
Generally healthier
Pre-ESKD options education

Table 4. Systematic Barriers to Home Dialysis

Educational Issues
Patient education regarding home therapies
Physician education
Dialysis staff education

Governmental Issues
Frequency of clinic visit requirements
Reimbursement strategies for dialysis accesses
Home care partner support
Accreditation and certification of home dialysis units
Requirements for home visits by training staff
Availability of "state of the art" equipment/solutions

Business Practices of Dialysis Providers
Availability of solutions and equipment
Deliveries
Pharmacy
Business conflicts with patient care
Laboratory services
Continuous quality improvement strategies
Home dialysis unit independence
Physical environment
Staffing

Table 5. Steps in Developing the Life Plan For End-stage Kidney Disease

Step 1	Discuss with patient what a Life Plan is and why it is essential for optimal outcomes
Step 2	Discuss how age, medical status, comorbidity, and choice of replacement therapy can affect survival
Step 3	Ask patient's goals and priorities
Step 4	Discuss patient actions that can improve outcomes
Step 5	Develop a patient/provider contract for living well with CKD
Step 6	Chart the course
Step 7	Monitor, measure, and adjust therapy

Table 6. Transition Points in Dialysis

PD Transfer to HD	HD Transfer to PD
Recurrent infection	Recurrent volume excess
Catheter malfunction	Angio access failure
Ultrafiltration failure	Hypercoaguble
Solute removal failure	Malnutrition
Psychological burnout	Hypertension
Activity of daily living failure	Loss of transportation
Overwhelming co-morbidities	
Peritoneal membrane disrupting surgery	
Uncontrolled diabetes	
Excessive obese weight gain	
Hypotension	
Malnutrition	

Steps in developing a Life Plan (Table 5) should be individualized. Describing its general features and importance is essential. How age, medical status, social situation, co-morbidities and choice of therapy affect decisions is often of benefit but our experience has been that very few patients favor life expectancy over quality. Nonetheless, one must be prepared to answer this line of inquiry. Find out the patient's priorities and goals, immediate and long term. Asking what the patient wants to achieve in the future makes them understand that in fact there is a future despite having kidney failure. Discuss actions the patient and family must take to achieve the goals and improve outcomes. If necessary, develop a patient/provider contract for living well with CKD. Chart the progress by monitoring, measuring and adjusting as needed. This may be as simple as escalating dialysis dose in a patient utilizing incremental dialysis. Alternatively, it may be as complex as an entire modality transfer. The integrated care concept requires physician (team) expertise in all modalities and the Life Plan concept requires anticipation of risks. The pre-emptive transfer of a PD patient with progressive ultra-filtration failure to hemodialysis is started by the elective creation of a proper HD access while still undergoing PD. Recognition of transition points while undergoing one modality is crucial to lead to the success of the next modality. Examples of such transition points are given in Table 6. In fact, we believe that transition points are so important that the modality change should be labeled as modality transfer or transition. The term modality failure has negative connotations that imply something about behavior when nothing behavioral has occurred. An example is failed HD arteriovenous access. The failed access may lead to a transition to PD, so why label HD a failure? Patients with ESKD face enough obstacles without being labeled failures. So the word of choice is transitions.

Roadblocks to effective communication abound. Firstly, effective communication is given a low priority because often the discussions include unpleasant topics and the time needed for closure is quite unpredictable. So rather than primarily dedicate a session just for such discussions, one avoids them altogether. These topics can be as equally uncomfortable for the patient as for the provider, but avoidance and denial only leads to further miscommunication later. Secondly, some providers feel threatened or challenged by well-informed patients and their families. In this age of electronic information, such providers must transcend this concern and learn to adapt. Thirdly, communication skills may be lacking by provider or patient and that is why more than one discipline is involved in the team approach. It is not so much about what we say as to how we say it. One team member may have a better rapport than another and this should be exploited for maximal communication benefit. Lastly, one might resent the time needed for effective communication because our current health delivery system does not value it. Again, dedicated sessions and staff can overcome this obstacle.

Conclusion

An integrated care approach to end-stage kidney disease brings out the best performance by patients and providers. It is based on forthright discussions, education, empowerment and shared decision making. It utilizes a team approach including multidisciplinary professionals and family/friends. Its goals are to define and deliver success as the patient sees it. It requires competency in all aspects of ESKD care and in communication among all the team's participants. Lastly, this approach results in the most derived pleasure for its participants.

References

[1]   Morton R, Tong A, Howard K et al. The views of patients and carers in treatment decision making for chronic kidney disease: systematic review and thematic synthesis of qualitative studies. BMJ. 2010;340:c112.

[2]   Murtagh F, Marsh J, Donohoe P et al. Dialysis or not? A comparative survival study of patients over 75 years with chronic kidney disease stage 5. Nephrol Dial Transplant. 2007;22:1955-1962.

[3]   Visser A, Dijkstra G, Kuiper D et al. Accepting or declining dialysis: considerations taken into account by elderly patients with end-stage renal disease. J Nephrol. 2009;22:794-799.

[4]   Stack A. Determinants of Modality Selection among Incident US Dialysis Patients: Results from a National Study. J Am Soc Nephrol. 2002 May 13;5:1279-87.

[5] Miskulin D, Meyer K, Athienites NV. et al. Comorbidity and other factors associated with modality selection in incident dialysis patients: The CHOICE study. Am J Kidney Dis. 2002 Feb;39(2):324-36.

[6] Golper TA, Saxena AB, Piraino B et al. Systematic barriers to the effective delivery of home dialysis in the US. 2011, Am J Kid Dis. (in press).

[7] Yeoh H, Tiquia H, Abcar A. et al. Impact of predialysiscare on clinical Outcomes. Hemodial Int. 2003 Oct; 7;338-341.

[8] Devins G, Mendelssohn D, Barre P et al. Predialysispsychoeducational intervention extends survival in CKD: A 20-Year Follow-Up. Am J Kidney Dis. 2005 Dec;46:1088-1098.

[9] Golper, TA. Patient education: Can it maximize the success of therapy? Nephrol Dial Transplant. 2006;16:20-24.

In: Issues in Dialysis
Editor: Stephen Z. Fadem

ISBN: 978-1-62417-576-3
© 2013 Nova Science Publishers, Inc.

Chapter III

Accept this Kidney or Continue Dialysis? A Strategic Approach to Donor Options

Amy L. Friedman[*]
SUNY Upstate Medical University, Syracuse, New York, US

Abstract

Facing high mortality on dialysis, patients and their providers must recognize the need to approach the limited supply of donor kidneys in a very strategic manner. A focus on the intrinsic quality of every potential donor kidney, together with optimization of how it is handled through the obligatory transplant process that necessarily entails ischemia and reperfusion and, therefore, acute kidney injury, is appropriate. With fully informed consent, patients confronting long waiting times or high mortality rates, particularly those with diabetes, or older than 40 years, should consider the use of Expanded Criteria Donor (ECD) kidneys, or organs with low, but increased risk of disease transmission, in order to obviate the otherwise, potentially insurmountable wait.

Introduction

Fifty eight years ago Joseph Murray and his Boston team performed the first successful organ transplant in a human being, transferring the kidney from a healthy twenty three year old man into his ill, identical twin brother, whose renal failure would otherwise have been fatal. [1] Through the ensuing years, progressive developments in science as a whole, and in medical skills and knowledge in general, as well as within the most specific fields directly

---

[*] E-mail: friedmaa@upstate.edu.

impacting transplantation such as immunobiology, have generated enormous changes both in the scope of who is considered a realistic transplant candidate and in which organ will be considered for transplantation. Indeed, transplant outcomes have become so predictably good that this once novel, virtually unimaginable therapy has become the cost effective standard of care for many patients with endstage renal disease (ESRD) in the United States (U.S.) and is therefore a required element of consideration within every patient's annually performed management plan. Yet, the sad reality is that the majority of qualified candidates seeking kidney transplantation do not succeed in attaining their goal. In fact, more patients than ever before; 4,841 in 2010, died while on the active waiting list for a kidney in the U.S., simply because there were insufficient usable organs available for transplantation. During that same year, only 16,085 kidney transplants were performed throughout the entire U.S. [2] With such a pressing demand for transplants serving as a driving force, every potentially suitable kidney must be carefully assessed to be certain that the opportunity to offer this life saving therapy to another patient is not missed.

What Is the Kidney Expected to Do?

Normal renal function usually represents the combined contribution of two organs, while most transplants provide only one. That single organ is also often impacted by multiple adverse factors such as nephrotoxic drugs, hypertension, etc. So, it is particularly important to set realistic expectations for the transplanted organ to fulfill (Table 1).

Table 1. What is the transplanted kidney expected to do ?

Primary Graft Function – no need for post-transplant dialysis
- Fluid/volume control
- Blood pressure control
- Acid/base control
- Potassium balance

Long-Term Graft Function – no need for long-term dialysis
- Fluid/volume control
- Blood pressure control
- Acid/base control
- Erythropoiesis
- Calcium regulation
- Proteinuria controlled
- Sleep cycle normal
- Energy level normal

Primary Graft Function is defined as whether or not the kidney ever functions well enough for dialysis to be stopped following transplantation. This is an important determination, since those patients whose deceased donor kidneys never function will likely qualify for reinstatement of all of the waiting time that was utilized for allocation of the kidney. In other words, UNOS policy recognizes that it would be unfair to penalize a patient who received a poor quality kidney that never functioned, by forcing them to start waiting all over again. [3] Delayed Graft Function (DGF) is also crisply defined within UNOS policies. Although there are three specific definitions, the most practical and widely accepted of these, is whether or not dialysis is required following transplantation. As always, dialysis may be indicated to emergently control volume, potassium, blood pressure, or acidosis, and more subjective indications are also similar to those utilized for all post-surgical patients. DGF increases cost and morbidity, and may also be associated with diminished long term graft survival as a result of increased allograft immunogenicity and increased risk of acute rejection. [4] Clearly, it is an outcome to be avoided, if possible.

Once the allograft has recovered from the acute insult of transplantation, a level of long-term function is established. Under the best of circumstances, fluid and blood pressure regulation are easily controlled, a normal diet is tolerated, normal erythropoiesis occurs, acidosis is controlled, significant proteinuria is absent, energy level is good, calcium metabolism is restored, sleep pattern is normal and dialysis is unnecessary. However, it is not uncommon for a kidney to fail to satisfy one or more of these specific functions in an individual patient. This is particularly true for those patients in whom other contributory factors such as obesity or heart failure are present. For nearly all registry and other scientific purposes, the definition of a functioning kidney transplant is survival without maintenance dialysis. If chronic dialysis is initiated, the start date is also considered the date of transplant allograft failure. The key outcome measures by which transplant programs are now measured are patient survival and graft survival at one and three years. These results are also available to the public.

How Good Is this Kidney?

If kidneys came with labels containing individualized "Kidney Quality"(KQ) scores, the decision about whether or not to accept a specific kidney offered for transplantation, as well as setting realistic expectations for all stakeholders, for how well it would subsequently function, would be greatly facilitated. However, there is no single measure of KQ that adequately assesses all aspects of kidney function or predicts post-transplant outcomes. As in the assessment of renal function in any patient, it would be optimal to have a basic data set including the donor's creatinine clearance, rate of 24-hour protein excretion, and urinalysis. These are mandatory elements in the assessment of a live donor, but may be individually unavailable or invalid in a deceased donor in whom a steady state is never attained.

The 1954 identical twin transplant was also the first live donor transplant. Today, all U.S. live kidney donor programs are required to have established selection criteria that donors must satisfy for acceptance. [5] In all cases, these will have identified excellent kidney function, because, of course, the inviolate principle is that no donor will be left with a single kidney that has less than excellent function. So, by definition, a live donor kidney should always be an excellent kidney, at the far end of the KQ spectrum (Figure 1). However, the reality of the organ shortage and pressure to satisfy the demand for transplants has resulted in the use of live donors of increasingly marginal suitability because of advanced age, mild or moderate hypertension, mild diabetes, mild or moderate obesity, or even cardiovascular disease. As expected, these efforts are controversial because of concern for the donor's long-term safety. The other obvious consequence is that even within the previously essentially perfect category of live donor kidneys, it is now necessary to inject a range of quality. Even live donor kidneys are not all equal.

Whether or not to use a specific kidney (from the transplant surgeon's perspective), or to accept a kidney (from the patient's perspective) remains a subjective judgment based in large part on an understanding of the prior health history impacting that specific organ and familiarity with the statistical post-transplant outcomes from similar kidneys. The demographic information of greatest importance includes age and history of cardiovascular disease. Hypertension and diabetes are often present, poorly characterized, and may or may not have affected the renal function. Further complicating the assessment of the impact of these diseases on a kidney that may be under consideration for transplantation, is the challenge that many patients who have been prescribed medications for treatment of diabetes and/or hypertension may have been variably compliant with those regimens. Ultimately, the degree to which that kidney had been exposed to, and damaged by a hypertensive or hyperglycemic environment is extremely difficult to predict solely from a potential donor's history. For this reason, the use of a pre-transplant biopsy is often relied upon (see below).

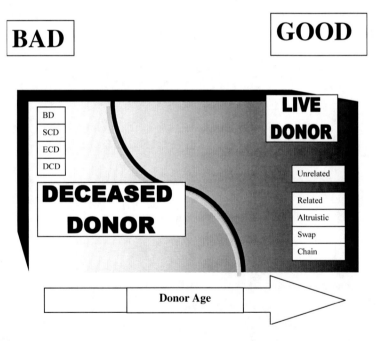

Figure 1. The kidney quality (kq)spectrum.

However, though helpful, biopsies also have limitations to their predictive value. For example, sampling error, resulting from a single sample not appropriately representing the entire kidney would certainly be an unfortunate reason to forego utilization of an appropriate kidney that might have saved a life. [6] Even the question of which biopsy technique should be utilized has not yet been resolved, for exactly that reason. Another key challenge to the use of biopsies for making the transplant or don't transplant decision, is the brief time frame available in which to complete and interpret them. Since many deceased donor organs are recovered in hospitals outside of transplant centers, pathologists with specific transplant expertise may not be immediately available to participate in the tissue preparation or biopsy interpretation, introducing considerable variation into the value of the biopsy upon which a key decision is being based.

Table 2. Kidney donor profile index (KDPI)

Factors included in the KDPI
- Donor Age (years)
- Donor Height
- Donor Weight
- Donor Ethnicity/Race
- Donor History of Hypertension
- Donor History of Diabetes
- Donor Cause of Death
- Donor Serum Creatinine
- Anti-Hepatitis C Virus Antibody
- Donor Meets DCD Criteria?

KDPI ranges from 0 to 1, which indicates that this donor's risk is greater than a percentage of all procured kidney donors (Based on a reference population consisting of all procured kidney donors in 2009. Procured kidney donors include donors from which at least one kidney was procured for the purposes of transplantation, though not necessarily transplanted. A value of 100% does not necessarily mean that no donors had a value exceeding this donor, but just that this donor's relative risk measure exceeds the 99th percentile risk measure.)

[http://optn.transplant.hrsa.gov/ContentDocuments/KDRI_KDPI_Calculator_v1-2.xls]

A new index, the Kidney Donor Profile Index (**KDPI**), (Table 2) combines multiple donor factors into a single number that summarizes the risk of graft failure after kidney transplant, has been developed for use in assessment of organ offers and for statistical analysis following transplantation. Since, as noted above, each of the factors it incorporates has limitations, the overall index will still be of limited value. It is likely that it will be more valuable for exclusion of poor quality kidneys, than for the specific selection of those organs which are acceptable. The **KDPI** will be incorporated into U.S. organ allocation within the next several years. [7]

Table 3. Protective strategies for the donor kidney

- Cold temperature
- Speed
- Pulsatile Pump Perfusion vs. Static Cold Storage
- Heparin
- Excellent surgical technique.

How Well Was the Kidney Treated?

Any kidney that is transplanted sustains significant injury, regardless of who donated it, since the transfer from one host to another required interim disruption of its blood flow, as well as two operations with significant technical manipulations. The key objective in transplantation is to ameliorate as much of the requisite damage as possible, including the ischemia and reperfusion injury, and ranging from the visible (e.g., laceration or thrombosis of a major renal vessel) to the level of the gene (e.g., role of the ICAM1 and VCAM1 gene polymorphisms on DGF and acute kidney allograft rejection). [8] Today, the main strategies for renal protection during this process include speed, cold temperature, heparin to prevent thrombosis, pulsatile pump perfusion versus static cold storage [9] to protect marginal organs, and, of course, excellent surgical technique (Table 3).

Modern kidney transplantation relies on the use of cold perfusion solution directly through the renal artery to flush blood out of the organ and to rapidly cool the kidney, thereby initiating the period of cold ischemia which ends when the kidney is subsequently removed from cold protection. In live kidney donation, the cold flush is placed directly into the renal artery. In deceased organ donation, the cold flush flows through an aortic cannula, while sterile ice slush is applied directly onto the kidneys. This time period is measured, reported to UNOS, and used for multiple statistical analyses. In fact, program specific reports including these data collected by time period, not by individual case, are publicly available at the Scientific Registry of Transplant Recipients website. [10]

Warm Ischemia refers to the period of time initiated by removal of the kidney from protective cold (termination of Cold Ischemia), and concluded by restoration of blood flow to the kidney (opening vascular clamps) which is also measured, reported and tracked. During this more vulnerable period, the organ has less protection, though many surgeons will try to keep the kidney as cold as possible by wrapping it in ice packs, etc. During this period the vascular anastomoses are performed. Though little has been written about the surgical issues occurring during this period, it should be clear that many factors including the patient's body habitus, vascular disease in the recipient and/or donor vessels, as well as a learning curve for the surgeon(s) may impact this measure. At the SUNY Upstate Medical University transplant program, an academic teaching program without a transplant surgical fellowship, the attending transplant surgeons permit individual residents to perform as much of these anastomoses as they are individually capable of doing, without compromising a goal warm ischemic time of 40 minutes. This measure is tracked as an over part of our Transplant Quality program (Figure 2).

In reality, cost containment concerns frequently play a pivotal role in the outcome for organs that might have been accepted for transplantation if they had been treated optimally. For illustration, deceased donor kidneys are usually transported by commercial airline flights within the U.S., in contrast to deceased donor hearts or livers for which airplanes are chartered at significantly greater cost. Awaiting available flights, as well as airplane pilots who agree to transport the well packaged organs (individual pilots have the prerogative to decline) introduces significant delay into this process, in order to control cost. No public data are available regarding how many kidneys may have been discarded because of these delays.

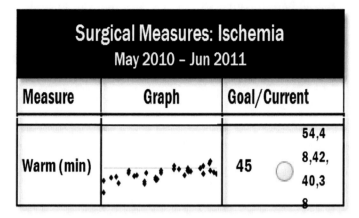

Each point equals the measure for one transplant. Current goal is ≤ 45 minutes.

Figure 2. Suny Upstate Medical University kidney transplant program. Quality Assessment, Performance Improvement (QAPI) measure – warm ischemia.

Transplant Jargon - Which Type of Kidney Is it?

There is an important distinction between KQ and the way a kidney donor is classified, because the mechanism of donation strongly affects the transplant related outcomes, specifically including Delayed Graft Function (DGF) and Long-Term Graft Survival.

Live Donor

As noted above, the live donor has been the gold standard in kidney transplantation. As in the 1954 identical twin transplant, the donor has fully assessed, excellent function and is in an optimal, steady state of health. Objectivity and at least a minimal level of protection from the recipient's potentially conflicting interests are attained through Live Donor Advocacy, now formally required at all U.S. live donor transplant programs. [11]

The live donor organ itself is technically protected through the systematic approach to conduct of the donor nephrectomy until the intentional initiation of the period of Cold Ischemia (actually, cold was not used during the ischemic period in the 1954 transplant). The length of Cold Ischemia is also minimized by appropriate adjustments to the donor and recipient operating schedules.

Development of the laparoscopic donor nephrectomy introduced a new concern because of the technically greater challenge in rapidly accomplishing initiation of Cold Ischemia. [12] While vascular clamps were individually applied to the renal vein and renal artery, each of which was then rapidly transected to separate the kidney in the traditional, open donor nephrectomy, the same techniques could not be utilized laparoscopically. Application of vascular clips, now known to be linked to multiple donor mortalities [13], or of a vascular stapler, is significantly more cumbersome and time consuming. Early in the development of this approach, some authors reported significant rates of delayed graft function and other technical complications that have, for the most part, now been overcome.

Evolutionary improvements in histocompatibility methods as well as in the pharmacotherapy of immunosuppression have combined to make other dramatic changes in live kidney donation appropriate. While that first transplant was feasible only because of the absence of an immune response between the genetically identical donor and host, results are now predictably excellent between live related (genetically related) as well as live unrelated (genetically unrelated) pairs. [14] For this reason, altruistic donors who have volunteered to donate to an unidentified person, and have been carefully psychiatrically and psychosocially evaluated, may be utilized. [15] Finally, to accomplish transplantation for patients who would not otherwise be able to have transplants, logistically challenging swaps and sequential chains between multiple pairs and sets of donor-recipient pairs are now being undertaken to overcome ABO blood type barriers and high levels of anti-human leukocyte antigen antibodies. [16] In these circumstances, either the donor or the donor's extirpated kidney must travel to the geographic locale in which the matched recipient resides. In the former circumstance, the human donor suffers from undergoing a major operation remote from home. In the latter, the live donor kidney has significant prolongation of Cold Ischemia. Either option is sub-optimal, but may be tolerable for the fully informed, for whom appropriate expectations are set. For these reasons, the era of live donor kidney transplantation has truly entered a new paradigm.

Deceased Donor

The crucial distinctions between a kidney from a live donor versus an organ from a deceased donor are: 1) the lack of elective scheduling, 2) the adverse consequences of whichever acute processes have caused the donor's death, 3) the absence of a steady state of good health and renal function, and 4) the frequent need to optimize function of multiple organs, not only the kidneys. Although 2 and 3 may seem to be inconsequentially different, in fact, they often represent the conceptual focus of whether or not the kidneys from a specific donor should be transplanted. It is also important to acknowledge that 4) often generates substantial inconvenience and adverse impact specifically from the renal perspective. This concept is readily illustrated by the example of a cardiac transplant team's requirement for cardiac catheterization in order to determine whether or not to transplant the heart. Unfortunately, this use of intravenous contrast, particularly during a period of pre-existing hypotension and/or vasopressor requirement, may compound acute kidney injury.

Brain Death (BD)

Deceased organ donation cannot legally proceed in the absence of a formal, legal declaration of death. To be clear, the procurement of both kidneys for the purpose of transplantation, from one human being who has not previously been declared to be dead, would be homicide. In fact, the planned, controlled cessation of cardiac function, coincident with complete exsanguination accomplished by delivery of cold perfusate into the abdominal and thoracic viscera through an aortic cannula delivering perfusate for replacement of the patient's blood volume, could not sound more like "cold blooded murder"! But, these are precisely the technical tenets of organ recovery when brain death has been declared. The surgeon's ability to preserve blood flow to the kidneys (and all other organs during the multi-organ procurement), until the moment that Cold Ischemia is intentionally initiated, mitigates recovery associated acute kidney injury.

Donation After Circulatory Death (DCD)

Many patients who have sustained severe neurologic injury either do not reach the stage of brain death, or are never formally declared brain dead despite having actually met the clinical criteria for this condition. In each of these two circumstances, organ procurement cannot be undertaken despite a patient's pre-existent consent for donation, or a family's wish (and permission) to do so. However, artificial support may be withdrawn with the expectation that death will ensue from circulatory arrest. After comprehensive review, the Institute of Medicine has fully supported approaching the family following the decision to withdraw support, to seek consent for organ donation if 1) heart activity ceases within one hour and, 2) a period of five minutes is waited and, 3) a physician independent of the transplant team declares death and, 4) heparin has been administered prior to cessation of circulation and, 5) organ recovery occurs immediately and, 6) the patient returns to the ICU if heart activity does not cease within one hour. [17] Kidneys recovered from DCD donors sustain additional warm ischemia while the circulatory system fails and before cold ischemia is initiated. Since DCD kidneys must recover from the collective acute kidney injury resulting from the donor's acute illness as well as the DCD process itself, a more restrictive range of KQ organs is generally accepted. Even among those transplants, the rate of DGF is substantially increased, although the long-term outcomes have been excellent, as should be expected due to the high KQ. Overall encouraging results have led to a nearly tenfold increase in DCD kidney donors from 1999 up to a high of 1306 kidneys in 2008 in the U.S. [18]

In 1954, Murray and his pioneer cohort could not have imagined the wide spectrum of deceased donors from whom, out of sheer desperation, we now consider using organs. For clarity, the most desirable deceased donor is now defined as the Standard Criteria Donor (SCD). [19] But, as shown in Table 4, there is significant variation in the patient demographics even within the SCD category. Accordingly, the associated risks of Primary Non-Function (due to technical issues), DGF, and Patient and Graft Survival all exhibit wide variance. At one extreme of the SCD category, for example, are kidneys from pediatric donors less than two or three years. These small organs have fabulous quality parenchyma but very small blood vessels and are therefore at significantly increased risk of thrombosis. To obviate this risk, they are often transplanted as two En Bloc kidneys, still attached to the donor aorta and vena cava that are used to create large anastomoses with the recipient vasculature. Such organs may be technically challenging to position without the kidneys twisting (imagine a two headed lollipop) so that all of the vessels remain patent. Not surprisingly, En Bloc pediatric kidneys are associated with an increased rate of thrombosis and primary failure. [20] An offer of such En Bloc organs would therefore require prospective discussion with a potential recipient as part of the informed consent process.

Table 4. Standard criteria (SCD) vs. Expanded criteria donor (ECD).

	SCD	ECD
Age < 50 years	+	-
Age = 50-59 years and 2 of following: death from CVA, Hypertension, Creatinine > 1.5	-	+
Age ≥ 60 years	-	+
Delayed Graft Function	+	+++
Patient Survival – Short Term	+++	++
Graft Survival – Short Term	+++	++
Patient Survival – Long Term	+++	+
Graft Survival – Long Term	+++	+

The least demographically desirable deceased donors are now called Expanded Criteria Donors (ECD). As expected, the intrinsically lower KQ of the ECD kidney, combined with the logistics of deceased organ donation, leads to substantially diminished outcomes when compared to SCD organs. Transplant surgeons, well aware of that issue, are therefore generally conservative about which ECD kidneys they will accept for transplantation. And, for those that are accepted and transplanted, a particular emphasis on optimization of all other conditions of how the kidney is treated, particularly Cold Ischemia and, increasingly, the use of pulsatile perfusion, is undertaken. This subtle point is generally not fully elaborated in studies comparing outcomes between ECD and SCD kidneys. To be clear, the expected rate of DGF is significantly higher following ECD than SCD transplantation, driven principally by differentially better KQ for the latter. But, this rate is also affected by the overall health of the host into whom it has been transplanted. In general, as will be discussed below, ECD recipients are significantly older and sicker than SCD recipients, undoubtedly also contributing to the increased rate of DGF. Both long-term Graft Survival and Patient Survival are significantly better for SCD versus ECD kidneys. Again, all three factors, including the KQ, the way the kidney is treated, and the overall health of the allograft's host contribute to this differential advantage.

Matching Patients and Kidneys

There is no question that, given a choice, no transplant surgeon would ever opt to offer any patient an ECD organ, and no patient would ever preferentially select an ECD kidney. But, with a rising proportion of patients failing to survive on the waiting list, and sustained high rates of mortality on maintenance dialysis, there simply is no alternative to the use of those ECD kidneys. Those marginal organs that can be expected to function sufficiently well to support patients' lives without dialysis, with a good enough quality of life to fulfill the expectations of the patient and family, and for long enough to justify the investment of the necessary resources, must be utilized. There is also no doubt that, given an alternative source of organs with acceptable KQ, no surgeon would ever agree to perform a live donor nephrectomy, thereby subjecting a healthy individual to the immediate risks of surgery as well as the long-term consequences of life with only a single kidney. Again, the problem is that such an endless source of high KQ organs simply does not exist. Without the use of live donor kidneys, many additional, appropriate transplant candidates would die. Our challenge is to identify potentially appropriate scenarios in which to consider the use of each type of kidney, and to propose doing so to the relevant stakeholders in a transparent manner, permitting them to participate as informed partners, to the extent to which they are capable of doing so. In the past, many of these choices were made in a paternalistic manner that is no longer appropriate. Merion et. al. retrospectively analyzed the outcomes of 109,127 ESRD patients added to the U.S. kidney waiting list between January 1995 and December 2002 and demonstrated that the excess ECD recipient mortality in the perioperative period limited the survival advantage afforded by ECD transplantation to those candidates older than 40 years, in locations with long waiting times, or with diabetes. [21] This strategy is quite representative of the current consensus about appropriate utilization of ECD kidneys.

Transplant candidates themselves evince the complete spectrum of comfort and acquiescence to the use of a live donor's kidney. For example, some parents share a preformed and immutable decision to decline a kidney offered by their own child. Yet, in some cases, grandparents in their seventh and eighth decades have accepted kidneys from grandchildren in their twenties. More commonly encountered is the challenge posed by candidates who are unwilling to accept offers from live donors within their own family, yet comfortable moving forward with the offer from an individual with substantially less emotional connection, and no genetic relationship at all, such as a friend or solicited, volunteer donor. Such scenarios clearly demonstrate the importance of the live donor advocacy requirement.

When a suitable live donor is either unavailable or unacceptable to the candidate, the only option for transplantation remains deceased donor organ allocation through the national waiting list. The massive disparity between the volume of candidates hoping to receive organs and the available kidneys should motivate all stakeholders to carefully consider the strategic approach to the waiting list, without denial of the severity of the shortage. The stakes are very high. For many patients who decide to accept only the highest quality organs, (SCD), death will arrive before a kidney. Though this is a tough message to deliver, and must certainly be extremely difficult to hear, such a communication is exactly what must transpire between the transplant program and the candidates it serves. Each patient should then be offered an individualized approach based on an overall assessment combining the factors shown in Figure 2: including the patient's likely lifespan on dialysis, the level of difficulty in identification of a compatible donor, and the projected Graft Survival of the specific organ type. As time passes without transplantation, this approach must be reassessed intermittently to determine whether new live donors have become available (or the candidate has become more accepting of a previously declined offer), changes in the medical condition merit reconsideration of previously unacceptable strategies (e.g., has a recent coronary artery bypass grafting procedure induced the patient to accept an ECD kidney?), or to clarify miscomprehension about complex issues that were previously reviewed.

Currently, many transplant programs including SUNY Upstate Medical University, use an additional informed consent process and form specifically for ECD kidneys. Patients are educated about the benefits of using an ECD kidney (relatively rapid transplantation; ECD listing is in addition to, not in lieu of, SCD listing), as well as the risks (e.g., higher DGF rate; lower Patient Survival rate; lower Graft Survival rate; risk of antibody formation) so that they

High Risk Donors

Another, less common, strategy to hasten access to a deceased donor kidney is the use of an organ from a donor at low but increased, risk of transmitting an infectious disease or malignant cell to the recipient. The reality is that no human organ can be transplanted with complete obviation of such risks. In fact, multiple infections are known to be commonly transmitted, including Cytomegalovirus and the Epstein Barr virus, each of which can also be associated with substantial adverse consequences. The strategic decision therefore becomes a question of whether or not any additional risk, above that which is already recognized, is acceptable in order to accomplish transplantation. If it is considered acceptable, the threshold of how much additional risk is tolerable, must be determined. As an example, transplant candidates with pre-existing infection with the Hepatitis C virus who receive education about the outcomes of kidney transplantation from Hepatitis C infected donors (i.e., results from donors with Hepatitis C match results from donors without Hepatitis C), often decide to accept such kidneys and are therefore listed accordingly. Since relatively few candidates on the national waiting list agree to accept Hepatitis C positive kidneys, the waiting time for SCD organs is often substantially shortened, with excellent outcomes. [22] Similar strategies have been successful for patients with Hepatitis B infection, and are now being advocated by some for HIV infected candidates. Such approaches benefit not only these specific recipients, for whom the waiting time for otherwise high quality organs is shortened, but also the other candidates on the waiting list through expansion of the pool of acceptable donor kidneys. These are win-win strategies, provided that all stakeholders fully comprehend the issues.

A similar concept applies to donors with a history of malignancy other than squamous or basal cell skin cancer. While active metastatic cells of any type obviously preclude safe transplantation, a history of a prior, now resolved cancer without current evidence of disease, or occasionally, a very locally confined tumor with a behavior pattern that is not typically aggressive, may have low enough associated risk of disease transmission to be considered tolerable in some cases. Such an approach is illustrated by the increasingly assertive approach to renal cell carcinoma. Cautious use of a deceased donor's contralateral organ, or even the remnant ipsilateral kidney following resection of an early stage lesion at the back table, has gained the support of some transplant programs. [23] While the development of true informed consent from a recipient who chooses to pursue this approach may be difficult within the rapid time constraints of deceased organ donation, it is much more feasible within the slower, more systematic context of live kidney donation. Thus, a potential recipient without available alternate live donors may prudently opt to accept a donor's remnant kidney, regardless of whether a frozen section diagnosis indicates that a small, resected lesion was benign or malignant.

Less clearly defined risk is associated with human behaviors that are known to increase rates of infections transmitted through sexual activity and exposure to blood. Though it is acknowledged to be an imperfect one, a current definition of increased behavioral risk by a donor is the Centers for Disease Control High Risk (CDC High Risk), (Table 5). Thus far, careful surveillance of outcomes of kidney transplants from CDC High Risk donors have shown a two year median survival that is no different than the non-high risk cohort. [24]

The patient who is thriving on dialysis may have little inclination to consider any increased risk of disease transmission, or to settle for an ECD kidney. Such a patient is likely to survive the long wait for an optimal quality kidney. On the other hand, to a patient who is medically deteriorating or running out of dialysis access, or whose age is associated with a shorter than average life expectancy, any of these strategies may be very appealing and/or appropriate.

Table 5. Centers for Disease Control high risk donor

- Men who have had sex with another man in the preceding 5 years
- Persons who report nonmedical intravenous, intramuscular, or subcutaneous injection of drugs in the preceding 5 years
- Persons with hemophilia or related clotting disorders who have received human derived clotting factor concentrates
- Persons who have engaged in sex in exchange for money or drugs in the preceding 5 years
- Persons who have had sex in preceding 12 months with any person described in i-iv above or with a person known or suspected to have HIV infection
- Persons who have been exposed in the preceding 12 months to known or suspected HIV-infected blood through percutaneous inoculation or through contact with an open wound, nonintact skin, or mucous membrane
- Inmates of correctional systems

Matching Kidneys and Expectations

The approach that has been meticulously emphasized throughout this chapter is the use of decision algorithms that incorporate careful identification of available alternatives, comprehensive education about each option together with its strengths and weaknesses, and the measurement of outcomes to determine whether they meet expectations that were carefully and prospectively developed. Transparency is essential to satisfy these objectives, and applies equally to all stakeholders. Thus, use of an organ, such as a DCD kidney, that has a particularly high risk of DGF, should be reviewed in advance with the patient, the referring nephrologist, the transplant administrator, and the transplant team. Unless DGF is expected (but, obviously not hoped for!), the patient may be disappointed to learn that continued dialysis is required following the transplant, leading to low patient satisfaction scores. An unprepared nephrologist may not protect the patient's outpatient dialysis slot with the adverse consequence of a prolonged length of stay in the hospital (if a new outpatient dialysis arrangement is required), and diminished patient satisfaction. The transplant administrator and other team members may not recognize the need to collectively optimize all other methods of treating the kidney, and to address all other sources of patient dissatisfaction. Similarly, they may view the DGF as a potentially avoidable, poor outcome rather than a predictable consequence of the use of a DCD organ.

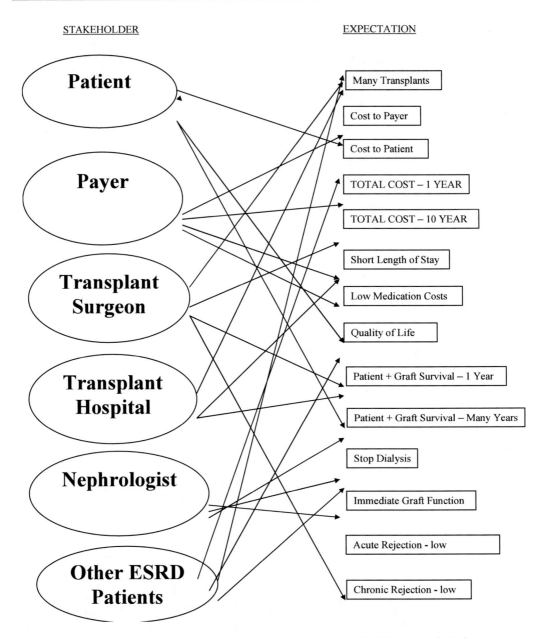

Figure 3. Links between stakeholders expectations and their perspectives in kidney transplantation.

In other words, it is essential for the transplant program to develop reasonable outcome expectations among all stakeholders, and to carefully measure and track those outcomes in order to improve performance, as appropriate. Accomplishment of these objectives can be ethically and emotionally challenging for virtually all who personally interact with the human beings involved, and is best approached through transparency and sensitivity.

Conclusion

The various stakeholders in kidney transplantation have disparate expectations linked to their own perspectives, an issue that is often underemphasized despite its substantial relevance (Figure 3). While a copious supply of high kidney quality organs that are associated with a low rate of delayed graft function, and high rates of long-term patient and graft survival (e.g., from either live donors or standard criteria donors, brain death deceased donors) would likely satisfy everyone's requirements, this currently remains an unrealized fantasy. Until research breakthroughs succeed in overcoming the barriers to tolerance of animal organs or clinically applicable bioengineered organs become available as needed, it is the prudent and strategic consideration of the practically available donor options that remain the ESRD patient's best hope for undergoing a life saving kidney transplant before time runs out. Careful outcome tracking is underway and suggests that these approaches continue to be reasonable and appropriate. Finally, patients and other participants in the process must be fully informed in order to best comprehend, recognize and appreciate the strengths, weaknesses and costs of every strategy.

References

[1] Merrill JP, Murray JE, Harrison JH, Guild WR. Successful homotransplantation of the human kidney between identical twins. JAMA. 1956;160(4):277-82.

[2] Removal reasons by year. Removed from the waiting list: January, 1995 – April 30, 2011 for Organ = Kidney, Based on OPTN data as of July 22, 2011. [cited 26 Jul 2011]. Available from: http://optn.transplant.hrsa.gov/latestData/rptData.asp

[3] UNOS Policy 3.2.4.2 Waiting Time Reinstatement for Kidney Recipients. [cited 23 Nov 2011]. Available from: http://optn.transplant.hrsa.gov/PoliciesandBy+ laws2/policies/pdfs/policy_4.pdf

[4] Perico N, Cattaneo D, Sayegh MH, Remuzzi G. Delayed graft function in kidney transplantation. Lancet. 2004;364(9447):1814-27.

[5] Department of Health and Human Services. Centers for Medicare & Medicaid Services. Medicare program; Hospital Conditions of Participation: Requirements for Approval and Re-Approval of Transplant Centers To Perform Organ Transplants; Final Rule. 482.90 Condition of participation: Patient and living donor selection. Federal Register. 2007;72(61): 15202.

[6] Yushkov Y, Dikman S, Alvarez-Casas J, Giudice A, Hoffman A, Goldstein MJ. Optimized technique in needle biopsy protocol shown to be of greater sensitivity and accuracy compared to wedge biopsy. Transplant Proc. 2010;42(7):2493-7.

[7] U.S. Department of Health & Human Services. OPTN resources/ allocation calculators. KDPI Calculator. [cited 26 Jul 2011]. Available from : http://optn.transplant.hrsa. gov/resources/allocationcalculators.asp?index=80

[8] Kloda K, Domanski L, Pawlik A, Kurzawski M, Safranow K, Ciechanowski K. Effect of the ICAM1 and VCAM1 gene polymorphisms on delayed graft function and acute kidney allograft rejection. Ann Transplant. 2010;15(4):15-20.

[9] Moers C, Smits JM, Mathis MH, Treckmann J, van Gelder F, Napieralski BP, et. al. Machine perfusion or cold storage in deceased-donor kidney transplantation. N Engl J Med. 2009;360(1):7-19.

[10] Scientific Registry of Transplant Recipients. Find a Transplant Center. [cited 26 Jul 2011]. Available from: http://www.srtr.org/csr/current/Centers/Default.aspx

[11] Department of Health and Human Services. Centers for Medicare & Medicaid Services. Medicare program; Hospital Conditions ofg Participation : Requirements for Approval and Re-Approval of Transplant Centers To Perform Organ Transplants; Final Rule. 482.98 Condition of participation: Human resources. Federal Register. 2007;72(61):15203.

[12] Ratner LE, Ciseck LJ, Moore RG, Cigarroa FG, Kaufman HS, Kavoussi LR. Laparoscopic live donor nephrectomy. Transplant. 1995;60(9):1047-9.

[13] Friedman AL, Peters TG, Jones KW, Boulware LE, Ratner LE. Fatal and nonfatal hemorrhagic complications of living kidney donation. Ann Surg. 2006;243(1):126-30.

[14] Terasaki PI, Cecka JM, Gjertson DW, Takemoto S. High survival rates of kidney transplants from spousal and living unrelated donors. New Engl J Med. 1995;333(6):333-6.

[15] Spital A. Evolution of attitudes at U.S. transplant centers toward kidney donation by friends and altruistic strangers. Transplant. 2000;69(8):1728-31.

[16] Segev DL, Gentry SE, Warren DS, Reeb B, Montgomery RA. Kidney paired donation and optimizing the use of live donor organs. JAMA. 2006;293(15):1883-90.

[17] Herdman R, Study Director. Non-Heart-Beating Organ Transplantation. Medical and ethical issues in procurement. Washington: National Academy Press; 1997.

[18] OPTN/SRTR Annual Report. Chapter II. Organ Donation and Utilization in the United States, 1999-2008. [cited 26 Jul 2011]. Available from : http://optn.transplant.hrsa.gov/ar2009/Chapter_II_AR_CD.htm?cp=3#17

[19] UNOS Policy 3.5.1 Definition of Expanded Criteria Donor and Standard Donor. [cited 26 Jul 2011]. Available from : http://optn.transplant.hrsa.gov/PoliciesandBylaws2/policies/pdfs/policy_7.pdf

[20] Thomusch O, Tittelbach-Helmrich D, Meyer S, Drognitz O, Pisarski P. Twenty-year graft survival and graft function analysis by a matched pair study between pediatric en bloc kidney and deceased adult donors grafts. Transplant. 2009;88(7):920-5.

[21] Merion RM, Ashby VB, Wolfe RA, Distant DA, Hulbert-Shearon TE, Metzger RA, et. al. Deceased-donor characteristics and the survival benefit of kidney transplantation. JAMA. 2005;294(21):2726-33.

[22] Brown KL, El-Amm JM, Doshi MD, Singh A, Morawski K, Cincotta E, Siddiqui F, et. al. Intermediate-term outcomes of hepatitis C-positive compared with hepatitis C-negative deceased-donor renal allograft recipients. Am J Surg. 2008;195(3):298-302.

[23] Ghafari A. Transplantation of a kidney with a renal cell carcinoma after living donation: a case report. Transplant Proc. 2007;39(5):1660-1.

[24] Duan KI, Englesbe MJ, Volk ML. Centers for disease control «high-risk» donors and kidney utilization. Am J Transplant. 2010;10(2):416-20.

In: Issues in Dialysis
Editor: Stephen Z. Fadem

ISBN: 978-1-62417-576-3
© 2013 Nova Science Publishers, Inc.

Chapter IV

Dialysis at Home, the Seattle Experience

Christopher R. Blagg[*]
University of Washington, Seattle, Washington, US
Northwest Kidney Centers, Seattle, Washington, US

Abstract

Home hemodialysis was first used in Boston, Seattle and London in 1964, primarily as a means of allowing a few more patients to be treated by dialysis with the then very limited availability of this treatment and its high cost. At the University of Washington in Seattle three times a week dialysis in the home during the day or evening was usual until after Stanley Shaldon in London reported the first use of overnight home hemodialysis in late 1964. It soon became obvious that home hemodialysis provided as good or better patient survival, less morbidity, better quality of life and greater opportunity for rehabilitation than center dialysis and it was adopted as the required treatment for all Seattle patients so more patients could be treated. By 1972, there were some 10,000 dialysis patients in the United States, of whom about 40 percent were on home hemodialysis. At the same time home peritoneal dialysis was being developed, also at the University of Washington.

This chapter describes in some detail Seattle's role in both home hemodialysis and peritoneal dialysis over the years, as well as the reasons for the decline of home hemodialysis in the United States following introduction of the Medicare End-Stage Renal Disease Program in 1973 and the increased role of peritoneal dialysis. It also comments on the more recent use of more frequent home hemodialysis during the day or overnight, the development of new technologies specifically designed for safe hemodialysis in the home and the resulting gradual recrudescence of home dialysis in the United States.

---

[*] Address for Correspondence: Christopher R. Blagg, MD. 2427 84th Avenue SE, Mercer Island, WA 98040; Phone 206-234-8791; Fax 206-230-4916.

Introduction

Hemodialysis for chronic renal failure first became possible when Belding Scribner and Wayne Quinton developed the Teflon arteriovenous shunt at the University of Washington in Seattle and reported on this at the sixth annual meeting of the American Society for Artificial Internal Organs (ASAIO) in Chicago in April 1960. [1,2] By the end of 1960, four patients were living at home and coming in to be treated for 20 to 24 hours every 5 to 7 days at University Hospital in Seattle. The treatment worked, but it soon became obvious that it was expensive, at least $10,000 a year, and the hospital administration refused to allow Scribner to start more patients because of concern about how they would be supported when research funding ended. As a result Scribner, James Haviland and the King County Medical Society established the Seattle Artificial Kidney Center (SAKC) in January 1962 as the first free-standing dialysis unit in the world. [3] The non-profit community-supported center became famous when Life magazine published an article by Shana Alexander in its November 9th 1962 issue titled "They Decide Who Lives, Who Dies: Medical miracle and a moral burden of a small committee." This described the Center, its patients, and the lay committee that made the final selection of patients because of the very limited funds and space available. [4]

The Early History of Home Hemodialysis

The first mention of home hemodialysis was at the 1961 meeting of the ASAIO. Willem Kolff complimented Scribner for the work he had started and presented him with a cartoon showing a patient attached to a dialysis machine rushing to the railway station, noting that "Undoubtedly, we all want our artificial kidneys at home, and this will happen if you're a little late" Later at the same meeting, Charles Kirby, a cardiac surgeon, in his presidential address noted that "Perhaps what we need is a home dialysis unit to be placed by the patient's bedside, so that he can plug himself in for an eight-hour hour period once or twice a week." [5]

Credit for the first use of home hemodialysis in a patient with chronic renal failure goes to John Merrill and colleagues at the Peter Bent Brigham Hospital in Boston when, in late 1963, they sent a carefully selected patient home with a twin-coil dialysis machine. A physician and a nurse went to the home twice a week to do dialysis, but soon it was seen there was no need to have a physician present. The next step was to train the wife to treat her husband, so eliminating the need for a nurse to be present during the treatment. [6,7] Three more patients were sent home during the next year. The cost was estimated as $5,000 -$7,000 a year.

Meanwhile in Seattle in 1963, Scribner and his team began a very fruitful relationship with Albert "Les" Babb, professor of nuclear and chemical engineering at the University of Washington. Their cooperation led to the first use of proportioning pumps to mix water and concentrated electrolyte solutions to prepare dialysate on-line continuously in a machine to serve the four station dialysis unit at the University Hospital. This eliminated the need to make dialysate in a basement laboratory by mixing water and dry chemicals in a 380 liter stainless steel tank using a canoe paddle to stir the mixture; the extremely heavy tank was then taken up to the fifth floor of the hospital to a patient's bedside. Dialysate was recirculated to the tank during dialysis, requiring the dialysate temperature be maintained at 20° C to avoid excessive bacterial growth in the tank. The proportioning pump system allowed dialysate to be pumped through the dialyzer and then discarded – single pass dialysate flow – allowing the dialysate temperature to be 37° C and eliminating the need for blood rewarming, so shortening the blood lines and allowing increased blood flow rates so mass transfer of urea and creatinine was-improved throughout the dialysis. [8,9]

Early in 1964, soon after the proportioning system was installed at the hospital, a 15 year-old patient of Scribner's was developing renal failure but was ineligible for treatment at the SAKC because she was below the then minimum acceptable age of 18. Because Babb knew her father, Scribner pressured him to have his team develop a miniature single-patient version of their proportioning system that would incorporate monitoring and fail-safe devices to make it suitable for dialysis at home. This machine was also the prototype for almost all dialysis machines in use today.

The patient and her mother were trained to do dialysis using the shunt and the low-resistance Kiil dialyzer that did not need a blood pump, and went home in June 1964 using the single–patient machine, [10] (Figure 1) She survived for four years on home hemodialysis without serious problems, completing her last two years of high school and two years at university before dying from complications of systemic lupus erythematosus. A second patient was trained a month later with a home dialysis system using batch mixing of dialysate in a large tank that was made by the Sweden Freezer Manufacturing Company in Seattle. Both these devices were designed to need minimal maintenance and startup and shutdown time and incorporated programmed sterilize-rinse-normalize cycles and appropriate monitoring.

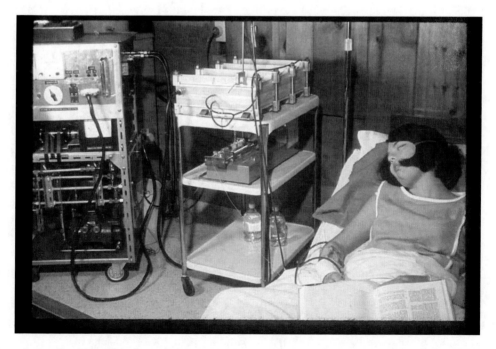

Figure 1. Caroline Helm dialyzing at home, 1965 (Photo courtesy of the University of Washington).

The patients dialyzed two or three times a week in the evening for 6 to 8 hours using standard Kiil dialyzers and 3% acetic acid as the post-assembly sterilizing agent for dialyzer, connectors and tubing. Periodic formalin treatment was used to control the growth of *Bacillus subtilis*.

In 1963, Stanley Shaldon and colleagues at the Royal Free Hospital in London had started a program in which patients did self-care dialysis in a hospital unit, [11] and in September 1964 began a program of home hemodialysis using a setup similar to that developed in Seattle. To Shaldon goes credit for the first use of overnight (nocturnal) unattended hemodialysis at home in October 1964. [12] He described this at a meeting in Seattle in December of that year [13] and based on this information the University of Washington first began to use nocturnal home hemodialysis in Seattle in 1965, using a blood-in-effluent monitor, a drip bulb pressure monitor and a digital blood pressure monitor.

During 1965, the Seattle Artificial Kidney Center became concerned about the University's growing home hemodialysis program because in the event of a change in a patient's situation treatment would have to be continued in the center. Consequently it was planned to build some kind of long-term financial reserve into acceptance into the University's home dialysis program.

By early 1966, equipment and monitoring had been further developed and the University of Washington program had eight patients dialyzing eight to ten hours three times a week at home, seven of them on commercially available equipment, and five of them dialyzing overnight. At that time, the equipment cost between $7,000 and $10,000, the cost of home remodeling was about $1,000, training averaged about two months and cost about $1,800, and yearly expenses including supplies, recannulations, blood transfusions, laboratory tests, equipment service and physician costs, were about $4,000. [14]

At the 1966 Third International Congress of Nephrology in Washington DC, Scribner said "In my opinion the future of chronic dialysis lies in the home" and discussed the advantages and disadvantages of home hemodialysis. [15] Advantages included lesser cost and personnel needs, dialysis at night was becoming relatively easy and allowed normal work and leisure hours, the risk of hepatitis and other infections common in a center was avoided, and experience had shown remote home dialysis could be supervised by a physician practicing hundreds of miles from a home dialysis training unit. Home dialysis had the potential for more frequent and more intense treatment, so further reducing complications and allowing elimination of dietary protein restriction and liberalization of salt restriction. A patient on self-dialysis at home developed a much healthier attitude towards their disease and its treatment than the patient on center dialysis. Nevertheless, treatment was demanding and minor technical failures and other problems took time, but these issues would be improved with time. Dialysis at home also imposed stress on the patient and family, particularly if there was a lack of emotional stability in the home. As a result, not all patients would be suitable candidates for this treatment. For those not able to treat themselves at home, he suggested the development of a self-care center as had been done by Shaldon.

In the summer of 1966 home hemodialysis was adopted by the SAKC as a means of treating more patients with the available funds and shortly thereafter the SAKC went on to institute a policy that all patients must dialyze at home. As a result over the next several years some 90 percent of Seattle patients were on home hemodialysis three times a week, mostly overnight, and generally well rehabilitated.

Another early program was established by Kolff and Nosé at the Cleveland Clinic in 1966 using coil dialyzers immersed in Maytag washing machines. [16] They soon had to change to the Baxter twin coil system as the Maytag Corporation expressed grave concern about their potential liability.

The success of the University of Washington's home hemodialysis program at a time when dialysis was unavailable at most U.S. centers and abroad led to the Division of Nephrology establishing a remote home hemodialysis program. This trained and supported 52 patients, their families and their physicians from elsewhere in the U.S. and as far away as India, Chile, the Philippines and the Sudan. [17]

Results with Conventional Three Times Weekly Home Hemodialysis

Experience gained with conventional three times a week home hemodialysis is very pertinent to more frequent and longer hemodialysis today as these are generally done at home.

Over the years, three times a week conventional home hemodialysis and three times a week 6 to 8 hour dialysis have been shown to provide better patient survival than three times a week center hemodialysis. [18-26] This undoubtedly relates in part to longer dialysis than is available in the typical center setting, better blood pressure control [27], and to patient selection. The criticism has often been made that none of these studies was a randomized controlled trial (RCT); all were uncontrolled or observational comparisons. The segment of the recently completed National Institutes of Health RCT to compare nightly home hemodialysis with conventional center hemodialysis [28] had serious recruitment problems and was too small to provide data on patient survival. Even if such a trial were to be completed there are likely to be incomparable life style-dependent variables that will prevent conclusions with certainty. [29] A recent editorial suggests that the cost, ethical issues when comparing dialysis modalities and the question whether the findings will reflect the real world make it unlikely that such a large scale RCT will be undertaken. [30] Interestingly, Bradford Hill, the originator of the RCT, in his 1965 Heberden Oration to the Royal College of Physicians of London noted that "Any belief that the controlled trial is the only way would mean not that the pendulum had swung too far but that it had come right off the hook" [31] and in his 2008 Harveian Oration to the same institution Sir Michael Rawlins, Chair of the UK's National Institute for Health and Clinical Excellence (NICE) suggested that RCTs have been placed on "an undeserved pedestal" and called for a broader approach to testing clinical interventions. [32]

Studies of quality of life, rehabilitation and ability to work in home hemodialysis patients also have shown these to be significantly better than in conventional center dialysis patients and more closely approach those of patients with a successful kidney transplant. [33-35] In 1967, the Washington State Department of Vocational Rehabilitation began to pay the SAKC to train and equip patients for home hemodialysis and to provide ongoing treatment support because of the excellent rehabilitation and lower cost associated with this treatment.

From a patient's viewpoint the advantages of home hemodialysis soon became obvious. It encouraged patient independence, responsibility and confidence, freed patients from the center and enforced socialization, eliminated the need for three times a week travel to a center, allowed them to set their own schedule and to dialyze longer than in center, was more comfortable and convenient, reduced the risk of infection and, most significantly, cost less than dialysis in a center. [36] The disadvantages included the need for space for equipment and supplies, most patients using early equipment needed the presence or some assistance from a family member or other individual during dialysis, modification of domestic electricity and plumbing were required, utility bills increased, and dialysis in the home impacted on family life generally.

Very early on we recognized that patients dialyzing in the center soon become dependent on their doctor, nurse and machine, and that when patients lose control of factors that may gratify or hurt them they eventually may be reduced to what Seligman called "learned helplessness." [37] As Scribner often reiterated, involvement of patients in their own care is important for those with any chronic disease, and particularly for those on chronic dialysis. [38] Attitudes of physicians and staff are important in fostering independence in all dialysis patients and in educating patients about the benefits and safety of dialysis in the home, (including peritoneal dialysis). Dialysis should begin early, and so it is important that patients are seen well ahead of time to learn about their treatment options and to have a fistula placed.

Potential Candidates

Almost any patient who is motivated, compliant and able to learn and wishes to be considered for this treatment is a potential candidate. Contraindications include severe cardiovascular disease, instability during dialysis, contraindications to use of heparin, and blindness unless a helper is available. The patient must have suitable living accommodation. Generally, even if a patient is capable of carrying out the whole dialysis themself it is preferable that someone else be in the home, although with modern developments in communication this is less of a necessity. Age in itself is not a contraindication.

As to intelligence, a clinical psychologist studied the intelligence quotients of 100 consecutive patients successfully trained for home hemodialysis at the SAKC. The average IQ of the group was 103 ± 16.2, ranging from 76 to 147, compared with a normal IQ of 100 ± 15.0. [39]

An unpublished study in 2001 compared demographic characteristics of home hemodialysis patients in the Northwest Kidney Center (NKC) program (the SAKC had been renamed) with those of all Washington state and all U.S. dialysis patients. The home hemodialysis patients had a very similar age distribution, a slightly greater proportion of males, and a similar distribution of diabetics as the State and national groups (38% vs. 37% vs. 39%). The major difference was the significantly lower number of black patients and the lower frequency of hypertension as a cause of renal failure in the Seattle home patients compared with national figures, reflecting the lesser proportion of blacks in the general population in the Northwest United States.

Requirements for Home Hemodialysis

These include blood access that is easy to use, treatment hours and ultrafiltration rate prescribed to provide adequate dialysis while minimizing symptoms during and between treatments, cautious use of antihypertensive medications, and dialysis equipment designed for easy and safe use by a patient in the home. Patients must provide monthly blood samples to the laboratory for analysis, the results of which are reported to the patient, their nephrologist and training staff. They must also provide a log of details of each dialysis to the nephrologist, training staff, and to the facility which requires this information for billing purposes. While in the past this was done using paper log sheets, with modern technology much better communication is possible. Real time monitoring is not necessary but may be useful during the first three to six months at home, although probably not essential thereafter.

Before a patient is accepted for training their home should be surveyed to check the adequacy of electricity, water supply and drainage, and availability of a telephone outlet close to where the machine will be installed. Necessary water treatment must be decided on based on analysis of the local water. There must be space for the machine by the bedside or next to a dialysis chair, and space to store supplies. If the patient is accepted for treatment any necessary electrical or plumbing changes can be done.

General requirements for a successful home dialysis program are understanding and support from all who have contact with the patient, a high quality training program run by dedicated experienced teaching staff who understand the need to foster patient independence, one of whom is available on call at all times to handle questions about problems. Technical maintenance and repair staff must also be available to handle equipment problems promptly. Other supporting services must include social work and dietary support for patient and family and, most importantly, access to rehabilitation services. Patients must be encouraged to resume work, school and other everyday activities and to exercise regularly. There should be ongoing education and reinforcement of patient and family as well as physicians and facility staff so they will encourage the use of all forms of home dialysis The patient should be seen by their nephrologist at least once every two months.

Concerns about Home Hemodialysis

Patients, particularly new patients, have many concerns about home hemodialysis. A study of 173 Canadian in-center dialysis patients looked at factors they associated with the attitude "patients should not perform dialysis without being supervised by a nurse". The commonest were lack of satisfactory explanation of treatment options, belief that patients should only dialyze under direct supervision, fears of failure to do dialysis adequately, fear of social isolation; fear of needles, and concern about lack of space in the home. A negative attitude was related to age, fear of poor care, needle phobia, fear of change, fear of social isolation and unwillingness to remain awake during dialysis. [40] A more recent study showed similar concerns – fear of self-cannulation, fear of a catastrophic event, and concern about the potential burden on the family. [41] Needle phobia is one of the most significant issues and it is best to teach the patient to stick themself before starting actual home dialysis training.

A 2002 study of 1,074 hemodialysis patients and 1,175 peritoneal dialysis patients using USRDS data found that only about 20 percent of new patients had been told about home hemodialysis as an option. [42] Many U.S. patients report similar experiences even though facilities had been required to inform all patients about the options of transplantation and home dialysis from the start of the Medicare Program. The recent new Conditions of Coverage require much more specific evidence from the facility that patients have been educated about these options and that, if the unit itself does not provide a treatment requested by the patient they have been informed where they can obtain training for home hemodialysis or peritoneal dialysis. The Medicare surveyors will review the data on this requirement at their routine visits.

Facility concerns include whether home hemodialysis is cost effective. The cost of training is high, of the order of $4,000 to $6,000 and still inadequately reimbursed. Even with the per dialysis margin it may take a year or so to make up the cost and in any case home dialysis patients are among the best transplant candidates. Machines and water treatment equipment are expensive and so many programs elect to lease the equipment together with technical support and provision of supplies. Setting up an effective home hemodialysis training and support program requires specialized staff and it is ridiculous to expect 5,000 or so U.S, dialysis units can each set up such a program. The best approach would be to regionalize home dialysis training centers. It remains to be seen whether the recently implemented bundling will be more effective in encouraging home dialysis than the composite rate reimbursement of the last 30 years.

Many nephrologists are also concerned about patient safety and the adequacy of patient support from home hemodialysis programs, but this reflects lack of exposure to home hemodialysis (and to outpatient dialysis generally) in most fellowship training programs in the United States.

What Happened to Home Hemodialysis in the United States?

Following introduction of the Medicare ESRD Program in 1973 the percentage of patients treated by home hemodialysis in the United States declined from about 40 percent of all dialysis patients to a low point of less than 0.5 percent of patients, although this was partly offset with the growth in the use of peritoneal dialysis that began in the late 1970s. There were many reasons for the decline, including the rapid increase in diabetic and elderly patients following universal entitlement, proliferation of dialysis centers, especially for-profit centers, problems with reimbursement and other reasons. [43] Initially reimbursement for home dialysis was grossly inadequate while payment to facilities for outpatient dialysis was very generous. For example, if a facility purchased a machine for home dialysis the supplier had to be paid in full, but Medicare only reimbursed 80% of this in 24 payments over the next two years and did not pay for delivery and installation. Some of the supplies, including syringes, , tape, bandages, alcohol wipes, povidone-iodine and underpads were not covered in the home as they were not regarded as needed for "effective operation of a home dialysis machine. "As a result of the negative impact of issues like these, legislation was introduced several years later to reimburse home hemodialysis on a three times a week per dialysis basis at 70% of the rate for center dialysis. Nevertheless, home dialysis continued to decline and so in 1981 Congress passed legislation to pay the same for both center and home dialysis – the composite rate. Again this failed to increase the use of home dialysis which continued to decline nationally.

Home Hemodialysis in Seattle

At the start of the Medicare ESRD Program in 1973, the Northwest Kidney Center had 199 dialysis patients, 163 (82%) of who were on home hemodialysis, 18 (9%) on home peritoneal dialysis and 18 on center hemodialysis. Despite the changes in the patient population resulting from entitlement and the shortcomings in reimbursement 95% of 554 patients were on home dialysis at the end of 1980. The number of patients on home hemodialysis fell gradually thereafter while the number of patients on peritoneal dialysis gradually increased, so that at the end of 2010 54 (3.9%) of 1,390 patients were on home hemodialysis and 165 (11.9%) were on peritoneal dialysis. Even so, the Northwest Kidney Centers had the largest home hemodialysis program in the United States until a year or two ago.

Over the years, the Northwest Kidney Center developed two innovations to help its home hemodialysis program. The first, in 1972, was development of a program using videotapes filmed at the center to educate new patients about their disease and their treatment options. This was used in addition to the usual meetings with physicians, nurses, social workers, nutritionists and others and enabled patients to study individually and in groups. [44]

The second was the suggestion by Dr. Eschbach to establish what was called the orientation unit. [45] This opened in 1981, consisting of six individual patient rooms in an area adjacent to the home hemodialysis training unit and directed by the nurse who ran the home training program. All new patients were admitted to this unit for their first six to eight weeks of outpatient dialysis, whether they were potential candidates for home dialysis or not, and were exposed to one-on-one and group teaching by staff on all aspects of treatment. Caroline Davis, then head of the Health Care Financing Administration, visited the Center shortly after the unit was established and was so impressed that she arranged a reimbursement exception for unit. The unit continued to operate until the later 1990s, by which time the Center had five satellite units around King County and transportation and other issues were making it more arduous for patients to have to come downtown to dialyze for the first few weeks of their treatment. As a result home hemodialysis numbers declined.

Another home hemodialysis- related activity at the Center was involvement with the Aksys Company of Lincolnshire, Illinois, that had developed a completely new very patient-friendly machine, the PHD System. This was designed for more frequent, short, so-called "daily" hemodialysis in the home. NKC was the first unit to use it September 1999 and provided 13 of the 23 patients included in studies that led to FDA approval of the device in March 2002. This was a 52 L batch system that prepared truly ultrapure, biocompatible and endotoxin-free dialysate. Patient effort was minimal as the system automatically cleaned the whole extracorporeal circuit between dialyses, sanitized it with hot water, and prepared dialysate for the next treatment. Ultimately NKC treated 52 patients who dialyzed five or six times a week, some of them overnight. Those who already experienced conventional hemodialysis commented on their improved well-being, energy, activity, improved mental outlook and quality of life and the lightening of their complexion. [46] Unfortunately the company went bankrupt in 2006 but fortunately for our patients the NxStage machine had become available in 2005. This is a smaller and more readily portable device. The majority of NKC home hemodialysis patients now use the NxStage machine for more frequent dialysis, although some still use a conventional hemodialysis machine for three times a week overnight hemodialysis. The availability of the NxStage device has been a major factor in increasing the number of home hemodialysis patients nationally to more than 6,000. Several other new home hemodialysis machines are under development in the U.S. and abroad and will become available over the next few years.

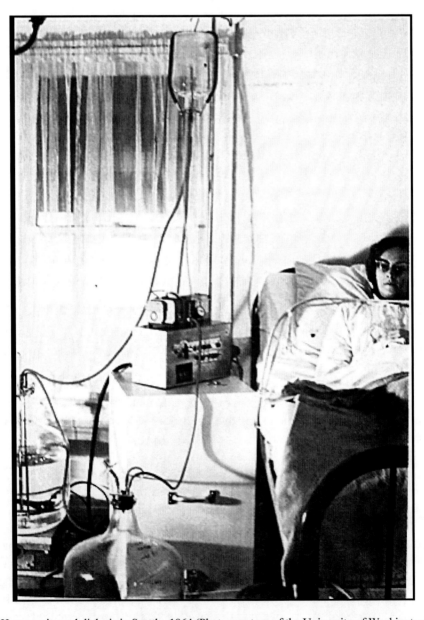

Figure 2. Home peritoneal dialysis in Seattle, 1964 (Photo courtesy of the University of Washington).

History of Peritoneal Dialysis in Seattle

It is often forgotten that Seattle played a significant role in the development of peritoneal dialysis both in the center and at home. In the late 1950s, Fred Boen, a Dutch physician, wrote a classic thesis on the dynamics of peritoneal dialysis. As a result, in 1961 Scribner invited him to come to Seattle to establish a peritoneal dialysis program at the University of Washington. The following year Boen reported development of a peritoneal dialysis cycling machine using 40 liter carboys of sterile dialysate for use in the hospital and a patient who had been treated with this device 2 or 3 times a week for 12 weeks. [47] Over the next two years Boen and his colleagues modified and improved this machine and showed that insertion of a cannula into the peritoneal cavity for each dialysis and removing it after treatment greatly reduced the risk of infection that had been so common using currently available indwelling peritoneal "buttons", They reported on two patients, one of whom had been on peritoneal dialysis for two years. [48]

In 1965 he reported on the first patient on home peritoneal dialysis in the U.S. who had started outpatient peritoneal dialysis in March 1964 and after six weeks of training went home in May 1964. [49] (Figure 2). Hypertension was controlled with 20 to 22 hours of dialysis twice a week and medication. She used the same automated cycling equipment that had been used in hospital and was treated by intermittent puncture with a physician visiting her home before the start of each dialysis. During dialysis she had no or minimal discomfort, was able to sit up in bed, and could turn on her side while asleep. Constant monitoring was not necessary and when her husband was at work she and her five-year-old son were alone at home with a telephone at her bedside. Dialysate was prepared in the hospital in 40 L and 20 L bottles and shipped to the patient's home once a month; about 60 L of dialysate was exchanged during each dialysis. Bacterial and asbestos filters were used to prepare the dialysate and no infections or pyrogenic reactions had been seen. The cost of supplies for one year of home peritoneal dialysis was $2,640, not including one and a quarter hours of physician time to insert the catheter for each treatment.

Henry Tenckhoff joined Boen in 1964 and took charge of the peritoneal dialysis program in 1967 when Boen returned to Europe. Because the repeated puncture technique did not lend itself readily to home use it was important to develop in an implanted device for safe intermittent use. A new device would have to be inherently safe from a bacteriological standpoint without the need for antibiotic prophylaxis, reliable in its irrigation properties, and physical and psychological inconvenience to the patient should be minimal. None of the previously used indwelling access devices had met these criteria although Russell Palmer in Vancouver BC, who had first done home peroitoneal dialysis shortly before Boen, had worked with Wayne Quinton and developed an indwelling Silastic catheter for peritoneal dialysis. [50] This also was prone to leakage and infection but Tenckhoff developed a modification that used Dacron felt cuffs below the skin and outside the peritoneum to anchor the catheter and tissue growth into the cuffs closed the sinus tract around the catheter against bacterial invasion. In 1968 he reported the results of the catheters implanted in six patients for periods ranging from 14 to 4 months for a total of 47 patient months and an average of 7.8 months, during which 464 dialysis were performed with frequent cultures of peritoneal fluid. [51] On only two occasions were positive cultures for staph aureus found, one without any associated clinical signs or symptoms and one in a patient who developed signs and symptoms of peritonitis eight and half months after the catheter was placed. This patient was treated with antibiotics, admitted to hospital for removal of the catheter, recovered and a new catheter was placed. The Tenckhoff catheter and the use of a closed system with dialysate in large containers minimized infection and further data from more than 900 peritoneal dialyses performed on eight patients over a total of 127 patient months showed positive peritoneal cultures in less than 0.5% of treatments. Since then the Tenckhoff catheter or its modifications have become used worldwide for peritoneal access.

With development of a safe peritoneal access device the remaining problem obstructing wider use of peritoneal dialysis was the need for large quantities of sterile dialysate. Tenckhoff and his colleagues worked to develop a system that was simple, safe, and required less maintenance. In 1969 they described two prototype devices for preparing sterile dialysate. [52] One proportioned pre-sterilized pure water with sterile concentrate at a rate of 20 to 1 using a roller proportioning pump; the other was batch preparation mixing sterile concentrate with an appropriate amount of pure water in a tank and heat sterilizing the entire mixture in a pressure boiler. Both systems required ready supplies of high purity water and of concentrate free from the impurities frequently encountered in hemodialysis concentrates.

The batch system used a pressure boiler of stainless steel with a highly polished inside surface and equipped with automatic controls and safety features. Based on previous experience, 80 L of dialysate would be sufficient for a single dialysis for most home patients. The tank took about 3 hours to heat up to the sterilizing temperature of 124° C and a pressure of 18 p.s.i. and this was maintained for 45 minutes. It then took about 15 to 18 hours to cool down to the operating temperature of 38 ± 1° C. The whole operation from initial activation of the fill cycle was fully automatic. A prototype system had been tested clinically in hospital and had performed entirely satisfactorily for dialyses lasting from 10 to 18 hours.

The proportioning method used sorbitol concentrate for reasons of cost and convenience and because this did not cause corrosion and leaching of metals. However the system was more complex and costly as well as slightly more expensive to run because of the addition of the roller proportioning pump. This method was being studied and appeared to be satisfactory. Approximate cost of one dialysis with the proportioning method was estimated at $15.43 and $12.95 for the batch method. Inclusion of a disposable conductivity cell would increase the cost by about $1.50.

In 1969, the Seattle Artificial Kidney Center reviewed the experience with home peritoneal dialysis at the University of Washington and concluded this had been shown to be an acceptable and effective treatment. As a result, the decision was made that the Center would support this treatment as an alternative to home hemodialysis in suitable patients.

In 1970, Tenckhoff and Curtis reported on 19 patients maintained on peritoneal dialysis for up to four years for a total of 25 patient years during which they performed 3,001 dialyses. Sixteen of them self-dialyzed at home. [53] There were 16 episodes of peritonitis, all of which were cured, and the incidence of peritonitis was 0.59% of all dialyses performed with indwelling catheters. There were three deaths. In general, patients were well and rehabilitated although three were limited in activities by pre-existing severe cardiac disease. This experience showed peritoneal dialysis was an acceptable alternative to hemodialysis and in certain circumstances might be the preferable mode of treatment, such as in patients living alone, those with cardiovascular disease, children, and. since blood transfusions were not required routinely, might be preferable in patients who would not accept transfusions, and in those being maintained for renal transplantation.

The two systems of peritoneal dialysate preparation were developed commercially. The batch system using the pressure boiler was made by the Cobe Company of Denver Colorado, and the proportioning system was manufactured by the PhysioControl Company of Redmond, Washington. In 1972 Tenckhoff and his coworkers described their experience with the latter machine. [54] By 1976, the PhysioControl machine was proving so successful that there were 26 patients on home peritoneal dialysis, 226 on home hemodialysis, and 46 dialyzing in-center in the Northwest Kidney Center program (the Seattle Artificial Kidney Center had been renamed).) and consideration was being given to developing a second generation device.

This all changed after Popovich and Moncrieff described what they called a portable-wearable equilibrium peritoneal dialysis technique. This used 5 exchanges a day of 2 L of peritoneal dialysate, 7 days a week, and did not require a machine. [55] Baxter soon was making the dialysate, at first in 2 L bottles and then in 2 L plastic bags, and the name of the technique was changed to continuous ambulatory peritoneal dialysis (CAPD). Over the years this became the most widely used form of home dialysis. Even CAPD had a Seattle connection as Popovich had been an engineering fellow with Babb at the University of Washington and had worked there in dialysis research.

Currently the Northwest Kidney Centers has between 160 and 170 patients on CAPD and CCPD (Continuous Cycling Peritoneal Dialysis) as patients can be trained to do this treatment themselves within a week. It is an excellent first treatment for those new patients who elect to use it.

Nationally, the use of peritoneal dialysis grew slowly but steadily following the introduction of CAPD, and reached a maximum of 14% to 15% of U.S. dialysis patients in the early 1990s but since then has gradually declined for no obvious reason so that in 2008 it was 6.9%. [56] Peritoneal dialysis, like home hemodialysis, is a less-expensive form of treatment than center hemodialysis. Over the years the question has been whether peritoneal dialysis has as good a long-term outcome as center hemodialysis and there have been a number of comparisons of these outcomes using data from national registries and prospective cohort studies. There are many difficulties in comparing outcomes with two treatments when patient assignment is nonrandom. Most of the recent observational studies have shown that survival of hemodialysis and peritoneal dialysis patients is remarkably similar, at least for several years, suggesting there should be greater use of peritoneal dialysis, [57] particularly as peritoneal dialysis is a self-administered home treatment that has many of the other benefits of home hemodialysis.

Longer Hemodialysis and More Frequent Hemodialysis

When the SAKC opened in 1962 routine dialysis was twice weekly overnight for at least 12 hours – 24 hours or more per week, and the highly selected patients continued to work and were rehabilitated. Several years later most Seattle patients were dialyzing at home, 6 to 8 hours three times weekly, usually overnight for 18 to 24 hours a week. In the U.S. it was not until the 1970s and 1980s with disposable dialyzers, the proliferation of dialysis units and the belief that adequacy was best measured by Kt/V that three times a week dialysis, often for less than 3½ hours, became common and overnight conventional home hemodialysis almost disappeared. In 1996. Uldall and colleagues in Toronto reported on the results of slow nocturnal "nightly" home hemodialysis for 8 hours, 5 to 7 nights a week. [58] This revived interest in nocturnal home hemodialysis, particularly as excellent survival with minimal complications, fewer hospitalizations and greatly increased quality of life were reported. [59] In situations where nightly nocturnal home hemodialysis may be too expensive a good alternative is alternate night home hemodialysis. [60] Nocturnal hemodialysis in center three times weekly also has been shown to be much better than conventional dialysis [61] and is now been offered in a small number of dialysis units in the U.S. and elsewhere.

A simulation study in 1965 showed that more frequent hemodialysis would be most helpful in lowering the concentration of substances that moved slowly from the intracellular to the extracellular space [62] and in 1968 DePalma and colleagues started seven patients on 4 to 5 hours of dialysis 5 times a week using Kiil dialyzers and dialyser reuse, changing later to using an automatic home coil dialyzer system. Patients felt better, hypertension was more easily controlled, serum albumin level increased, and dietary restrictions could be eased. [63] This treatment was stopped for financial reasons after the Medicare program began. More frequent dialysis was used in a small number of patients after that, principally as a fourth treatment in the week for patients with serious complications or instability during dialysis. This changed in the 1990s when more frequent ("daily") treatment was becoming recognized as providing improvement in survival, patient well-being and quality of life. [64-66] Now both nightly and daily dialysis are increasing; in the United States. The percentage of dialysis patients treated by home hemodialysis reached a nadir of 0.57% in 2002 but there are now estimates that this is more than 1%.A factor in this is the recent development of new technology specifically designed for patient use in the home. Ideally, such equipment should be designed to increase the adequacy of dialysis, diminish morbidity, and make home hemodialysis simpler and safer for the patient, thus leading to the use of more frequent hemodialysis. [67]

Comment

The advantages of home hemodialysis and peritoneal dialysis have been known for more than 40 years but were largely ignored in the U.S. once the original financial problems were resolved by the ESRD Medicare Program. They were rediscovered over the last 15 years or so' with growing interest in longer and/or more frequent hemodialysis. In 2001 a survey of nephrologists in the U.S. and Canada showed that there was a general belief that 11 to 14 percent of patients should be treated by home hemodialysis and that use of peritoneal dialysis could be increased two- or three-fold over current practices. [68] Also, in 2007 6,595 physicians and nurses at five international conferences were asked what dialysis modality they considered the best; peritoneal dialysis was considered the best initial treatment for a planned start in a typical patient and the best treatment for long term use was considered to be home or self-care hemodialysis more than three times a week. [69] In addition, a couple of surveys of nephrologists asked what treatment they would choose for themselves if they had kidney failure and could not have a kidney transplant. The overwhelming majority said more frequent home hemodialysis, even though most nephrologists in the U.S. do not have any of their patients on this modality.

What is needed is a change of culture. All hemodialysis patients should be expected to do as much of their own care as they can and if possible to insert their own needles. Peritoneal dialysis must be an option for all new patients and at the same time home hemodialysis must also be offered and should also be offered at intervals thereafter to patients established on center hemodialysis or with failing peritoneal dialysis. The aim should be for as many dialysis patients as possible, including center patients, doing a significant amount of their own care. Maximum rehabilitation should be the goal in all patients. Nephrologists need to learn more about home dialysis so they can explain the possible alternatives to their patients and guide their choice.

As for patients, Scribner always said they should take as much responsibility for their own care as they can, and that the good dialysis patient knows as much or more about their care than their doctor. Knowledge helps in reducing patient fears and depression, makes it possible to face chronic illness more realistically and positively and provides the opportunity to select the best possible treatment for them.

Shortly before he died, Scribner sent the following message about the effects of more frequent dialysis to be read at a session about more frequent dialysis at the 2003 Annual Dialysis Conference in Seattle.

"The annual cost of dialysis will drop. Innovations and automation will make the task of self-dialysis simpler to comprehend and less work for the patient. The resulting healthy, well-nourished, normotensive hemodialysis patients will incur lesser additional health care costs than their sickly, malnourished, hypertensive counterparts on short three times weekly hemodialysis."

References

[1] Quinton W, Dillard D, Scribner BH. Cannulation of blood vessels for prolonged hemodialysis. Trans ASAIO. 1960;6:104-113.

[2] Scribner BH, Buri R, Caner JZ, Hegstrom R, Scribner BH. The treatment of chronic uremia by means of intermittent hemodialysis. A preliminary report. Trans ASAIO. 1960;6:114-122.

[3] Haviland J. Experiences in establishing a community artificial kidney center. Trans Am Clin Climatol Assoc. 1965;77:125-129.

[4] Alexander S. They Decide Who Lives, Who Dies: Medical miracle and a moral burden of a small committee. Life. 9 November 1962;19:102-125.

[5] Kirby C. Presidential address. Trans ASAIO. 1961;7:153-155.

[6] Merrill JP, Schupak E, Cameron E, Hampers CL. Hemodialysis in the home. JAMA. 1964;190:468-470.

[7] Hampers C, Merrill JP, Cameron E. Hemodialysis in the home: a family affair. Trans ASAIO. 1965;11:3-6.

[8] Fry D, Hoover PL. Single-pass dialysate flow for the Seattle pumpless hemodialysis system. Trans ASAIO. 1964;10:98-105.

[9] Grimsrud L, Cole JJ, Lehman GA, Babb AL, Scribner BH. A central system for the continuous preparation and distribution of hemodialysis fluid. Trans ASAIO. 1964;10:107-109.

[10] Curtis FK, Cole JJ, Fellows BJ, Tyler LL, Scribner BH. Hemodialysis in the home. Trans ASAIO. 1965;11:7-10.

[11] Shaldon S, Baillod R, Comty C, Oakley J, Sevitt L. 18 months experience with a nurse-patient operated chronic dialysis unit. Proc EDTA. 1964;1:235-238.

[12] Baillod RA, Comty C, Ilahi M, Konotey-Ahulu FID, Sevitt L, Shaldon S. Overnight hemodialysis in the home. Proc EDTA. 1965;2:99-103.

[13] Shaldon S. Experience to date with home hemodialysis. In: Scribner (ed). Proceedings of the Working Conference on Chronic Dialysis, Seattle, WA. University of Washington 1964; 66-69.

[14] Eschbach JW Jr, Wilson WE Jr, Peoples RW, Wakefield AW, Babb AL, Scribner BH. Unattended overnight home hemodialysis. Trans ASAIO. 1966;12:346-356.

[15] Scribner BH. Hemodialysis in the treatment of chronic uremia. Pro 3rd Int Congr Nephrol, Washington DC, 3:305-315, Karger, Basel/New York 1967.

[16] Kolff WJ. Kidney transplant or home dialysis. Postgrad Med. 1968;44:93-99.

[17] Blagg CR. Hickman RO, Eschbach JW, Scribner BH. Home hemodialysis: six years' experience. N Engl J Med. 1970;283:1126-1131.

[18] Mailloux LU, Kapikian N, Napolitano B, Mossey RT, Bellucci AG, Wilkes BM, Vernace MA, Miller IJ. Home dialysis patient outcomes during a 24-year period of time from 1970 through 1993. Adv Ren Replace Ther. 1996;3:112-9.

[19] Delano BG. Home hemodialysis offers excellent survival. Adv Ren Replace Ther. 1996;3:106-111.

[20] Arkouche W, Traeger J, Delawari E, Sibaï-Galland R, Abdullah E, Galland R, Leitienne P, Fouque D, Laville M. Twenty-five years of experience with out-center hemodialysis. Kidney Int. 1999;56:2269-2275.

[21] Covic A, Goldsmith DJ, Venning MC, Ackrill P. Long-hours home haemodialysis: the best renal replacement method? QJM. 1999;92:251-260.

[22] McGregor DO, Buttimore AL, Lynn KL. Home hemodialysis: excellent survival at less cost, but still underutilized. Kidney Int. 2000;57:2654-2655.

[23] Woods JD, Port FK, Stannard D, Blagg CR, Held PJ. Comparison of mortality with home hemodialysis and center hemodialysis: a national study. Kidney Int. 1996;49;1464-1470.

[24] Saner, E, Nitsch, D, Descoeudres, C, Frey FJ, Uehlinger DE. Outcome of home haemodialysis patients: A case-cohort study. Nephrol Dial Transplant. 2005;20:604.

[25] Saran RM, Bragg-Gresham R, Levin NW, Twardowski ZJ, Wizemann V, Saito A, Kimata N, Gillespie BW, Combe C, Bommer J, Akiba T, Mapes DL, Young EW, Port FK. Longer treatment time and slower ultrafiltration in hemodialysis: Association with reduced mortality in the DOPPS. Kidney Int. 2006;69:1222-1228.

[26] Marshall MR, Byrne BG, Kerr PG, McDonald SP. Association of hemodialysis dose and session length with mortality risk in Australian and New Zealand patients. Kidney Int. 2006;69:1229-1236.

[27] McGregor DO, Buttimore AL, Lynn KL, Nicholls MG, Jardine DL. A comparative study of blood pressure control with short in-center versus long home haemodialysis. Blood Purif. 2001;19:293-300.

[28] The FHN Trial Group. In-center hemodialysis six times per week versus three times a week. N Engl J Med. 2010;363:2287-2300.

[29] Agar JWM. International variation and trends in home hemodialysis. Adv Chron Kidney Dis. 2009;16:205-214.

[30] Harman C. Putting clinical trials on trial. Nat Rev Nephrol. 2009;5:301.

[31] Hill AB. Heberden Oration 1965: reflections on the controlled trial. Ann Rheum Dis. 1966;25:107–13.

[32] Rawlins Sir M. De Testimonio: On the evidence for decisions about the use of therapeutic interventions. Harveian Oration 2008, Royal College of Physicians, London.

[33] Evans RW, Manninen DL, Garrison LP Jr, Hart LG, Blagg CR, Gutman RA, Hull AR, Lowrie EG. The quality of life of patients with end –stage renal disease. N Engl J Med. 1985;312:553-559.

[34] Bremer BA, McCauley, Wrona RM, Johnson JP. Quality of life in end-stage renal disease. Am J Kidney Dis. 1989;13:200-209.

[35] Oberley E, Schattel D. Home hemodialysis survival, quality of life and rehabilitation. Adv Renal Replace Ther. 1996;3:147-15.

[36] Blagg CR, Cole JJ, Irvine G, Marr T, Pollard TL. How much should dialysis cost? In: Freeman RB editor. Proceedings of the Workshop on Dialysis and Transplantation, ASAIO, Seattle WA. Washington DC: Georgetown University Press for the American Society for Artificial Internal Organs 1972: 54-60.

[37] Seligman ME. Depression and learned helplessness. In: Friedman RJ, Katz MN editors. The Psychology of Depression; Contemporary Theory and Research. Washington DC: Halstead Press 1974; 83-111.

[38] Blagg CR, Scribner BH. Dialysis: medical, psychological, and economic problems unique to the dialysis patient. In Brenner BM, Rector FC, editors. The Kidney, 1st edn. Philadelphia: Saunders 1976: 1705-1744.

[39] Snow W, Clark M. Understanding patient learning and performance capabilities for home dialysis training. J Am Assoc Nephrol Nurses Tech. 1976;3:20-24.

[40] McLaughlin K, Manns B, Mortis G, Hons R, Taub K. Why patients with ESRD do not select self-care as a treatment option. Am J Kidney Dis. 2003;41:380-385.

[41] Caffazo JA, Leonard K, Easty AC, Rossos PG, Chan CT. Patient-perceived barriers to the adoption of nocturnal home hemodialysis. Clin J Am Soc Nephrol. 2009;4:694-695.

[42] Stack AG. Determinants of modality selection among incident U.S, dialysis patients. Results from a national study. J Am Soc Nephrol. 2002;13:1279-1287.

[43] Blagg CR. What went wrong with home hemodialysis in the United States and what can be done now? Hemodial Int. 2000;3:55-58.

[44] Stinson GW, Clark MF, Sawyer TK, Blagg CR. Home hemodialysis training in 3 weeks. Trans Am Soc Artif Intern Organs. 1972;18:66-69.

[45] Eschbach JW, Seymour M, Potts A, Clark M, Blagg CR. A hemodialysis orientation unit. Nephron. 1983;33:106-110.

[46] Blagg CR, Hutton J, Hynes J, Young B, Kjellstrand CM. The Northwest Kidney Centers' experience with the Aksys PHD system. Nephrol News Issues. 20:56-61,2006.

[47] Boen ST, Mulinari AS, Dillard DH, Scribner BH. Periodic peritoneal dialysis in the management of chronic uremia. Trans Am Soc Artif Intern Organs. 1962:8:256-262.

[48] Ben ST, Mion CM, Curtis FK, Shilipetar G. Periodic peritoneal dialysis using the repeated puncture technique and an automatic cycling machine. Trans Am Soc Artif Intern Organs. 1964;10:409-414.

[49] Tenckhoff H, Shilipetar G, Boen ST. One year's experience with home peritoneal dialysis. Trans Am Soc Artif Intern Organs. 1965;11:11-14.

[50] Palmer RA, Quinton WE, Gray JE. Prolonged peritoneal dialysis for chronic renal failure. Lancet. 1964;1:700-702.

[51] Tenckhoff H, Schechter H. A bacteriologically safe peritoneal access device. Trans Am Soc Artif Intern Organs. 1968;4:181-186.

[52] Tenckhoff H, Shilipetar G, Van Paaschen WH, Swanson E. A home peritoneal dialysate delivery system. Trans Am Soc Artif Intern Organs. 1969;15:103-107.

[53] Tenckhoff H, Curtis FK. Experience with maintenance peritoneal dialysis in the home. Trans Am Sic Artif Intern Organs. 1970;16:90-95.

[54] Tenckhoff H, Meston B, Shilipetar G. A simplified automatic peritoneal dialysis system. Trans Am Soc Artif Intern Organs. 1972;18(0):436-40.

[55] Popovich RP, Moncrief JW, Decherd JF, Bomar JB, Pyle WK. The definition of a novel portable –wearable equilibrium peritoneal technique. Abst Am Soc Artif Intern Organs. 1976;64.

[56] U.S, Renal Data Sysrem,USRDS2010 Annual Data Report. Atlas of Chronic Kidney Disease and End-Stage Renal Disease in the United States, National Institutes of Health, National Institute of Diabetes and Digestive and Kidney Diseases, Bethesda, MD, 2010. Table D1, p 428.

[57] Chiu YW, Jiwakanon S, Lukowsky L, Duong U, Kalantar-Zadeh K, Mehrotra R. An update on the comparisons of mortality outcomes of hemodialysis and peritoneal dialysis patients. Semin Nephrol. 2011;31:152-158.

[58] Uldall R, Ouwendyk M, Francoeur R, Wallace L, Sit W, Vas S, Pierratos A. Slow nocturnal home hemodialysis at the Wellesley Hospital. Adv Ren Replace Ther. 1996;3;133-136.

[59] Pauly RP, Maximova K, Coppens J et al. Patient and technique survival among a Canadian multicenter nocturnal home hemodialysis cohort. Clin J Am Soc Nephrol. 2010;10:1815-1820.

[60] Mahadevan K, Pellicano R, Reid A, Kerr P, Polkinghorne K, Agar J. Comparison of biochemical, hematological and volume parameters in two treatment schedules of nocturnal haemodialysis. Nephrology (Carlton). 2006;11:413-418.

[61] OK E, Duman S, Asci G, Tumuklu M, Onen Sertoz O, Kayikcioglu M, Toz H, Adam SM, Yilmaz M, Tonbul HZ, Ozkahya M, Long Dialysis Study Group. Comparison of 4- and 8-h dialysis sessions in thrice-weekly in-centre haemodialysis: a prospective, case-controlled study. Nephrol Dial Transplant. 2011;26:1287-1296.

[62] Bell RL, Curtis FK, Babb AL. Analog simulation of the patient-artificial kidney system. Trans Am Soc Artif Intern Organs. 1965;11:183-189.

[63] DePalma JR, Pecker EA, Maxwell MH. A new automatic coil dialyzer system for 'daily' dialysis. Proc Euro Dial Transpl Assoc. 1969;6:26-34 (Reprinted in Hemodial Int. 2004;8:19-23.

[64] Short daily haemodialysis: survival in 415 patients treated for 1006 patient years. Nephrol Dial Transplant. 2008;23:2183-3289.

[65] Culleton BF, Asola MR. The impact of short daily and nocturnal hemodialysis on quality of life, cardiovascular risk and survival. J Nephrol. 2011;405-415.

[66] Perl J, Chan CVT. Home hemodialysis, daily hemodialysis, and nocturnal hemodialysis: Core Curriculum 2009. Am J Kidney Dis. 2009;54:1171-1184.

[67] Kjellstrand CM, Kjellstrand P. The ideal home hemodialysis machine. Hemodial Int. 2008;12 Suppl 1:S33-S39.

[68] Mendelssohn DC, Mullaney SR, Jung B, Blake PG, Mehta RL. What do American nephrologists think about dialysis modality selection? Am J Kidney Dis. 2001;37:22-29.

[69] Ledebo I, Ronco C. The best dialysis therapy? Results from an international survey among nephrology professionals. NDT Plus. 2008;1:403-408.

In: Issues in Dialysis
Editor: Stephen Z. Fadem

ISBN: 978-1-62417-576-3
© 2013 Nova Science Publishers, Inc.

Chapter V

How do Clinical Outcomes of Automated Peritoneal Dialysis Compare with those of Continuous Ambulatory Peritoneal Dialysis?

Sunil V. Badve[1,2], Carmel M. Hawley[1,2] and David W. Johnson[1,2,*]
[1]Department of Nephrology, Princess Alexandra Hospital, Brisbane, Australia
[2]School of Medicine, University of Queensland, Brisbane, Australia

Abstract

As compared to hemodialysis, peritoneal dialysis (PD) is underutilized as a dialysis modality in patients affected by end-stage renal disease (ESRD). However, there is a disproportionate expansion in the utilization of automated PD (APD). Unfortunately, this marked expansion in APD has occurred at the expense of continuous ambulatory peritoneal dialysis (CAPD), even though APD is a more costly therapy. This begs the question as to whether outcomes on APD differ from those on CAPD and justify the disproportionate growth in APD utilization. The purpose of this article is to comprehensively review the studies comparing APD and CAPD outcomes, including mortality and technique failure, peritonitis rates, solute clearances, sodium removal and ultrafiltration, residual renal function decline, quality of life and cost. Furthermore, the role of APD is reviewed in specific patient sub-groups, such as high and low transporters, anuric patients, elderly patients and children.

---

* Address for Correspondence and Reprints: Professor David Johnson. Department of Nephrology, Level 2, ARTS Building, Princess Alexandra Hospital, Ipswich Road, Woolloongabba, Brisbane Qld 4102, Australia. Tel: +61 7 3176 5080, Fax: +61 7 3176 5480; Email: david_johnson@health.

Introduction

In spite of a growing number of dialysis patients, the proportion of patients receiving peritoneal dialysis (PD) has steadily declined by 22% in the USA between 2000 and 2007; and by 18% in Australia between 2001 and 2008. [1,2] During the same period, the proportion of PD patients receiving automated PD (APD) increased from 47% to 62% in the USA and from 28% to 57% in Australia, such that relative growth in the number of prevalent APD patients exceeded that of hemodialysis (HD) patients (see Figure 1). The marked expansion in the utilization of APD has occurred at the expense of continuous ambulatory peritoneal dialysis (CAPD). This begs the question as to whether the outcomes on APD differ from those on CAPD and justify the disproportionate growth in APD utilization. In this chapter, we will review the difference in various clinical outcomes between CAPD and APD.

Basic Differences between CAPD and APD

CAPD involves 3 to 5 manual exchanges of PD solutions (also referred to as dialysate) per day without the aid of a cycler machine. CAPD offers greater flexibility due to a wider range of dwell times. A typical dwell time on CAPD could be as short as 3-4 hours and as long as 12-14 hours. Thanks to its simplicity, patients can be trained in a relatively shorter period of time. On the other hand, APD involves use of a cycler machine to perform the PD exchanges. The term APD encompasses several PD therapies, such as nightly intermittent peritoneal dialysis (NIPD), continuous cyclic peritoneal dialysis (CCPD), or tidal peritoneal dialysis (nightly tidal PD or continuous tidal PD). In tidal PD, a constant volume of PD solution remains in the peritoneal cavity while an additional volume (known as the tidal volume) of PD solution is exchanged at each cycle. Usually, 3 to 8 exchanges are performed using the cycler over 7 to 10 hours overnight. During the daytime, depending on their clinical condition, patients are prescribed zero (as in NIPD) to 2 manual exchanges (as in CCPD) to enhance solute and fluid clearance. Since, less time is spent on performing manual daytime exchanges; APD therapy is popular among younger and working individuals. However, it is technically more demanding than CAPD and the required training period may be longer than that of CAPD. APD is also more expensive than CAPD as it requires more consumables.

Mortality

Only two randomized controlled trials (RCT) reported mortality outcomes between CAPD and APD (Table 1). [3,4] Bro and colleagues randomized 34 prevalent PD patients from 3 Danish units to receive either CAPD or APD. [3] Patients with low-average or low peritoneal membrane transport status were excluded. Nine patients dropped out of the trial before commencing peritoneal dialysis. There were no deaths among the remaining 25 patients at 6 months. This trial was limited by small sample size and short follow-up period. Since only prevalent PD patients and those with high and high-average membrane transport status were included in this trial, the external validity of this RCT was severely restricted. In the other RCT, de Fijter and colleagues recruited 97 incident patients with end-stage renal disease (ESRD). [4] A total of 15 patients dropped out of the trial before commencing dialysis - 6 patients due to death. Among the remaining 82 patients, 2 of 41 patients (4.9%) from the CAPD group died (follow-up 723 patient-months) and 4 of 41 patients (9.8%) from the APD group died (follow-up 688 patient-months). This study was limited by small sample size and lack of external validity due to single-center trial design. Meta-analysis of these 2 trials showed comparable mortality rates in CAPD and APD (risk ratio [RR] 1.49, 95% confidence intervals [CI] 0.51 - 4.37). [5]

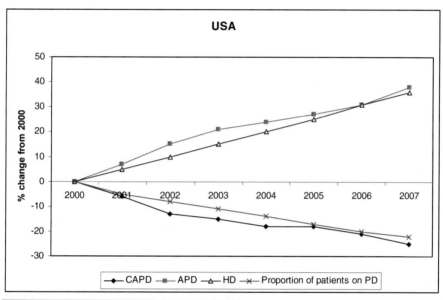

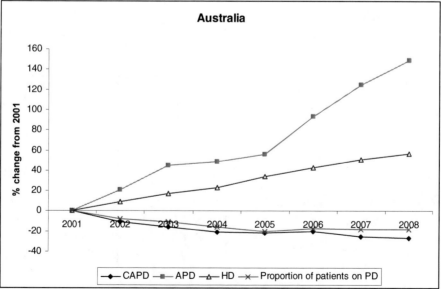

Figure 1. Percentage change in the number of prevalent patients on difference dialysis modalities in: Figure 1a- USA from 2000 and Figure 1b- Australia from 2001.

Table 1. Summary of difference in the mortality and technique failure rates between CAPD and APD

Study	Study design	n	Mortality	Technique failure
Bro 1999 [3]	RCT	25	No deaths during the 6-month follow-up	No deaths during the 6-month follow-up
de Fijter 1994 [4]	RCT	82	Number of deaths in CAPD group: 2/41, APD group: 4/41	Number of technique failures in CAPD group: 8/41, APD group: 4/41.
Guo 2003 [6]	Observational, Baxter database	32,135	1st year patient survival (P< 0.001)- CAPD: 78.5% (95%CI 77.6-79.3%) APD: 87.2% (95%CI 86.7-87.7%),	1st year technique survival (P< 0.001)- CAPD: 68.8% (95%CI 67.8-69.7%) APD: 81.3% (95%CI 80.7-81.9%), Adjusted HR for CAPD: 1.58, P<0.001 (APD as reference)
Badve 2008 [7]	Observational, National registry	4,128	Adjusted HR for APD: 1.03, 95% CI 0.86–1.24, P=0.723 (CAPD as reference)	Adjusted HR for APD: 1.08, 95% CI 0.91–1.27. (CAPD as reference)
Mehrotra 2009 [9]	Observational, National registry	66,381	Death rate: CAPD: 33%, APD 32.5%. Adjusted HR for APD: 1.03, 95% CI 0.99–1.06. (CAPD as reference)	Technique failure rate CAPD: 34.2%, APD: 32.3%. Adjusted HR for APD: 1.0, 95% CI 0.97–1.03. (CAPD as reference)
Michels 2009 [10]	Observational, National registry	649	Death rate: CAPD: 27%, APD 24%. Adjusted HR for APD: 1.09 (95% CI 0.65 to 1.83). (CAPD as reference)	Technique failure rate CAPD: 18%, APD: 25%. Adjusted HR for APD: 0.91 (95% CI 0.63 to 1.32). (CAPD as reference)
Sanchez 2008 [8]	Observational, Single-center	237	Patient survival at 1, 2, and 3 years: CAPD: 62%, 49%, and 42% APD: 82%, 62%, and 56% (P <0.001).	Technique survival at 1, 2 and 3 years: CAPD: 65%, 47%, and 42% APD: 76%, 56%, and 56% (P <0.001).

The paucity of adequately powered RCTs highlights difficulties in recruiting patients for such trials. In the absence of these trials, most of the evidence originates from observational studies. [6-10] Guo and colleagues reported clinical outcomes of 32,135 patients from the USA commencing PD between 1999 and 2001, using data from Baxter Healthcare Corporation. [6] Unadjusted 1-year survival was lower in patients treated with CAPD than APD (78% versus 87%, P <0.001). The authors reported a survival benefit in the APD group after adjusting for age and diabetic status.

We reported clinical outcomes in 4,128 incident PD patients from Australia and New Zealand using data from the Australia and New Zealand Dialysis and Transplant (ANZDATA) Registry. [7] Of these, 2,393 patients were treated with CAPD and the remaining 1,735 with APD. Compared to patients treated with CAPD, APD patients were more likely to be young (56 years versus 60 years), Caucasian (74% versus 68%), and were less likely to have baseline coronary artery disease (34% versus 40%) or diabetes (33% versus 41%). Overall follow-up was 6,981 patient-years. The mortality rate during APD treatment was comparable to that during CAPD treatment (unadjusted hazard ratio [UHR] 0.92, 95% CI 0.77–1.09, P=0.336). The multivariate analysis also showed comparable mortality in the 2 PD modalities (adjusted hazard ratio [AHR] 1.03, 95% CI 0.86–1.24, P=0.723).

Mehrotra and colleagues studied the effect of PD modality in 66,381 incident ESRD patients who started PD between 1996 and 2004 using data from the United States Renal Data System (USRDS). [9] Patients treated with APD were more likely to be younger, Caucasian, and less likely to have diabetes. The differences in these variables were of a small magnitude, but statistically significant. The median follow-up period for CAPD and APD patients was 18.3 and 17.6 months, respectively. All-cause mortality rates were similar in both the PD modalities on unadjusted and adjusted analyses. Similar results were reported by Michels and colleagues on 649 incident PD patients using the Netherlands Cooperative Study on the Adequacy of Dialysis (NECOSAD) data. Unadjusted and adjusted hazard ratios of mortality were 0.98 (95% CI 0.62–1.54) and 1.09 (95% CI 0.65 to 1.83), respectively. Sanchez and colleagues from Mexico reported their single-center experience of 237 incident PD patients (139 on CAPD and 98 on APD). [8] Total follow-up was 2,566 patient-months. Patient survival in the APD group was superior to the CAPD group. Patient survival at 1, 2, and 3 years were 82%, 62%, and 56%, respectively in the APD group and 62%, 49%, and 42%, respectively in the CAPD group (P <0.001).

Technique Failure

Technique failure is defined as completion of PD therapy and transfer to hemodialysis for an extended period of time (typically at least 1-3 months). RCT-based evidence on technique failure is sparse (Table 1). [3,4] In the RCT reported by Bro and colleagues, no patient from either group changed their PD modality during the short follow up period of 6 months. [3] In the other trial, 8 of 41 patients in the CAPD group and 4 of 41 in the APD group were permanently transferred to hemodialysis. [4]

In the ANZDATA Registry report, there was no significant difference in death-censored technique failure (defined as requirement of hemodialysis for >1 month) between the CAPD and APD groups. [7] The unadjusted and adjusted hazard ratios were 1.09 (95% CI 0.92–

1.30) and 1.08 (95% CI 0.91–1.27), respectively. In the Baxter Healthcare Corporation report, 1-year technique survival in CAPD patients was lower than APD patients (69% versus 81%, P< 0.001). [6] When age, gender, diabetes and origin of patient were adjusted for in a multivariate analysis, the risk of technique failure was 58% higher in CAPD patients. Mehrotra and colleagues defined death-censored technique failure as transfer to hemodialysis for greater than 60 days. [9] Unadjusted death-censored technique failure rate was slightly lower in APD patients than CAPD patients (32% versus 34%, P <0.001). However, in the multivariate analysis, there was no statistically significant difference in death-censored technique failure between the two PD modalities. In the NECOSAD study, 18% of CAPD patients and 25% of APD patients were transferred to hemodialysis for more than 3 months. [10] Unadjusted and adjusted hazard ratios of technique failure were 0.92 (95% CI 0.64–1.31) and 0.91 (95% CI 0.63 to 1.32), respectively. In the Mexican single-center study, technique survival at 1, 2 and 3 years were 76%, 56%, and 56%, respectively in the APD group and 65%, 47%, and 42%, respectively in the CAPD group. [8]

Peritonitis

There is conflicting evidence on comparing peritonitis rates between CAPD and APD, with some investigators reporting lower, [4,8,11,12] similar, [3,13-15] or higher [16] peritonitis rates in APD. In the de Fijter RCT, 54 peritonitis episodes were recorded in 25 patients (61%) CAPD patients, whereas 31 peritonitis episodes were recorded in 19 patients (46%) APD patients. [4] The observed difference in the peritonitis rates was 0.43 episodes per patient-year (95%CI 0.1 to 0.8; P = 0.03). Huang and colleagues from Taiwan followed 117 CAPD and 95 APD patients between 1993 and 2000. [11] They reported a lower incidence of peritonitis in APD patients compared with CAPD patients (1.22 episodes per 100 patient-months versus 2.28 episodes per 100 patient-months, P <0.001). Mean peritonitis-free survival in APD patients (50.9 ± 3.9 months) was better than CAPD patients (35.9 ± 2.7 months, P=0.079), but not statistically significant. In the Mexican study, APD was associated with a lower peritonitis rate than CAPD (1 in 16 patient-months versus 1 in 34 patient-months). [8] The possibility of a first peritonitis event during the first year was lower on APD than CAPD (21% versus 47%, P <0.001). In a single center retrospective study from Spain, Rodriguez-Carmona and colleagues observed that the peritonitis rate was higher in 213 CAPD patients (0.64 episodes/patient/year) compared to 115 APD patients (0.31 episodes/patient/year). Median survival to the first episode of peritonitis was better in APD than CAPD (24 versus 17 months, P=0.02). [12]

In the Bro RCT, 2 of 13 CAPD and 1 of 12 APD patients developed peritonitis. [3] Yishak and colleagues similarly reported comparable peritonitis rates in the two PD modalities (0.55 episodes per patient-year in CAPD and 0.57 episodes per patient-year in APD). [13] Akman and colleagues reported peritonitis rates in 212 pediatric PD patients from 12 centers in Turkey. [14] Mean age at initiation of dialysis was 10 years. The observed peritonitis rate in CAPD patients (1 in 15.6 patient-months) was similar to that found in APD patients (1 in 15.4 patient-months) with a relative risk of 1.01 (95%CI 0.78 to 1.30, P=NS). Golper and colleagues analysed peritonitis rates in prevalent PD patients from the Tri-State Renal Network 9. [16] Compared to 866 CAPD patients using a Y-set disconnect system, the peritonitis-free interval was inferior in 213 APD patients (14.9 vs 20.2 months), such that the relative risk for peritonitis with was 28% higher in APD patients.

The available evidence, which is predominantly based on observational and retrospective studies, needs to be interpreted cautiously. Although de Fijter and colleagues reported lower peritonitis rates with APD, this RCT was limited by small sample size and the use of a cycler machine that is no longer available. Moreover, the observed peritonitis rates may also have been variably affected by several center-specific factors (such as patient training, centre size, implementation of protocols for screening and treatment of *Staphylococcus aureus* nasal carriers, and regular auditing of infection rates) and patient-specific factors (such as compliance, age, diabetic status, hygiene, connection systems used, and previous peritonitis episodes). Furthermore, these studies were conducted at different time periods raising the possibility of vintage bias. The last 2 decades have witnessed a substantial change in PD practice in terms of connectology, cycler machines, solutions, adequacy targets, and guidelines for prevention and treatment of infections. Therefore, the results of some of these studies may not be generalizable to contemporary PD practice.

Solute Clearance

It is well known that small solute clearances can be increased on APD by manipulating the number of cycles, total cycler volume, and the amount of tidal volume. [17-19] However, this requires large volumes of dialysate with an attendant increased cost. Furthermore, undue focus on small solute clearance may lead to shorter dwell times, thereby contributing to poor clearance of middle and larger molecules. In a prospective sequential study, Rodriguez and colleagues compared small solute clearances between CAPD, CCPD, 50% tidal PD and 25% tidal PD in 45 PD patients. [18] Clearances of both urea and creatinine were significantly higher in all forms of APD than CAPD. Mean weekly Kt/V in the CAPD, CCPD, 50% tidal PD, and 25% tidal PD groups were 1.51 ± 0.32, 2.03 ± 0.39, 1.88 ± 0.35, and 1.80 ± 0.4, respectively. Similarly, mean creatinine clearances in the CAPD, CCPD, 50% tidal PD, and 25% tidal PD groups were 42.8 ± 9.95, 52.19 ± 11.11, 51.31 ± 13.35, and 49.17 ± 11.83 L/week/1.73 m^2, respectively. However, mean dwell times were considerably shorter in both the tidal PD groups (18.7 ± 9.28 minutes and 15 ± 6.9 minutes in 50% tidal PD and 25% tidal PD groups, respectively) compared to the CCPD group (56.6 ± 8.73 minutes). Data on middle molecule clearance were not reported. Furthermore, both the tidal PD regimens required larger night-time dialysate volumes (22.5 L and 17.8 L in the 50% tidal PD and 25% tidal PD groups, respectively).

In an open-label randomized controlled trial, Demetriou and colleagues randomized 18 PD patients with either high-average or low-average peritoneal membrane transport status to two APD regimens sequentially with a 7-day washout period. [20] The 2 APD regimens were a conventional APD with low nightly dialysate flow and one manual daytime exchange versus APD with high dialysate flow but without a manual daytime exchange. In both the regimens, the tidal volumes were 75% and icodextrin was used as the last fill. Compared to the low-flow dialysate regimen, high-flow APD was associated with increased creatinine clearance (8.56 ± 1.22 vs. 7.87 ± 1.04 L/treatment, P=0.011) and urea clearance (12.83 ± 1.98 vs. 11.68 ± 1.06 L/treatment, P=0.014). On the other hand, phosphate (7.74 ± 1.74 vs. $7.60 \pm$

1.94 L/treatment, P=0.78) and β2 microglobulin (1.10 ± 0.37 vs. 1.12 ± 0.41 L/treatment, P=0.68) clearances were similar between the 2 regimens, whilst the high-flow regimen was associated with 35-60% increases in cost. Although the investigators did not compare solute clearances between CAPD and APD, the results highlight the fact that APD regimens aimed at increasing small solute clearances have no beneficial effects on the clearance of middle and larger molecules and are expensive.

Direct comparisons of phosphate clearance between CAPD and APD have shown similar [21,22] or worse [23] peritoneal phosphate clearance on CAPD compared to APD. Juergensen and colleagues reported that increasing the number of APD cycles from 7 to 12 and the total cycler volume by 70% to 24 L improved peritoneal phosphate clearance by 19%. [24] The lack of separate analysis of membrane transport status and PD modality effect in these studies makes the interpretation difficult. Badve and colleagues analyzed small solute and phosphate clearances in 129 prevalent PD patients in a cross-sectional study. [25] Peritoneal Kt/V urea was higher in patients receiving CCPD than those receiving CAPD (1.86 ± 0.4 vs. 1.62 ± 0.3, P < 0.001), although there was no difference in peritoneal creatinine clearance between the two modalities (47 ± 12.8 vs. 44 ± 8.1 L/wk/1.73 m^2, P=0.11). When examined by PD modality alone, there was no significant difference in peritoneal phosphate clearance between those treated with CCPD or CAPD (38.3 ± 12 vs. 40.9 ± 10.4 L/wk/1.73 m^2, P=0.199). When peritoneal phosphate clearance by modality was examined for each membrane category, there was no significant difference in phosphate clearance between the modalities in the high transporters (49.5 ± 7.6 vs. 49.5 ± 7.6 L/wk/1.73 m^2, P=0.97). However, treatment with CAPD was associated with increased peritoneal phosphate clearance compared with CCPD among high-average transporters (42.4 ± 11.4 vs. 36.4 ± 8.3 L/wk/1.73 m^2, P=0.01) and low-average-low transporters (35.6 ± 5.9 vs. 28.9 ± 11 L/wk/1.73 m^2, P=0.034). Bernardo and colleagues reported similar findings in a retrospective cross-sectional study involving 264 PD patients. [26] Peritoneal phosphate clearance was comparable between CAPD and APD among high transporters (46.9 ± 12.6 vs. 48.1 ± 13 L/wk/1.73 m^2, P=0.76) and high-average transporters (39.3 ± 10.4 vs. 39.6 ± 9.3 L/wk/1.73 m^2, P=0.87). However, it was superior in CAPD to APD among low-average transporters (35.9 ± 7.8 vs. 31.6 ± 6.6 L/wk/1.73 m^2, P=0.006) and low transporters (33.9 ± 15.2 vs. 24.5 ± 9 L/wk/1.73 m^2, P=0.049).

In summary, small solute clearances can be easily maximized on APD by increasing the number of exchanges on the cycler machine, but at the cost of shorter dwell times, poorer middle molecule and phosphate clearances, and higher dialysate volumes. APD regimens that are focused too heavily on small solutes clearances are not cost-effective as targeting increased small solutes clearance does not offer confer a survival advantage in PD. [27]

Sodium Removal

In PD, sodium removal occurs predominantly by diffusion rather than convection. Sodium removal in APD is inferior to CAPD because the sieving of sodium is most pronounced during the initial phase of a dialysis dwell, and dwell times are usually shorter on APD. In one cross-sectional study, total sodium removal in 78 patients on APD was 91 mmol/day compared to 210 mmol/day in 63 CAPD patients (P<0.001). [28] On multivariate regression analysis, use of longer dwell during the night exchanges was associated with better sodium removal on APD (1.3 mmol/L/minute, 95%CI 0.4, 2.1; P= 0.004). The same trend persisted over a longitudinal follow up of 24 months. [29] Moreover, in 32 patients who switched from CAPD to APD, median sodium removal decreased from 192 to 92 mmol/day (P=0.02).

Boudville and colleagues also demonstrated low peritoneal sodium removal in 56 APD patients (mean peritoneal sodium removal 84.4 ± 67.7 mmol/day). [30] However, peritoneal sodium removal was greater in patients treated with icodextrin than those who were not treated with icodextrin (104.7 ± 75.5 vs. 64.0 ± 52.8 mmol/day, P= 0.023). On the other hand, in a cross-sectional study, Davison and colleagues reported comparable peritoneal sodium removal between 90 CAPD and 68 APD patients (66.1 ± 127.5 vs. 98.7 ± 82.0 mmol/day, P=0.069). [31]

Ultrafiltration

Data on comparative ultrafiltration volumes for CAPD and APD are both limited and conflicting, with studies variably showing inferior [28,29] or comparable [25,31] ultrafiltration on APD. In the cross-sectional study reported by Rodríguez–Carmona and colleagues, ultrafiltration was inferior in patients receiving APD compared with those receiving CAPD (907 ± 744 vs. 1367 ± 720 ml/day, P=0.001). [28] As with sodium removal, the same trend persisted on a longitudinal follow-up of 24 months. [29] In 32 patients whose PD modality was changed from CAPD to APD, median ultrafiltration volumes were not statistically different before and after the switch (1310 vs. 1067 ml/day, P=NS). [28] However, the use of icodextrin also increased from 25% to 53% after the change in modality and may have contributed to the observed increases in ultrafiltration on APD.

In the cross-sectional study reported by Badve and colleagues, median [interquartile range] ultrafiltration volumes were comparable in patients treated with CAPD versus APD (1.16 [0.63–1.45] vs. 0.99 [0.67–1.36] L/day, P=0.478). [25] Similarly, in another cross-sectional study, ultrafiltration volumes were 572 ± 1013 ml/day and 811 ± 661 ml/day (P=0.092) in CAPD and APD patients, respectively. [31]

Residual Renal Function

Preservation of residual renal function (RRF) is associated with improved patient survival in patients treated with PD. [32-36] RRF contributes substantially to clearances of middle molecules and protein-bound solutes. [37] A strong link exists between RRF and other clinical outcomes, including blood pressure control, [38] fluid balance, [39] phosphate balance, [40] left ventricular hypertrophy, [41] nutrition, [42] inflammation, [36,43] risk of peritonitis [44] and quality of life. [45] Therefore, there is a great focus on preservation of RRF in dialysis patients.

Hiroshige and colleagues studied the rate of decline in RRF in 18 incident PD patients, of which 8 were treated with NIPD and 5 each with CCPD and CAPD. [46] The rates of decline in renal creatinine clearance at 6 months after starting NIPD and CCPD were -0.29 and -0.34 mL/min/month, respectively, which were much greater than that of CAPD (+0.01

mL/min/month). Hufnagel and colleagues studied RRF in 12 CAPD and 18 APD (12 CCPD and 6 NIPD) patients over 12 months following commencement of maintenance PD. [47] The rate of decline in renal creatinine clearance was greater in APD patients than CAPD patients at 6 (-0.28 vs. -0.1 ml/min/month, P=0.04) and 12 (-0.26 vs. -0.13 ml/min/month, P=0.005) months. Rodríguez-Carmona prospectively followed 53 CAPD and 51 APD patients for at least 1 year (mean 28.9 months; range, 13 to 62 months). [29] At the end of the first year, 1 CAPD and 5 APD patients were anuric, and 5 CAPD (7.5%) and 11APD patients (21.7%) had a GFR <1 mL/min (P=0.04). Mean GFR at 24 months was lower in APD patients, and on multivariate regression, APD therapy was associated with a more rapid decline in RRF.

Michels and colleagues compared the rate of decline in RRF between 505 CAPD and 78 APD patients using the NECOSAD data. [48] The yearly decline of residual GFR was comparable between the CAPD and APD patients. However, on the intention-to-treat analysis, the risk of complete loss of RRF (defined as urine output <200 mL/day) was higher in APD patients than CAPD patients (adjusted HR 2.66, 95%CI 1.60 – 4.44). The results were unchanged on the as-treated analysis.

On the other hand, the rate of decline in the renal creatinine clearance over 24 months of follow up in a randomized controlled trial was similar between 13 CAPD and 11 CCPD patients (-0.07 vs. -0.08 ml/min/month). [49] Gallar and colleagues reported comparable RRF at baseline (6.1 ± 2.7 vs. 7.1 ± 1.5 ml/min) and 1 year (4.9 ± 4.4 vs. 5.5 ± 1.8 ml/min) in 11 CAPD and 9 APD patients. [50] Roszkowska–Blaim and colleagues also reported comparable RRF at baseline and at 12 months in their pediatric patients. [51]

Quality of Life

McComb and colleagues evaluated health-related quality of life (HRQOL) using the RAND 36-item Health Survey 1.0 in 8 PD patients. [52] Questionnaires were administered before switching from CAPD to APD and then at 3 months later. No statistically significant improvements in HRQOL were observed during the 3-month follow-up period. In a multicenter study, de Wit and colleagues compared HRQOL between APD and CAPD using 4 HRQOL instruments (Short-Form 36, EuroQol EQ-5D, Standard Gamble, and Time Trade Off). [53] SF-36 scores were comparable between the 2 groups, except for Social functioning scores which were greater in APD patients than CAPD patients (79 ± 29 vs. 65 ± 33, P< 0.05). EuroQol EQ-5D scores were also comparable, except that CAPD patients were more anxious and/or depressed than APD patients (P<0.05). There were no statistically significant differences in the scores of the remaining HRQOL instruments between the 2 groups.

Michels and colleagues studied the quality of life in the prospective NECOSAD cohort of incident PD patients using the SF-36 and the Kidney Disease and Quality of Life Short Form (KDQOL-SF) questionnaires. [54] There were a total of 486 CAPD and 64 APD patients. The mental summary score showed a different pattern over time for patients on APD and on CAPD (P=0.03), this difference was no longer significant after adjusting for age, sex, comorbidity, primary kidney disease, and residual GFR (P=0.06). Only the role function emotional subscale remained significant on the multivariate adjustment (P=0.05).

The pattern of the physical summary score was not different between the PD modalities. In summary, this large and prospective study did not show any major differences in QoL on the SF-36 and the KDQOL-SF between CAPD and APD.

Cost

Treatment with APD requires increased quantities of consumables, including larger dialysate volumes. In the RCT reported by Bro and colleagues in 1999, the daily running costs of APD and CAPD were US $75 and $61, respectively. [3] They reported that in the absence of any benefit observed in their trial, APD therapy was 22.3% more expensive than CAPD. Baboolal and colleagues reported a more recent cost analysis from the UK. [55] Although, both the PD modalities were less expensive than in-center hemodialysis, the annual costs of APD and CAPD per patient were £ 21,655 and £ 15,570, respectively. Thus, the cost of CAPD is considerably lower than that of APD. In some countries, the pharmaceutical and device companies do not provide cycler machines free or at reduced cost, which would further increase the cost of APD.

APD in Selected Groups

High Transporters

Modelling studies suggest that ultrafiltration in high transporters should be maximized by prescription of short-dwell therapies, such as APD. [56] Consequently, the International Society of Peritoneal Dialysis (ISPD) Ad Hoc Committee on Ultrafiltration Management in Peritoneal Dialysis strongly recommends APD for the treatment of high transporters with impaired net ultrafiltration. [56] Johnson and colleagues reported mortality and technique failure among 628 PD patients with high transport membrane status using the ANZDATA Registry data. [57] There were 486 patients in the CAPD group and 142 in the APD group. The patients in the APD group were more likely to be younger (54.5 ± 19.3 vs. 59.1 ± 15.6 years, P=0.003), Caucasian (82% vs. 66%, P=0.006) and less likely to be diabetic (31% vs. 41%, P=0.03) and treated in a large PD centre (49% vs. 65%, P=0.004) than the CAPD group. Mean baseline D–P Cr 4h in the APD group was comparable to the CAPD group (0.88 ± 0.09 vs. 0.87 ± 0.07, P=0.151). Compared to CAPD, treatment with APD was associated with a 44% reduction in all-cause mortality (adjusted HR 0.56, 95%CI 0.35–0.87) on intention-to-treat analysis. The results were unchanged on an as-treated analysis. Death-censored technique failure was comparable between CAPD and APD (adjusted HR 0.88, 95% CI 0.64–1.21).

Low Transporters

In the ANZDATA Registry analysis reported by Johnson and colleagues, treatment with APD was associated with increased mortality (adjusted HR 2.19, 95%CI 1.02-4.70) in 196 low transporters compared with CAPD. [57] These results may potentially be explained by the fact that solute clearances of middle molecules and phosphate are time-dependent, such that the shorter dwell times associated with APD might substantially compromise such solute clearances. [25]

Anuric Patients

Anuric patients continue to pose several challenges in PD, especially with solute clearance and ultrafiltration. Bhaskaran and colleagues studied dialysis adequacy in 89 CAPD and 26 APD patients, who were anuric (urine output <100 mL/day or renal creatinine clearance <1 mL/min). [58] Mean weekly Kt/V urea in the CAPD and APD groups were 2.07 ± 0.31 and 2.6 ± 0.6, respectively. Mean creatinine clearances in CAPD and APD groups were 57.3 ± 8.5 and 65.7 ± 18.1 L/1.73 m^2/week, respectively. Fifty-seven percent and 81% of CAPD and APD patients achieved the contemporary target Kt/V urea of 2.0 and 2.2, respectively. They further reported that 35% of patients each from both the groups achieved the contemporary creatinine clearance target of 60 and 66 L/1.73 m^2/week, respectively. Following publication of the ADEMEX trial, the Kt/V urea target has now been revised to 1.7.

In the prospective, multicenter European APD Outcome Study (EAPOS), 177 anuric patients (urine output <100 mL/day or GFR <1 mL/min) on APD were followed for 2 years. [59] The APD prescription was adjusted at physician discretion to aim for creatinine clearance 60 L/1.73 m^2/week per and ultrafiltration 750 mL/day during the first 6 months. At 1-year, 78% and 74% patients achieved creatinine clearance and ultrafiltration targets, respectively, with 50% of patients using icodextrin. Notably, both urea and creatinine clearances did not predict survival, but ultrafiltration > 750 mL/day at baseline was associated with better survival (Risk ratio 0.45, P=0.0469). The investigators concluded that anuric patients can be successfully treated with APD. However, these results need to be interpreted with caution. The investigators analyzed longitudinal membrane function by solute transport ratio and ultrafiltration capacity. [60] The whole cohort experienced an increase in the solute transport ratio and decline in the ultrafiltration capacity. These changes were more pronounced in patients receiving high-glucose PD solutions.

In summary, with a carefully prescribed regimen, both CAPD and APD modalities are able to deliver adequate dialysis, defined by weekly Kt/V urea >1.7, in anuric patients. However, close monitoring is advocated for timely diagnosis of ultrafiltration failure.

Elderly Patients

Increasing numbers of elderly patients are commencing dialysis. In Australia, 45% of all patients commencing dialysis in 2008 were over 65 years of age. [2] The optimal dialysis modality in this patient population is not well studied. Kadambi and colleagues analyzed PD outcomes in 493 patients commencing maintenance PD in the New Haven CAPD unit between 1994 and 2000. [61] Out of these, 192 patients were older than 65 years and 92% were treated with APD. Although mortality rate was higher in elderly patients than younger patients, their rates of technique failure, peritonitis, and quality of life scores were not different than from younger patients.

Castrale and colleagues studied the clinical outcomes of elderly patients (age ≥ 75 years) using data from the French Language Peritoneal Dialysis Registry (RDPLF). [62] A total of 1,613 elderly patients commenced PD between 2000 and 2007. Of these, 1,435 (89%) were treated with CAPD and 178 (11%) were treated with APD. CAPD patients were older (82.1 ± 4.5 vs. 80.7 ± 4.4 years) and had a greater modified Charlson comorbidity index. In addition, CAPD patients were more frequently assisted by a nurse than APD patients (80% vs. 47%, P < 0.01). In spite of these differences, on the multivariate model, patient survival was better in APD patients than CAPD patients (adjusted HR 0.72, 95%CI 0.55 – 0.93). However, death-censored technique failure and peritonitis rates were comparable between the 2 PD modalities. Therefore, APD is a viable option for elderly patients.

Pediatric Patients

Fabian Velasco and colleagues reported their 3-year experience with APD in 458 children between 2003 and 2006 from Mexico. [63] PD modality was changed from CAPD to APD in these children. Following modality change, improvements in ultrafiltration (from 590 ± 340 to 846 ± 335 ml/day), presence of edema (from 67 to 8%), and requirement for antihypertensive medications (from 83 to 38%) were observed. In addition, peritonitis rates improved (from 1 episode in 35 patient-months to 1 episode in 47 patient-months) and the number of hospitalizations decreased (from 384 to 51). Chiu and colleagues also reported very low peritonitis rates (1 episode in 54.2 patient-months) in 30 children treated with APD. [64] Between 1992 and 2002, 65% of 4,150 index dialysis patients enrolled in the North American Pediatric Renal Transplant Cooperative Study (NAPRTCS) dialysis registry underwent PD. [65] Of these, 69% patients received APD. Median time to peritonitis was shorter for CAPD than APD (472 vs. 348 days, P=0.06) and fewer patients receiving APD developed peritonitis than CAPD at 1-year (44 vs. 51%). Thus, APD may be a preferred PD modality in children, considering 85% of 458 Mexican children treated with APD were attending school. [63]

Conclusions and Future Directions

Currently available evidence suggests that important clinical outcomes, such as mortality and technique failure are comparable between CAPD and APD. Most of the evidence originates from large observational registry studies as there have been only 2 small underpowered randomized controlled trials. Both of these randomized controlled trials were severely limited by a very small sample size (131 participants in total). Furthermore, both studies were conducted in the late 1980s and 1990s. PD apparatus has undergone significant improvement in many areas since then and the results of these studies may be not generalizable to the contemporary dialysis population. In comparison, the observational studies are larger, more inclusive and are more likely to represent 'real world' practice. However, these studies are limited by retrospective study design, indication bias, and reporting or recall bias. Consequently, in spite of adjusting for multiple variables, the possibility of residual confounding could not be excluded. Furthermore, data on adverse events has not been systematically captured.

Currently available evidence also does not favour either APD or CAPD with respect to peritonitis rates, solute clearances, ultrafiltration, residual renal function decline or quality of life. However, APD could be a favourable option for certain types of individuals. For example, APD offers a survival advantage for high transporters. Data on more children and adolescents attending schools with APD are encouraging. In the absence of strong evidence favouring one of the 2 PD modalities, we recommend that the selection of PD modality should be based on individual circumstances including, lifestyle considerations.

Ideally, an adequately powered randomized controlled trial is required to demonstrate the benefit of one PD modality over other. However, from the pragmatic point of view, it is unlikely that such a trial will ever be done. Difficulty in conducting such a trial is highlighted by the fact that only 2 small trials have been performed so far and further trials have not attempted in the last 10-15 years. Since most of the questions on the other clinical outcomes are unanswered, more research is required in this area. Future studies, whether interventional or observational, need to be conducted on a larger patient population and thus will require collaboration between multiple centres. In the absence of randomized controlled trials, there is a need to collect in depth data on a wide number of variables for adjusting in the multivariate models. Finally, the study interventions and research themes should be focused on the outcomes that are relevant from the patient's perspective and include cost-effectiveness analysis.

References

[1]   US Renal Data System, USRDS 2009 Annual Data Report: Atlas of End-Stage Renal Disease in the United States. Bethesda, MD: National Institutes of Health, National Institute of Diabetes and Digestive and Kidney Diseases, 2009.

[2]   ANZDATA Registry Report 2009. Adelaide, South Australia: Australia and New Zealand Dialysis and Transplant Registry, 2009.

[3]   Bro S, Bjorner JB, Tofte-Jensen P, et al. A prospective, randomized multicenter study comparing APD and CAPD treatment. Perit Dial Int. 1999;19:526-33.

[4]   de Fijter CW, Oe LP, Nauta JJ. Clinical efficacy and morbidity associated with continuous cyclic compared with continuous ambulatory peritoneal dialysis. Ann Intern Med. 1994;120:264-271.

[5]   Rabindranath KS, Adams J, Ali TZ, Daly C, Vale L, Macleod AM. Automated vs continuous ambulatory peritoneal dialysis: a systematic review of randomized controlled trials. Nephrol Dial Transplant. 2007;22:2991-8.

[6]   Guo A, Mujais S. Patient and technique survival on peritoneal dialysis in the United States: evaluation in large incident cohorts. Kidney Int. 2003:S3-12.

[7]   Badve SV, Hawley CM, McDonald SP, et al. Automated and continuous ambulatory peritoneal dialysis have similar outcomes. Kidney Int. 2008;73:480-8.

[8] Sanchez AR, Madonia C, Rascon-Pacheco RA. Improved patient//technique survival and peritonitis rates in patients treated with automated peritoneal dialysis when compared to continuous ambulatory peritoneal dialysis in a Mexican PD center. Kidney Int. 2008;73:S76-S80.

[9] Mehrotra R, Chiu YW, Kalantar-Zadeh K, Vonesh E. The outcomes of continuous ambulatory and automated peritoneal dialysis are similar. Kidney Int. 2009;76:97-107.

[10] Michels WM, Verduijn M, Boeschoten EW, Dekker FW, Krediet RT. Similar survival on automated peritoneal dialysis and continuous ambulatory peritoneal dialysis in a large prospective cohort. Clin J Am Soc Nephrol. 2009;4:943-9.

[11] Huang JW, Hung KY, Yen CJ, Wu KD, Tsai TJ. Comparison of infectious complications in peritoneal dialysis patients using either a twin-bag system or automated peritoneal dialysis. Nephrol Dial Transplant. 2001;16:604-7.

[12] Rodriguez-Carmona A, Perez Fontan M, Garcia Falcon T, Fernandez Rivera C, Valdes F. A comparative analysis on the incidence of peritonitis and exit-site infection in CAPD and automated peritoneal dialysis. Perit Dial Int. 1999;19:253-8.

[13] Yishak A, Bernardini J, Fried L. The outcome of peritonitis in patients on automated peritoneal dialysis. Adv Perit Dial. 2001;17:205-208.

[14] Akman S, Bakkaloglu SA, Ekim M, Sever L, Noyan A, Aksu N. Peritonitis rates and common microorganisms in continuous ambulatory peritoneal dialysis and automated peritoneal dialysis. Pediatr Int. 2009;51:246-9.

[15] Troidle LK, Gorban-Brennan N, Kliger AS, Finkelstein FO. Continuous cycler therapy, manual peritoneal dialysis therapy, and peritonitis. Adv Perit Dial. 1998;14:137-41.

[16] Golper TA, Brier ME, Bunke M, et al. Risk factors for peritonitis in long-term peritoneal dialysis: the Network 9 peritonitis and catheter survival studies. Academic Subcommittee of the Steering Committee of the Network 9 Peritonitis and Catheter Survival Studies. Am J Kidney Dis. 1996;28:428-36.

[17] Perez RA, Blake PG, McMurray S, Mupas L, Oreopoulos DG. What is the optimal frequency of cycling in automated peritoneal dialysis? Perit Dial Int. 2000;20:548-56.

[18] Rodriguez AM, Diaz NV, Cubillo LP. Automated peritoneal dialysis: a Spanish multicenter study. Nephrol Dial Transplant. 1998;13:2335-2340.

[19] Juergensen PH, Murphy AL, Kliger AS, Finkelstein FO. Increasing the dialysis volume and frequency in a fixed period of time in CPD patients: the effect on Kpt/V and creatinine clearance. Perit Dial Int. 2002;22:693-7.

[20] Demetriou D, Habicht A, Schillinger M, Horl WH, Vychytil A. Adequacy of automated peritoneal dialysis with and without manual daytime exchange: A randomized controlled trial. Kidney Int. 2006;70:1649-55.

[21] Sedlacek M, Dimaano F, Uribarri J. Relationship between phosphorus and creatinine clearance in peritoneal dialysis: clinical implications. Am J Kidney Dis. 2000;36:1020-4.

[22] Evenepoel P, Bammens B, Verbeke K, Vanrenterghem Y. Superior dialytic clearance of beta(2)-microglobulin and p-cresol by high-flux hemodialysis as compared to peritoneal dialysis. Kidney Int. 2006;70:794-9.

[23] Gallar P, Ortega O, Gutierrez M, et al. Influencing factors in the control of phosphorus in peritoneal dialysis. Therapeutic options. Nefrologia. 2000;20:355-61.

[24] Juergensen P, Eras J, McClure B, Kliger AS, Finkelstein FO. The impact of various cycling regimens on phosphorus removal in chronic peritoneal dialysis patients. Int J Artif Organs. 2005;28:1219-23.

[25] Badve SV, Zimmerman DL, Knoll GA, Burns KD, McCormick BB. Peritoneal Phosphate Clearance is Influenced by Peritoneal Dialysis Modality, Independent of Peritoneal Transport Characteristics. Clin J Am Soc Nephrol. 2008;3:1711-1717.

[26] Bernardo AP, Contesse SA, Bajo MA, et al. Peritoneal Membrane Phosphate Transport Status: A Cornerstone in Phosphate Handling in Peritoneal Dialysis. Clin J Am Soc Nephrol. 2011;6:591-597

[27] Paniagua R, Amato D, Vonesh E. Effects of increased peritoneal clearances on mortality rates in peritoneal dialysis: ADEMEX, a prospective, randomized, controlled trial. J Am Soc Nephrol. 2002;13:1307-1320.

[28] Rodriguez-Carmona A, Fontan MP. Sodium removal in patients undergoing CAPD and automated peritoneal dialysis. Perit Dial Int. 2002;22:705-13.

[29] Rodriguez-Carmona A, Perez-Fontan M, Garca-Naveiro R, Villaverde P, Peteiro J. Compared time profiles of ultrafiltration, sodium removal, and renal function in incident CAPD and automated peritoneal dialysis patients. Am J Kidney Dis. 2004;44:132-45.

[30] Boudville NC, Cordy P, Millman K, et al. Blood pressure, volume, and sodium control in an automated peritoneal dialysis population. Perit Dial Int. 2007;27:537-43.

[31] Davison SN, Jhangri GS, Jindal K, Pannu N. Comparison of volume overload with cycler-assisted versus continuous ambulatory peritoneal dialysis. Clin J Am Soc Nephrol. 2009;4:1044-1050.

[32] Bargman JM, Thorpe KE, Churchill DN. Relative contribution of residual renal function and peritoneal clearance to adequacy of dialysis: a reanalysis of the CANUSA study. J Am Soc Nephrol. 2001;12:2158-62.

[33] Jose AD-B, Edmund GL, Nancy LL, Zhang SMH, Xiaofei Z, Lazarus JM. Associates of mortality among peritoneal dialysis patients with special reference to peritoneal transport rates and solute clearance. Am. J. Kidney Dis. 1999;33:523-534.

[34] Rocco M, Soucie JM, Pastan S, McClellan WM. Peritoneal dialysis adequacy and risk of death. Kidney Int. 2000;58:446-57.

[35] Szeto CC, Wong TY, Leung CB, et al. Importance of dialysis adequacy in mortality and morbidity of chinese CAPD patients. Kidney Int. 2000;58:400-7.

[36] Wang AY, Wang M, Woo J, et al. Inflammation, residual kidney function, and cardiac hypertrophy are interrelated and combine adversely to enhance mortality and cardiovascular death risk of peritoneal dialysis patients. J Am Soc Nephrol. 2004;15:2186-94.

[37] Bammens B, Evenepoel P, Verbeke K, Vanrenterghem Y. Removal of middle molecules and protein-bound solutes by peritoneal dialysis and relation with uremic symptoms. Kidney Int. 2003;64:2238-43.

[38] Menon MK, Naimark DM, Bargman JM, Vas SI, Oreopoulos DG. Long-term blood pressure control in a cohort of peritoneal dialysis patients and its association with residual renal function. Nephrol Dial Transplant. 2001;16:2207-13.

[39] Konings CJ, Kooman JP, Schonck M, et al. Fluid status in CAPD patients is related to peritoneal transport and residual renal function: evidence from a longitudinal study. Nephrol Dial Transplant. 2003;18:797-803.

[40] Wang AY, Woo J, Sea MM, Law MC, Lui SF, Li PK. Hyperphosphatemia in Chinese peritoneal dialysis patients with and without residual kidney function: what are the implications? Am J Kidney Dis. 2004;43:712-20.

[41] Wang AY, Wang M, Woo J, et al. A novel association between residual renal function and left ventricular hypertrophy in peritoneal dialysis patients. Kidney Int. 2002;62:639-47.

[42] Wang AY, Sea MM, Ip R, et al. Independent effects of residual renal function and dialysis adequacy on actual dietary protein, calorie, and other nutrient intake in patients on continuous ambulatory peritoneal dialysis. J Am Soc Nephrol. 2001;12:2450-7.

[43] Chung SH, Heimburger O, Stenvinkel P, Qureshi AR, Lindholm B. Association between residual renal function, inflammation and patient survival in new peritoneal dialysis patients. Nephrol Dial Transplant. 2003;18:590-7.

[44] Han SH, Lee SC, Ahn SV, et al. Reduced residual renal function is a risk of peritonitis in continuous ambulatory peritoneal dialysis patients. Nephrol Dial Transplant. 2007;22:2653-8.

[45] Termorshuizen F, Korevaar JC, Dekker FW, van Manen JG, Boeschoten EW, Krediet RT. The relative importance of residual renal function compared with peritoneal clearance for patient survival and quality of life: an analysis of the Netherlands Cooperative Study on the Adequacy of Dialysis (NECOSAD)-2. Am J Kidney Dis. 2003;41:1293-302.

[46] Hiroshige K, Yuu K, Soejima M. Rapid decline of residual renal function in patients on automated peritoneal dialysis. Perit Dial Int. 1996;16:307-315.

[47] Hufnagel G, Michel C, Queffeuloe G. The influence of automated peritoneal dialysis on the decrease in residual renal function. Nephrol Dial Transplant. 1999;14:1224-1228.

[48] Michels WM, Verduijn M, Grootendorst DC, et al. Decline in Residual Renal Function in Automated Compared with Continuous Ambulatory Peritoneal Dialysis. Clin J Am Soc Nephrol. 2011.

[49] de Fijter CW, ter Wee PM, Donker AJ. The influence of automated peritoneal dialysis on the decrease in residual renal function. Nephrol Dial Transplant. 2000;15:1094-6.

[50] Gallar P, Ortega O, Carreno A. Rate of decline in residual renal function is equal in CAPD and automated peritoneal dialysis patients. Perit Dial Int. 2000;20:803-805.

[51] Roszkowska-Blaim M, Skrzypczyk P, Drozdz D, Pietrzyk JA. Residual renal function in children treated with continuous ambulatory peritoneal dialysis or automated peritoneal dialysis--a preliminary study. Adv Perit Dial. 2009;25:103-9.

[52] McComb J, Morton AR, Singer MA. Impact of portable APD on patient perception of health-related quality of life. Adv Perit Dial. 1997;13:137-140.

[53] de Wit GA, Merkus MP, Krediet RT, de Charro FT. A comparison of quality of life of patients on automated and continuous ambulatory peritoneal dialysis. Perit Dial Int. 2001;21:306-12.

[54] Michels WM, van Dijk S, Verduijn M, et al. Quality of Life in Automated and Continuous Ambulatoryperitoneal Dialysis. Perit Dial Int. 2011 February;31:138-147.

[55] Baboolal K, McEwan P, Sondhi S, Spiewanowski P, Wechowski J, Wilson K. The cost of renal dialysis in a UK setting--a multicentre study. Nephrol Dial Transplant. 2008;23:1982-9.

[56] Mujais S, Nolph K, Gokal R. Evaluation and management of ultrafiltration problems in peritoneal dialysis. International Society for Peritoneal Dialysis Ad Hoc Committee on Ultrafiltration Management in Peritoneal Dialysis. Perit Dial Int. 2000;20:S5-S21.

[57] Johnson DW, Hawley CM, McDonald SP, et al. Superior survival of high transporters treated with automated versus continuous ambulatory peritoneal dialysis. Nephrol Dial Transplant. 2010 Jun;25(6):1973-9. Epub 2010 Jan 22.

[58] Bhaskaran S, Schaubel DE, Jassal SV, et al. The effect of small solute clearances on survival of anuric peritoneal dialysis patients. Perit Dial Int. 2000;20:181-7.

[59] Brown EA, Davies SJ, Rutherford P, et al. Survival of functionally anuric patients on automated peritoneal dialysis: the European APD Outcome Study. J Am Soc Nephrol. 2003;14:2948-57.

[60] Davies SJ, Brown EA, Frandsen NE, et al. Longitudinal membrane function in functionally anuric patients treated with APD: data from EAPOS on the effects of glucose and icodextrin prescription. Kidney Int. 2005;67:1609-15.

[61] Kadambi P, Troidle L, Gorban-Brennan N, Kliger AS, Finkelstein FO. APD in the elderly. Semin Dial. 2002;15:430-3.

[62] Castrale C, Evans D, Verger C, et al. Peritoneal dialysis in elderly patients: report from the French Peritoneal Dialysis Registry (RDPLF). Nephrol Dial Transplant. 2010;25:255-62.

[63] Fabian Velasco R, Lagunas Munoz J, Sanchez Saavedra V, et al. Automated peritoneal dialysis as the modality of choice: a single-center, 3-year experience with 458 children in Mexico. Pediatr Nephrol. 2008;23:465-71.

[64] Chiu MC, Tong PC, Lai WM, Lau SC. Peritonitis and exit-site infection in pediatric automated peritoneal dialysis. Perit Dial Int. 2008;28 Suppl 3:S179-82.

[65] Fine RN, Ho M. The role of APD in the management of pediatric patients: a report of the North American Pediatric Renal Transplant Cooperative Study. Semin Dial. 2002;15:427-429.

In: Issues in Dialysis
Editor: Stephen Z. Fadem

ISBN: 978-1-62417-576-3
© 2013 Nova Science Publishers, Inc.

Chapter VI

Intensified Hemodialysis Programs for Children and Adolescents

Julia Thumfart and Dominik Müller
Department of Pediatric Nephrology, Charité
Augustenburger Platz, Berlin, Germany

Abstract

Early renal transplantation is the method of choice for end stage renal disease in childhood and adolescence. However, average waiting time for kidney transplantation exceeds several years. Even more important, morbidity and mortality are extremely high in this group of patients. Additionally, in childhood and adolescence, school attendance and social rehabilitation is poor.

Studies in adults have shown that neither a modest increase of dialysis dosage delivered nor the use of high-flux filters can improve long term outcome. Therefore, intensified hemodialysis programs have been developed by varying modalities of dialysis (short daily, nocturnal intermittent or at home) in order to improve not only physical but also psychosocial conditions. For adult dialysis patients it has been demonstrated that such programs significantly improve uremia associated biochemical parameters as well as blood pressure control, nutritional status and quality of life. In the light of these advantages, intensified hemodialysis programs have preliminary been also adopted to pediatric hemodialysis programs. Although only few centers provide intensified programs, like in adults, uremia associated parameters improve dramatically. Medication, like phosphate-binders, erythropoietin and antihypertensive agents can be reduced. Fluid limitations and dietary restrictions can be lifted. Hospitalizations due to intradialytic problems are reduced. Likewise, social rehabilitation greatly improves.

In summary, as discussed in this chapter, intensified hemodialysis programs in childhood and adolescence are a promising option to improve uremia-associated symptoms and provide unprecedented psychosocial rehabilitation.

Introduction

The method of choice for renal replacement therapy in children and adolescents with end stage renal disease (ESRD) is early renal transplantation. However average waiting time on the transplantation list is actually more than two years. [1] This situation is worsened because morbidity and mortality is extremely high in young dialysis patients. [2,3] Mortality rates in children with renal replacement therapy are 30 times as high when compared to healthy controls. [4] Among young dialysis patients mortality risk is 4 times as high as for children with functional renal graft. [5] Additionally, social rehabilitation and quality of life are poor. Therefore, time on dialysis should not only be considered as a bridge to transplantation. Rather, dialysis modalities should be improved to provide adequate therapy to attenuate medical and social consequences of end stage renal disease.

Conventional hemodialysis is performed for 4-5 hours 3 times per week. In pediatric patients ESRD is associated with renal osteopathy, malnutrition, poor growth and insufficient weight gain. Conventional dialysis programs are unable to reduce these complications of chronic renal insufficiency; rather, they become even worse. Disturbance in Calcium-Phosphate-metabolism is poorly controllable on conventional dialysis. Patients have to obey strict dietary restrictions even when taking medications like phosphate and potassium binders.

It has been shown that alteration of the vascular system due to chronic renal insufficiency are responsible for the extremely high morbidity and mortality rate in patients with childhood onset renal failure. [3,6] During dialysis treatment uremic vasculopathy progresses. Whether these alterations in the vascular system are reversible after kidney transplantation, remains uncertain.

Table 1. Comparison of the common forms of hemodialysis in children and adolescents. SDHD short daily hemodialysis; NIHD nocturnal intermittent hemodialysis; NHHD nocturnal home hemodialysis

Modality	Location	Dialysis sessions per week	Duration (h)	Control of phosphate balance	Control of fluid balance	Social rehabilitation	Comment
Con-ventional	centre	3	4 – 5	poor	poor	poor	standardized
SDHD	centre	5 - 6	2 – 3	excellent	very good	modest	undisturbed sleep at home
NIHD	centre	3	8	good	very good	very good	continuous school attendance
NHHD	home	5 - 6	8	excellent	excellent	good	demanding claim on patient and parents

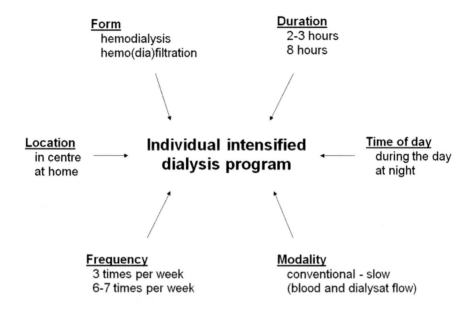

Figure 1. Different modalities of intensified hemodialysis for achieving for each patient the most suitable dialysis program.

Additionally, during conventional hemodialysis social life is extremely restricted. Full school attendance is only possible every other day. Even though teachers are working on the dialysis ward, the social environment of school is missing. These circumstances are major aspects for the poor quality of life under conventional dialysis treatment in childhood and adolescence.

In order to overcome these problems, alternative programs have been developed.

In adults, the Hemodialysis Study group (HEMO) has shown that patients on conventional hemodialysis neither a modest increase of Kt/V nor the use of high-flux filters are able to reduce mortality rates. [7] Similar results have been shown for adult patients on peritoneal dialysis. [8] For those reasons focus has been centered on dialysis time leading to intensified dialysis programs that means elongating of overall dialysis time (see Figure 1).

The following chapter focuses on intensified hemodialysis programs in adults. Thereafter we will discuss data on intensified hemodialysis programs in children and adolescents. (see Table 1)

Intensified Hemodialysis Programs in Adults

General Aspects

First reports on intensified hemodialysis programs appeared about 40 years ago, when an intensified program was established in Tassin, France. [9] Patients were treated with long slow hemodialysis (24 to 30 hours per week) and were followed up to 10 years. Blood pressure control was achieved by a strict maintenance of dry weight (with addition of a low salt diet, but without the use of antihypertensive medication). Overall survival rate was 85%

after ten years. Despite this impressive survival rate other centres in Europe or North America did not promptly adopt this concept.

From the late Nineties on, increasingly more reports on intensified dialysis programs appeared. Intensification of dialysis reduces mortality rate significantly. [10] Intensification of hemodialysis is reached by increasing dialysis time (>5 hours/session) or frequency (>4 times/week) (see Figure 1). Basically, there are 3 different modalities of intensified dialysis programs: short daily hemodialysis (2 to 3 hours 5 to 7 days per week), nocturnal intermittent hemodialysis (8 hours 3 days per week) and daily nocturnal hemodialysis (6 to 8 hours 5 to 7 days per week). These different programs can be performed either at home or in the dialysis centre. Usually daily nocturnal hemodialysis is conducted at home as nocturnal home hemodialysis (NHHD), whereas short daily hemodialysis (SDHD) and nocturnal intermittent hemodialysis (NIHD) are performed in the dialysis centre or at home. [11] All these different forms of intensified hemodialysis increase Kt/V considerably. Weekly single pool Kt/V with intensified programs is 4.5 – 9, whereas weekly single pool Kt/V with conventional dialysis is 3.6 – 4. [12] Expectedly intensified dialysis programs increase not only Kt/V, but also clearance of middle sized molecules. Ultrafiltration rate per hour can be lowered when compared with conventional dialysis, thus making this approach especially attractive for cardiovascular instable patients. High ultrafiltration rates are associated with high mortality rate. [13] There is an international quotidian dialysis register that collects data from all form of intensified dialysis. The aim of this register is to analyse outcome in a large cohort of patients under different forms of intensified dialysis. [11] Most of the published studies up to now include a small cohort of patients. In the majority of cases there are only patients included with one of the different forms of intensified dialysis. These studies will be discussed in the following chapters.

Short Daily Hemodialysis (SDHD)

First experiences with SDHS were gained over 30 years ago. [14] But like for all forms of intensified hemodialysis widespread application was only reported in the last decade. In adults SDHD is performed at home as often as in the dialysis centre. [11] A metaanalysis identified 25 studies on SDHD. [15] Each study contained five or more patients on SDHD (1.5 – 3 hours on 5 – 7 days per week). 10 of 11 studies showed improvement of blood pressure, left ventricular hypertrophy decreased in 4 studies. Kjellstrand et al. reported on 415 patients treated by SDHD for 29 (+/- 31) months at home or in the dialysis centre. [16] 10-year survival was 42% (+/- 9%). Survival was compared with matched patients from the United States Renal Data System (USRDS) Data Report: Survival of the SDHD patients was 2-3 times than that of the matched US hemodialysis patients. Survival of patients dialyzing daily at home was similar to that of age-matched recipients of deceased donor renal transplants. Yuen et al. reported that phosphorus levels decreased after converting patients from conventional hemodialysis to SDHD with the same dosage of phosphate binders. [17] Another study could show that SDHD improved phosphorus control by increasing dialytic phosphorus removal while maintaining nutritional status and reducing the use of phosphate binders. [18] SDHD also is associated with improved nutritional status and reduced markers of inflammation. [19,20] Quality of life greatly improved after switching from conventional dialysis to SDHD. [21]

Nocturnal Intermittent Hemodialysis (NIHD)

Because of the long dialysis time intermittent long hemodialysis is usually conducted at night. It can be performed at home or in the dialysis centre. Troidle et al. reported on 16 patients who switched from conventional hemodialysis to NIHD. Kt/V per session increased from 1.2 (+/- 0.16) to 2.6 (+/- 0.65). Serum phosphorus levels were reduced (5.3 versus 4.4 mg/dl). [22] Bugeja et al. reported that median serum phosphorus levels decreased from 5.9 to 3.7 mg/dl after switching to NIHD. [23] The mean number of antihypertensive drugs declined from 2.0 to 1.5 (p<0.05) during the course of NIHD, and the mean daily dosage of phosphate binders declined from 6.2 to 4.9 at study end (p<0.05). [23] Luik et al. could also demonstrate that blood pressure values are significantly lower after switching to NIHD. [24] In a prospective controlled trial the hospitalization rate was one-fourth of that observed in patients treated with four-hour conventional hemodialysis. Mortality rate was reduced by 78 percent. [25]

Nocturnal Home Hemodialysis (NHHD)

NHHD is mostly performed in countries like Canada or Australia where distances to the next dialysis centre are unacceptable long. In most cases blood and dialysate flow are reduced (slow nocturnal dialysis). [26,27] Lindsay et al. compared NHHD with conventional hemodialysis and SDHD. [28] NHHD patients showed significantly lower phosphorus levels than SDHD and matched control patients on conventional hemodialysis therapy. Phosphate-binder use by NHHD patients was significantly reduced. Patients on SDHD and NHHD showed decrease in calcium x phosphate product with significantly lower values for NHHD patients (38.11 mg^2/dl^2) compared with SDHD (53.99 mg^2/dl^2) and conventional dialysis patients (52.51 mg^2/dl^2). [28] Culleton et al. reported in the only randomized controlled trial that, compared with conventional hemodialysis, NHHD improved left ventricular mass, reduced the need for blood pressure medications and improved selected measures of quality of life. [29] Global quality of life was significantly better in NHHD patients. [30] These findings were affirmed in other trials. [31-35] In woman NHHD is associated with a return to fertility and many successful pregnancies have been reported. [36]

Intensified Dialysis Programs in Children and Adolescents

General Aspects

Intensified dialysis programs for children and adolescents are established in very few centres worldwide. [37] These programs are rather expensive in childhood. Children are much more demanding on dialysis like adults. Therefore one specialized dialysis nurse takes care of maximum 3 patients. Guidelines of different pediatric nephrology associations stipulate that it is mandatory for pediatric nephrologist to stay in the dialysis centre. It is obvious that such programs require additional financial resources but also save costs. Compared with the higher costs of prolonged dialysis time, there are savings of medications and hospitalization due to intradialytic complications. Currently, for nocturnal dialysis programs the dialysis centre gets reimbursed for only one "conventional" day, while SDHD gets financed every single day.

For children and adolescents intensified dialysis programs in the dialysis centre are more suitable at least in urban areas. Home dialysis requires from the patient and the parents a great amount of time, accuracy and responsibility. Especially nocturnal dialysis often disturbs the sleep of the whole family. Most parents cannot continuously provide home dialysis on a high professional level like pediatric dialysis centres do.

Pediatric SDHD

This concept was initiated by Fischbach et al. in France 2002 as daily in centre hemodiafiltration. [38] Like in adults positive effects of intensification of hemodialysis were impressive. At start of SDHD, diet intake due to medical prescription and limited appetite was restrictive with limitation in water, salt, potassium and proteins; only 2 of 12 children were free of antihypertensive drugs, all received phosphate and potassium binders. After switching to SDHD, diet was free and protein intake higher. 10 of 12 children were free of antihypertensive drugs, only 4 of 12 received potassium binders, 1 of 12 received phosphate binders. [39] Usually growth retardation is a frequent problem in children on chronic dialysis despite therapy with recombinant human growth hormone. Fischbach et al. showed that SDHD promotes catch-up growth. [40,41] The authors speculate that the improved response to recombinant human growth hormone is the result of less malnutrition and cachexia. [40] More trials on SDHD are not available up to now. Advances of SDHD are that patients can be seen by the medical staff every day and can sleep at home, which is mainly important for younger children. For older children who attend school, social rehabilitation in school environment can be difficult. Even the patients follow some courses in the dialysis centre, they miss most of the courses in school. The consequences of SDHD have on social rehabilitation and quality of life is examined currently.

Pediatric NIHD

This concept was initiated 2005 in Berlin, Germany. [42] This program combines medical advances of intensified dialysis and social rehabilitation due to nocturnal dialysis sessions. NIHD is especially suitable for metropolitan areas where distances to the dialysis centre are short. Up to now 16 patients were included in a prospective trial. [42] After switching from conventional dialysis to NIHD single pool Kt/V increased from 1.74 to 2.15 per session. Serum phosphorus levels decreased while phosphate binders could be reduced. Dietary restrictions could be lifted. 2 patients even needed to get phosphorus substitution. Two patients had left ventricular hypertrophy on conventional dialysis, which resolved after 6 months on NIHD. Antihypertensive drugs could be reduced. Hospitalization rates due to dialytic problems decreased. Days absent from school decreased from 37 per 6 month to 12 after switching to NIHD.

Pediatric NHHD

Geary et al. established a NHHD program in Canada. [43,44] Clearance of small and middle sized molecules is optimal. Patients have no fluid or dietary restriction after switching to NHHD. Like patients on NIHD some patients even needs phosphorus substitution. NHHD claims from the patient and the parents a great amount of time, accuracy and responsibility. In rural areas where distances to the dialysis centre a long it is a suitable option.

Conclusion

It has been shown in many trials that all forms of intensified dialysis (SDHD, NIHD and NHHD) overmatch conventional hemodialysis. These trials had mostly a small number of patients. For achieving more objective data an international register has been created where patients from the three different programs are enrolled. Data of this registry will help to determine the advantages and disadvantages of each program for the individual patient. Such a registry should also be created for pediatric patients to provide an insight in the medical and psychosocial consequences of intensified dialysis in these young patients.

References

[1] Oosterlee A RAe. Eurotransplant annual report 2009. 2009.
[2] Groothoff JW, Gruppen MP, Offringa M, Hutten J, Lilien MR, Van De Kar NJ, Wolff ED, Davin JC, Heymans HS. Mortality and causes of death of end-stage renal disease in children: A dutch cohort study. Kidney Int. 2002;61:621-629.
[3] Oh J, Wunsch R, Turzer M, Bahner M, Raggi P, Querfeld U, Mehls O, Schaefer F. Advanced coronary and carotid arteriopathy in young adults with childhood-onset chronic renal failure. Circ. 2002;106:100-105.
[4] Kramer A, Stel VS, Tizard J, Verrina E, Ronnholm K, Palsson R, Maxwell H, Jager KJ. Characteristics and survival of young adults who started renal replacement therapy during childhood. Nephrol Dial Transplant. 2009;24:926-933.
[5] McDonald SP, Craig JC. Long-term survival of children with end-stage renal disease. N Engl J Med. 2004;350:2654-2662.
[6] Brancaccio D, Bellasi A, Cozzolino M, Galassi A, Gallieni M. Arterial accelerated aging in dialysis patients: The clinical impact of vascular calcification. Curr Vasc Pharmacol. 2009;7:374-380.
[7] Eknoyan G, Beck GJ, Cheung AK, Daugirdas JT, Greene T, Kusek JW, Allon M, Bailey J, Delmez JA, Depner TA, Dwyer JT, Levey AS, Levin NW, Milford E, Ornt DB, Rocco MV, Schulman G, Schwab SJ, Teehan BP, Toto R. Effect of dialysis dose and membrane flux in maintenance hemodialysis. N Engl J Med. 2002;347:2010-2019.
[8] Paniagua R, Amato D, Vonesh E, Correa-Rotter R, Ramos A, Moran J, Mujais S. Effects of increased peritoneal clearances on mortality rates in peritoneal dialysis: Ademex, a prospective, randomized, controlled trial. J Am Soc Nephrol. 2002;13:1307-1320.

[9] Charra B, Calemard E, Cuche M, Laurent G. Control of hypertension and prolonged survival on maintenance hemodialysis. Nephron. 1983;33:96-99.

[10] Chertow GM, Levin NW, Beck GJ, Depner TA, Eggers PW, Gassman JJ, Gorodetskaya I, Greene T, James S, Larive B, Lindsay RM, Mehta RL, Miller B, Ornt DB, Rajagopalan S, Rastogi A, Rocco MV, Schiller B, Sergeyeva O, Schulman G, Ting GO, Unruh ML, Star RA, Kliger AS. In-center hemodialysis six times per week versus three times per week. N Engl J Med. 2010 Dec 9;363:2287-2300.

[11] Nesrallah GE, Suri RS, Moist LM, Cuerden M, Groeneweg KE, Hakim R, Ofsthun NJ, McDonald SP, Hawley C, Caskey FJ, Couchoud C, Awaraji C, Lindsay RM. International quotidian dialysis registry: Annual report 2009. Hemodial Int. 2009;13:240-249.

[12] McFarlane PA. More of the same: Improving outcomes through intensive hemodialysis. Semin Dial. 2009;22:598-602.

[13] Movilli E, Gaggia P, Zubani R, Camerini C, Vizzardi V, Parrinello G, Savoldi S, Fischer MS, Londrino F, Cancarini G. Association between high ultrafiltration rates and mortality in uraemic patients on regular haemodialysis. A 5-year prospective observational multicentre study. Nephrol Dial Transplant. 2007;22:3547-3552.

[14] Bonomini V, Mioli V, Albertazzi A, Scolari P. Daily-dialysis programme: Indications and results. Proc Eur Dial Transplant Assoc. 1972;9:44-52.

[15] Suri RS, Nesrallah GE, Mainra R, Garg AX, Lindsay RM, Greene T, Daugirdas JT. Daily hemodialysis: A systematic review. Clin J Am Soc Nephrol. 2006;1:33-42.

[16] Kjellstrand CM, Buoncristiani U, Ting G, Traeger J, Piccoli GB, Sibai-Galland R, Young BA, Blagg CR. Short daily haemodialysis: Survival in 415 patients treated for 1006 patient-years. Nephrol Dial Transplant. 2008;23:3283-3289.

[17] Yuen D, Richardson RM, Chan CT. Improvements in phosphate control with short daily in-center hemodialysis. Clin Nephrol. 2005;64:364-370.

[18] Ayus JC, Achinger SG, Mizani MR, Chertow GM, Furmaga W, Lee S, Rodriguez F. Phosphorus balance and mineral metabolism with 3 h daily hemodialysis. Kidney Int. 2007;71:336-342.

[19] Galland R, Traeger J, Arkouche W, Delawari E, Fouque D. Short daily hemodialysis and nutritional status. Am J Kidney Dis. 2001;37:S95-98.

[20] Ayus JC, Mizani MR, Achinger SG, Thadhani R, Go AS, Lee S. Effects of short daily versus conventional hemodialysis on left ventricular hypertrophy and inflammatory markers: A prospective, controlled study. J Am Soc Nephrol. 2005;16:2778-2788.

[21] Reynolds JT, Homel P, Cantey L, Evans E, Harding P, Gotch F, Wuerth D, Finkelstein S, Levin N, Kliger A, Simon DB, Finkelstein FO. A one-year trial of in-center daily hemodialysis with an emphasis on quality of life. Blood Purif. 2004;22:320-328.

[22] Troidle L, Hotchkiss M, Finkelstein F. A thrice weekly in-center nocturnal hemodialysis program. Adv Chronic Kidney Dis. 2007;14:244-248.

[23] Bugeja A, Dacouris N, Thomas A, Marticorena R, McFarlane P, Donnelly S, Goldstein M. In-center nocturnal hemodialysis: Another option in the management of chronic kidney disease. Clin J Am Soc Nephrol. 2009;4:778-783.

[24] Luik AJ, Charra B, Katzarski K, Habets J, Cheriex EC, Menheere PP, Laurent G, Bergstrom J, Leunissen KM. Blood pressure control and hemodynamic changes in patients on long time dialysis treatment. Blood Purif. 1998;16:197-209.

[25] Ok E DS, Asci G, Yilmaz M, Sertoz OO, Toz H, Adam SM, Basci A, Ozkahya M. Eight-hour nocturnal in-center hemodialysis provides survival benefit over four-hour conventional hemodialysis. J Am Soc Nephrol. 2008;19:71A.

[26] Komenda P, Chan C, Pauly RP, Levin A, Copland M, Pierratos A, Sood MM. The evaluation of a successful home hemodialysis program: Establishing a prospective framework for quality. Clin Nephrol. 2009;71:467-474.

[27] Lindsay RM, Leitch R, Heidenheim AP, Kortas C. The London daily/nocturnal hemodialysis study--study design, morbidity, and mortality results. Am J Kidney Dis. 2003;42:5-12.

[28] Lindsay RM, Alhejaili F, Nesrallah G, Leitch R, Clement L, Heidenheim AP, Kortas C. Calcium and phosphate balance with quotidian hemodialysis. Am J Kidney Dis. 2003;42:24-29.

[29] Culleton BF, Walsh M, Klarenbach SW, Mortis G, Scott-Douglas N, Quinn RR, Tonelli M, Donnelly S, Friedrich MG, Kumar A, Mahallati H, Hemmelgarn BR, Manns BJ. Effect of frequent nocturnal hemodialysis vs conventional hemodialysis on left ventricular mass and quality of life: A randomized controlled trial. JAMA. 2007;298:1291-1299.

[30] McFarlane PA, Bayoumi AM, Pierratos A, Redelmeier DA. The quality of life and cost utility of home nocturnal and conventional in-center hemodialysis. Kidney Int. 2003;64:1004-1011.

[31] Chan CT, Jain V, Picton P, Pierratos A, Floras JS. Nocturnal hemodialysis increases arterial baroreflex sensitivity and compliance and normalizes blood pressure of hypertensive patients with end-stage renal disease. Kidney Int. 2005;68:338-344.

[32] Chan CT, Notarius CF, Merlocco AC, Floras JS. Improvement in exercise duration and capacity after conversion to nocturnal home haemodialysis. Nephrol Dial Transplant. 2007;22:3285-3291.

[33] Pierratos A. New approaches to hemodialysis. Annu Rev Med. 2004;55:179-189.

[34] Pierratos A. Daily nocturnal home hemodialysis. Kidney Int. 2004;65:1975-1986.

[35] Pierratos A, McFarlane P, Chan CT. Quotidian dialysis--update 2005. Curr Opin Nephrol Hypertens. 2005;14:119-124.

[36] Barua M, Hladunewich M, Keunen J, Pierratos A, McFarlane P, Sood M, Chan CT. Successful pregnancies on nocturnal home hemodialysis. Clin J Am Soc Nephrol. 2008;3:392-396.

[37] Muller D, Zimmering M, Chan CT, McFarlane PA, Pierratos A, Querfeld U. Intensified hemodialysis regimens: Neglected treatment options for children and adolescents. Pediatr Nephrol. 2008;23:1729-1736.

[38] Fischbach M, Terzic J, Laugel V, Dheu C, Menouer S, Helms P, Livolsi A. Daily on-line haemodiafiltration: A pilot trial in children. Nephrol Dial Transplant. 2004;19:2360-2367.

[39] Fischbach M, Dheu C, Seuge L, Menouer S, Terzic J. In-center daily on-line hemodiafiltration: A 4-year experience in children. Clin Nephrol. 2008;69:279-284.

[40] Fischbach M, Terzic J, Menouer S, Dheu C, Seuge L, Zalosczic A. Daily on line haemodiafiltration promotes catch-up growth in children on chronic dialysis. Nephrol Dial Transplant. 25:867-873.

[41] Fischbach M, Terzic J, Menouer S, Dheu C, Soskin S, Helmstetter A, Burger MC. Intensified and daily hemodialysis in children might improve statural growth. Pediatr Nephrol. 2006;21:1746-1752.

[42] Hoppe A vPC, Linke U, Kahler C, Booß M, Braunauer-Kohlberg R, Hofmann K, Joachimasky P, Hirte I, Schley S, Utsch B, Thumfart J, Briese S, Gellermann J, Zimmering, Querfeld U, Müller D. A hopital-based intermittent nocturnal hemodialysis program for children and adolescents. The Journal of Pediatrics. 2010, in press

[43] Geary DF, Piva E, Gajaria M, Tyrrel J, Picone G, Harvey E. Development of a nocturnal home hemodialysis (nhhd) program for children. Semin Dial. 2004;17:115-117.

[44] Geary DF, Piva E, Tyrrell J, Gajaria MJ, Picone G, Keating LE, Harvey EA. Home nocturnal hemodialysis in children. J Pediatr. 2005;147:383-387.

In: Issues in Dialysis
Editor: Stephen Z. Fadem

ISBN: 978-1-62417-576-3
© 2013 Nova Science Publishers, Inc.

Chapter VII

The Wearable Artificial Kidney: A Paradigm Change in the Treatment of ESRD

Victor Gura
Cedars Sinai Medical Center, Beverly Hills, California, US
Clinical Associate Professor, David Geffen School of Medicine at UCLA,
Beverly Hills, California, US

Abstract

Conventional dialysis may not be practical to meet the needs of a worldwide expanding population. It is disproportionately costly, yet fraught with complications and morbidities that interfere with patient lifestyle. Home dialysis is a viable alternative, but hemodialysis still requires a stable home environment and the cannulation of an arteriovenous access, and thus has not gained wide acceptance. Peritoneal dialysis has also not been widely accepted. A continuously wearable artificial kidney that provides constant dialysis may show promise in greatly improving adequacy and volume control while decreasing the patient "pill burden" and enabling patients sufficient freedom to remain employed and live an active lifestyle.

Introduction

As the population of dialysis patients increases worldwide, the costs and strains to the population will be enormous. In the US the healthcare costs of Medicare recipients on dialysis are disproportionately high, approximately 10 fold higher than the costs of beneficiaries not undergoing ESRD therapy. [1,2,3]

As former undeveloped countries prosper, their food consumption begins to mirror that of the western countries causing a pandemic of increased hypertension, diabetes and obesity.

These, in turn, fuel a variety of co-morbidities, among which is chronic kidney disease (CKD), which all too often advances to end stage renal disease (ESRD). ESRD is more prevalent as the population ages. Thus, as life span is globally prolonged, patients live long enough to develop CKD and require ESRD in growing numbers. [4,5] This is highlighted in Figure 1.

Yet the outcomes of the treatment of End Stage Renal Disease (ESRD) remain disappointing despite the disproportionate resources allocated by society to maintain their therapy. Yearly mortality in some countries is 10 to 12% whereas in the US, mortality exceeds 20%. [6] If data were available it would not be surprising to learn that in some underdeveloped countries where the few that can afford any dialysis get treated twice a week at best and sporadically at worst, mortality is, in all likelihood, much worse.

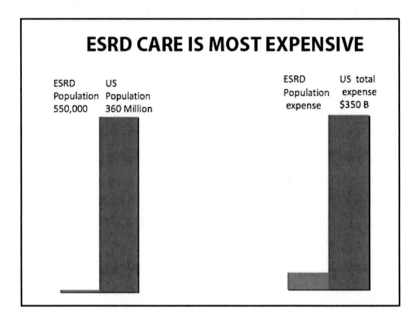

Figure 1. The expense of dialysis per capita, is substantially higher than for the rest of the population.

Table 1. Despite expense, the quality of life for ESRD patients is poor

Complications associated with dialysis		
• Blunt and massive changes in fluid balance • Sudden changes in electrolyte concentration and pH • Insufficient clearance of "middle molecules" • Insufficient phosphorus removal • Poor removal of protein bound toxins • Poorly controlled hypertension	• Endothelial dysfunction • Left Ventricular hypertrophy • Hemodynamic instability • Arrhythmia • Cerebrovascular disease • Anemia • Sleep apnea • Hyperparathyroidism • Pill burden • Myocardial "stunning"	• Coronary disease • Neurological deficit • Post dialysis fatigue • Fluid restriction • Salt restriction • Restrictive diet • Poor sleep • Depression • Disability • Tethered to a machine • Pain

In addition, as demonstrated in Table 1, the quality of life of ESRD patients is dramatically worsened by numerous complications, limitations on life style, the "pill burden" of numerous drugs they require to swallow and pay for, and the lengthy hours they must spend tethered to a large machine make their life quite miserable. [7]

Frequent hospitalizations due to infections, vascular access problems, heart disease and stroke, create a considerable hardship for not only the patient, but family members. In many dialysis patients the quality of life is compromised. Intermittent dialysis may often be accompanied by weakness and fatigue following each treatment. Many patients report they are exhausted and unable to function for many hours after each treatment. Hence, unemployment is high in the in center hemodialysis population. Dietary limitations are challenging, as patients are restricted in their intake of foods high in potassium, sodium and phosphorus. The attendant association with cardiovascular disease and diabetes imposes further dietary limitations. Hence, food is often bland and tasteless. A secondary hardship is that families with several members must specially prepare diets for the individual undergoing dialysis. This imposes economic hardships on many families, already challenged by the high costs of transportation and medications, and who are faced with the dilemma of disability. Fluid limitations and salt imbalance lead to frequently insatiable thirst that results in fluid overload with serious hemodynamic consequences; these patients require removal of large amounts of fluid in annon-physiological amount of time. The challenge of keeping volume in control has been demonstrated to result in a high morbidity and mortality. [8]

During the last decade mounting evidence has emerged that more frequent and longer dialysis can in fact improve outcomes in ESRD patients and reduce costs. It seems that the nephrology community has had a "monoclonal fixation" on dialysis regimens that are 9 to 12 hours per week. Data is emerging that many of the untoward effects of dialysis can be in fact improved or eliminated with daily or more frequent dialysis. [9] Furthermore, recent randomized controlled studies have provided conclusive evidence that in fact daily dialysis can improve outcomes and reduce mortality in the ESRD population. [10]

However, daily dialysis is largely unfeasible in the vast majority of ESRD patients, as society cannot sustain the capital requirements to construct more dialysis units. Furthermore, there is not sufficient nursing or technical personnel to provide twice as much dialysis as provided today. In addition, there are not adequate financial resources worldwide to fund this amount of therapy. Lastly, it is not clear at all that patients will accept being required to spend more time tied down to large, stationary dialysis machines, as this detracts from their freedom to use their time for working or their activities of daily life.

Home dialysis is a welcome yet limited solution to some of these problems, as it poses many obstacles that few patients and their families can overcome. To qualify for home hemodialysis, one must have a suitable home environment, adequate electrical wiring and a water-resistant surface for the machine. Water drainage must meet municipal codes. Often, one must obtain permission from a landlord to adapt and modify the site for care. [11]

Despite that the concept of home dialysis has been available for decades, it has remained a very limited option that very few patients and families are willing to consider. The main obstacles to its mass adoption have been the reluctance of many patients to insert their own needles, the lack of professional supervision if "something goes wrong", and the numerous logistic problems posed by the space, water and electrical requirements posed by the large size of the equipment, and its lack of portability.

Wearable Kidneys – Issues and Solutions

Given the scarcity of resources and presently available solutions it is incumbent upon the nephrology community to redouble its efforts to find cost effective ways of delivering more affordable longer and more frequent dialysis. The search for a feasible answer to this question has provided the impetus to miniaturize a dialysis device and make it small enough for patients to wear continuously. The reasoning was that the wearable kidney should be thought of in the same light as the native kidney, a permanent part of the body, and functional constantly. Ideal renal replacement therapy should be continuous. [12,13]

Continuous renal replacement therapy (CRRT) allows for such a time scheme, but so far it has only been possible in a hospital critical care setting. To date, delivering continuous dialysis 24 hours a day, 7 days a week requires CRRT machines that are not only unsuitable to treat ESRD patients but they require disproportionate nursing time, making their use in chronic units unaffordable and impractical. Also, conventional equipment is heavy, requires a wall electrical outlet and utilizes several gallons of water. The ideal device must be independent of fixed water and energy resources, and must be small and light weight. Undertaking the task to design a wearable artificial kidney (WAK) required miniaturizing the device to the point that it would be small and light enough to be worn constantly by the patient. This posed several major technical challenges: [14]

1. *Energy supply:* Since the equipment must be wearable, conventional electrical wall outlet connectors are not practical. Thus, batteries that can power all the components of the device must be used. However such batteries have to be small and light and last for a reasonable period of time yet they cannot be too heavy as to impede the patient's ability to ambulate.

2. *Water Supply:* Convention dialysis machines use about 40 gallons of fresh water per treatment. This magnitude of fluid load would make the WAK impossible to use. Sorbent system dialysis has been used for decades in REDY machines, greatly reducing the amount of water required to generate dialysate. The same sorbents were configured to enhance the task of regenerating dialysate so that only 375 ml of water were necessary to clear sufficient amounts of undesired toxins. Also, no dialysis device in the US market uses intravenous quality water for dialysate. The AAMI standards require bacteria levels of< 200 cfu/ml and endotoxin levels of<0.2 EU. The dialysate circuit of the WAK is initially primed with 375 ml of 0.45% normal saline intravenous fluid and the tubing and sorbent system are gamma sterilized, therefore eliminating the controversy on the use of non-sterile and impure water.

3. *Electrolytes and acid-base management:* The WAK was designed to supply sufficient bicarbonate and maintain adequate electrolyte balance.

4. *Ultrafiltration:* It is evident that while insufficient fluid removal during dialysis results in hypertension and congestive heart failure, rapid removal of large amounts of fluid invariably results in hemodynamic instability and ultimately in increased cardiovascular morbidity and mortality.

5. *Ergonomics:* The wearable equipment has to be light weight and ergonomically adapted to the body contour so that it can be worn continuously without impinging on the patient's ability to sleep, ambulate work or perform activities of daily life.

6. *Flow patterns and convection:* To achieve blood and dialysate flow through a dialyzer, current machines use several heavy pumps that require 110 or 220 V electricity. In order to improve the efficiency of the pumps and obtain better clearances with less weight and power a double channel pump for both blood and dialysate was created. As pulsatile flow has been shown to increase convective transfer across membranes, opposite phase pulsations were created in the blood and dialysate compartments conferring to the WAK improved clearances with a single pump using much less energy and weight. Also the intermittent changes in the direction of the transmembrane pressure gradients create a "push pull" exchange between blood and dialysate representing a novel way of hemodiafiltration. [14] The effective removal of beta 2 microglobulins in our human trials is most likely due to the improved efficiency afforded by this flow pattern. [15] We have also shown that the pulsatile flow of the dialysate improves the adsorptive performance of the sorbents. [14]

7. *Body comfort:* in order for patients to accept the need to wear the WAK, it must be adapt to the body contour without interfering with the patient's mobility and comfort and avoid creating an excessive weight burden on the patient's body. We therefore opted for a belt form as the most ergonomic way of accomplishing these objectives.

8. *Blood access:* Vascular access remains a problem not only for the WAK but for all forms of dialysis. The use of arteriovenous fistulae is now promoted by many as the preferred form of vascular access for hemodialysis mostly due to its much lower rate of infection. Opponents of fistulae have pointed to increased hemodynamic complications of AV shunting including cardiomegaly and CHF.

As for the WAK, the use of an arteriovenous access with needles held in place with adhesive tape poses an unacceptable risk of disconnection. Needles may become dislodged as the patient moves and this may result in blood loss. With respect to the WAK, catheters are connected to the device and the connectors locked in a way that will render disconnection close to impossible. Moreover, the WAK has built in wetness sensors that, in case of disconnection and blood loss will shut down the device and trigger an alarm.

Arguably, the use of catheters makes the device prone to promote infections. However, it has been shown that strict observance of aseptic technique during connection and disconnection of catheters greatly mitigates the risk of infection. Additionally, the design of the WAK makes the risk of infection even lower, namely that any manipulation or opening of the blood circuit of the WAK will be done in strict observance of the same aseptic precautions that are the standard of care for any surgical procedure.

Also, the use of catheters as practiced today, results in the creation of a column of fluid in the lumen of the catheter that will remain stagnant for 48 to 72 hours. In the event a bacterium enters such column, it will be allowed to fester and multiply unchecked by white cells and antibodies as there is no blood circulation for so many hours. In contrast, the continuous and pulsatile flow of blood in the WAK ensure that in the unlikely event that a bacterium enters the lumen of the catheter, it would be immediately washed out and exposed to white cells and antibodies. Ultimately, of course the improved outcomes brought about by these factors are yet to be proven in practice.

Early Studies

As these issues were addressed, the first prototypes emerged from our laboratory and trialed in pigs we determined first the capability of the device to effectively remove fluid overload and showed that the device can ultra-filter up to 700 ml/hour from fluid overloaded animals. In a human trial designed to confirm the results in fluid overloaded humans120 to 288 ml/hr were removed with no complications. [16,17] In additional trials uremic pigs underwent dialysis with the WAK and the device delivered a urea clearance of 37 ± 7.3 ml/min and a creatinine clearance of 27 ± 4.0 ml min. [14]

Table 2. Economic impact of the WAK
(Wearable Artificial Kidney) on ESRD patient issues

Economic Impact of the WAK on Patient Issues		
PROBLEM	**SOLUTION**	**ECONOMIC IMPACT**
Diet too restrictive	No food restrictions, including salt, potassium and phosphorus	
Fluid overload	Steady removal of fluid prevents pulmonary edema, peripheral edema and bloating	No hospitalization for pulmonary edema or fluid overload
Anemia	Less inflammation and red cell loss, better nutrition. Reduced ESA use	Reduced ESA utilization and reduced iron infusions
Bone disease	No hyperphosphatema. Less hyperparathyroidism?	Phosphate binders are usually not required. May require less cinacalcet
Hypertension	No fluid or sodium accumulation	Decreased blood pressure medications
Hypotensive episodes	Physiological removal rate of fluid. No blunt blood pressure decrease	No saline infusions during dialysis
Heart disease	Less hypertension. Steady electrolytes. Less arrhythmias and sudden death?	Decreased hospitalization and drug utilization
Cerebrovascular events	Less hypertension.	Decreased hospitalization, rehabilitation and drug utilization

Table 3. The impact of the WAK on dialysis value

Impact on Dialysis Value Chain		
STAKE HOLDER	**VALUE PROPOSITION**	**ECONOMIC IMPACT**
Patient	Improved quality of life Decreased mortality Decreased expense 16 times more dialysis	To many benefits to determine economic value
Physicians	Increased satisfaction and gratification Increased practice size	Increased demand for physician services
Dialysis providers	Reduced operating costs Eliminate physical barriers to expansion	Increased profit margin by > 25%
Payors Government Private Insurers	Decreased medication consumption Decreased hospitalization and surgery Decreased transportation costs	Potential savings of as much as 10 billion dollars

In patients with ESRD the WAK delivered urea clearance of22.7 +5.2 ml/min and a creatinine clearance of20.7+4.8 ml/min. [18] In addition the phosphorus removed in 8 hours was 445.2 ± 325.9 mg and the amount of beta 2 microglobulin (β2M) removed during the same period was 99.8 ± 63.1 mg. [15] No hemolysis, electrolyte imbalances or hemodynamic changes were observed in any patient. The patients expressed no discomfort pain or any untoward effect and were able to ambulate and sleep while undergoing dialysis with the WAK. Although these preliminary data indicate that the WAK is safe and efficient much more is needed to elucidate its clinical performance.

Potential Benefits

While perhaps not all patients will accept the WAK, the potential impact of the WAK on the life of ESRD patients that do is far reaching. (Table 2) The quality of life for ESRD patients should improve and hopefully so should lifespan.

The expected impact on the economic burden to society is not less significant as all stakeholders in the dialysis world should see positive results from implementing the WAK (Table 3):

1. *Patients*: The costs of dialysis therapy are often hidden in the fact that they often must receive disability benefits. The burdens of therapy outlined above make it all too often for them to continue working. While many patients who begin dialysis therapy are elderly and have reached retirement age, others who start dialysis have attendant co-morbidities that preclude them from being gainfully employed.

However, for many others, the opportunity to reduce the dialysis burden will enable them to become gainfully engaged in productive work or employment as a taxpayer rather than the recipient of disability benefits. Moreover, many of their expenses associated with transportation and purchase of drugs and ancillary services would disappear. Nevertheless, intangible improvements in their lives are immeasurable.

2. *Physicians:* The gratification of caring for patients who have optimized their lifestyle and reduced their dialysis burden is high. It should likewise be highly rewarding to care for patients undergoing WAK therapy.

3. *Dialysis Services Operators:* Providers of dialysis services would still remain necessary to deliver care to ESRD patients with the WAK. Although it is envisioned that there will be a need for providers to maintain a sterile environment where the dialyzers would be replaced, one can expect substantial savings in nursing and technician labor, utilities as well as "brick and mortar" expenses. Furthermore, there would no longer be the need for capital expenditures to construct more dialysis units in order to accommodate the growth of the ESRD population. In societies where peritoneal dialysis has become widely accepted, costs have sharply diminished, and this would also be expected with widespread use of the WAK. [1]

4. *Payers:* Emerging data on daily dialysis indicate that daily dialysis results in reduced need for ESAs. Many patients on daily dialysis do not require phosphate binders. Also, the use of antihypertensive medications would be greatly reduced. As the WAK delivers 16 times more dialysis time than currently used dialysis schemes, incremental clearances and better fluid removal, it stands to reason that similar saving would be achieved. In addition the reduction in hospitalizations as a result of cardiovascular disease and stroke and a decrease in surgical interventions would also reduce the health care costs. Transportation costs and associated challenges would shrink as patients would no longer require thrice weekly transportation to a dialysis facility.

Conclusion

In conclusion, ESRD is costly, and threatens to be a worsening dilemma. Outcomes and burdens associated with present ESRD therapy are less than optimal. A wearable artificial kidney may increase freedom, volume control, adequacy, pill burden, and quality of life. It will enable patients to liberalize their diets and volume intake. This translates to the potential of enabling patients to have a more optimal lifestyle. The WAK has been shown to be feasible on bench, animal and human subjects. The data also provide preliminary indications that the WAK is safe and efficient. It is thus promising that the WAK will reduce costs, improve quality of life and decrease mortality in ESRD patients.

References

[1] Li PK, Cheung WL, Lui SL, Blagg C, et al. Increasing home based dialysis therapies to tackle dialysis burden around the world: a position statement on dialysis economics from the 2nd Congress of the International Society for Hemodialysis. Economics in the Second Congress of the International Society for Hemodialysis (ISHD 2009). Nephrol. 2011;16(1):53-6.1440-1797.

[2] Held PJ, Garcia JR, Pauly MV, Cahn MA. Price of dialysis, unit staffing, and length of dialysis treatment. Am J Kidney Dis. 1990;15:441-450.

[3] Lysaght MJ. Maintenance dialysis population dynamics: current trends and long-term implications. J Am Soc Nephrol. 2002;13:37–40.

[4] Hamer RA and El Nahas AM. The burden of chronic kidney disease. BMJ. 2006;332:563.

[5] Hossain MP, Goyder EC, Rigby JE, El Nahas M. CKD and poverty: A growing global challenge. Am J Kidney Dis. 2009;53:166–174.

[6] Canaud B, Tong L, Tentori F, et al. Clinical Practices and Outcomes in Elderly Hemodialysis Patients: Results from the Dialysis Outcomes and Practice Patterns Study (DOPPS). Clin J Am Soc Nephrol. 2011;6(7):1651-1662.

[7] Chiu YW, Teitelbaum I, Misra M, et al. Pill Burden, Adherence, Hyperphosphatemia, and Quality of Life in Maintenance Dialysis Patients. Clin J Am Soc Nephrol. 2009;4:(6)1089-1096.

[8] Kimmel PL, Varela MP, Peterson RA, et al. Interdialytic weight gain and survival in hemodialysis patients: effects of duration of ESRD and diabetes mellitus. Kidney Int. 2000;57:1141–115.

[9] Kjellstrand CM, Buoncristiani U, Ting G, et al. Short daily haemodialysis: survival in 415 patients treated for 1006 patient-years. Nephrol Dial Transplant. 2008;23:3283–3289.

[10] Chertow GM, Levin NW, Beck GJ et al. In-center hemodialysis six times per week versus three times per week. N Engl J Med. 2010;363(24):2287-300.

[11] Mehrabian S, Morgan D, Schlaeper C et al. Equipment and water treatment considerations for the provision of quotidian home hemodialysis. Am J Kidney Dis. 2003;42(1 Suppl):66-70.

[12] Gura V, Beizai M, Ezon C, Polaschegg HD. Continuous renal replacement therapy for end-stage renal disease. The wearable artificial kidney (WAK). Contrib Nephrol. 2005;149:325-33.

[13] Gura V, Ronco C, Davenport A. The wearable artificial kidney, why and how: from holy grail to reality. Semin Dial. 2009;22(1):13-7.

[14] Gura V, Macy AS, Beizai M, Ezon C, Golper TA. Technical breakthroughs in the wearable artificial kidney (WAK). Clin J Am Soc Nephrol. 2009;4(9):1441-8.

[15] Gura V, Davenport A, Beizai M, Ezon C, Ronco C. Beta2-microglobulin and phosphate clearances using a wearable artificial kidney: a pilot study. Am J Kidney Dis. 2009;54(1):104-11.

[16] Gura V, Beizai M, Ezon C, Rambod E. Continuous renal replacement therapy for congestive heart failure: the wearable continuous ultrafiltration system. ASAIO J. 2006;52(1):59-61.

[17] Gura V, Ronco C, Nalesso F, Brendolan A, Beizai M, Ezon C, Davenport A, Rambod E. A wearable hemofilter for continuous ambulatory ultrafiltration. Kidney Int. 2008;73(4):497-502.

[18] Davenport A, Gura V, Ronco C, Beizai M, Ezon C, Rambod E. A wearable haemodialysis device for patients with end-stage renal failure: a pilot study. Lancet. 2007;15;370(9604):2005-10.

In: Issues in Dialysis
Editor: Stephen Z. Fadem

ISBN: 978-1-62417-576-3
© 2013 Nova Science Publishers, Inc.

Chapter VIII

Is Dialysis Ever an Inappropriate Therapy?

Susan Higley Bray
Clinical Associate Professor of Medicine,
Drexel University College of Medicine, Philadelphia, Pennsylvania, US

Abstract

Although dialysis has been shown to prolong life in patients afflicted with end stage kidney disease, the question of its appropriateness in some situations has been raised. Issues affecting the provision of dialysis include multiple comorbidities as well as the presence of undiagnosed and undertreated pain. Some data strongly suggest that in patients with advanced age and multiple comorbidities, therapy with dialysis may offer no benefit over solid medical management. The Renal Physicians Association has created a stepwise system and set of tools for determining and assessing whether patients are potentially not suitable candidates for dialysis. In circumstances in which dialysis is unlikely to benefit the patient, and the patient or designee and family have shared with the provider in the decision making process, alternate palliative care can and should be offered.

Introduction

Both hemodialysis and peritoneal dialysis have proven to be effective in prolonging life and improving quality of life for over fifty years. In the 1960s, many of the patients who needed dialysis never received it because it was unavailable in their region, or they lacked the funds. In Seattle, dialysis was initially only offered between the ages of 18 and 45 – The selection process by which dialysis was rationed created an outcry that was heard by Congress which ultimately created legislation to cover its care; following the implementation of the legislation dialysis became widely available. (See Chapter 1)

Current health care costs are beyond our control, and we once again face the dilemma of whether to ration critical services. CMS estimates that the national health expenditure percentage of our gross domestic product is now 17.6%. [1] A large percentage of Medicare funding is from general revenue, not payroll taxes; and recent reports suggest our Medicare system is not sustainable. [2] In the December, 2010 *New Yorker*, Atul Gawande pointed out that twenty-five percent of all health care spending by Medicare is for five percent of patients in their final year of life, mostly for care in the final months. [3] Regarding kidney disease, the relatively small percent of the dialysis population consumes a disproportionate percentage of the Medicare budget; and has already led to strict dialysis payment reform. [4,5]

Since 1973, the age of incident dialysis patients has substantially increased; it is now 62.2 years. [5] Many patients now requiring dialysis are concurrently afflicted with other comorbidities, especially diabetes and hypertension, making it more and more difficult to maintain an acceptable health related quality of life (HRQOL). Yet, decisions about choices that involve the finality of death are extremely difficult for patients, their families and their doctors. A treatment that may be ideal for one's condition may not be appropriate for the given circumstance.

The principles of maintaining well-being require us not only to apply therapy and treatment that is appropriate for a disease or condition, but also to do so within the context of the patient's needs, preferences and expectations. This chapter discusses basic principles that will guide physicians when faced with these difficult dilemmas.

The Principle of Autonomy

Dialysis is a life-sustaining therapy, which by definition is a medical treatment that serves to prolong life without reversing the underlying medical condition. Often physicians presume they have the right to decide which severe acute kidney injury (AKI) or end stage renal disease (ESRD) patient receives dialysis? Is it always necessary that patients who require dialytic intervention *must* undergo dialytic intervention? Is the Nephrologist required to order the intervention? Must the patient accept the decision?

Patients have the autonomous right to decide, if they have decision-making capacity, the capability to understand, communicate and reason to accept or refuse treatment. Patients are entitled to make decisions with which others disagree. [3,6,7] Thus, the first imperative is that all options are first discussed with patients, including that of not dialyzing at all or of withdrawing from dialysis, or perhaps attempting a time-limited trial of dialysis. [12]

Changing the way end-of-life is treated in our country and in our American culture will take time and effort and constitutes a major paradigm shift. In studies looking at end of life issues, two important demographic facts have potential influence on the perceptions of end-of-life: ethnicity and religious affiliation. [3,17] Allowing death to occur naturally, without dialytic intervention, remains, and should always remain, the autonomous right of every patient. The bioethical principles of autonomy allow that patients who are competent have the right to refuse treatment. We, as physicians, respect their dignity and autonomy when we acknowledge their freely chosen choice. [3,6,7] The principle is not altered when the result of withholding or withdrawing dialysis leads to the patient's foreseeable death. [6] The decision to forgo therapy is not contrary to the bioethical principles of beneficence or nonmaleficence.

Given that patients have the right to autonomy further obligates physicians to assure that they are well informed, and can make an appropriate decision. All too often, patients or their care givers insist upon "doing everything."

Doing Everything

Death, today, finally comes after a long, expensive medical struggle and patients are long past the point of coherence and awareness and the ability to have last words with their loved ones. The obligation to offer treatment (dialysis) should not include the obligation to impose the therapy treatment. Often "everything" includes so much technologic intervention that there is little to no touch by family members, or mental clarity in the patient. This actually may lead to more suffering at the end of life. In addition to suffering, the cost of prolonging a fading life, both financially and emotionally, is high and getting worse. [3,6,8] Yet many caregivers decide to make an all out effort to prolong the patient's life, even if it means sacrificing quality. [3]

In shared decision making, caregivers, patients (if competent) and the physician have an opportunity to review the prognosis, burdens and benefits, as well as the alternatives. This is done within the context of an awareness of the patient's needs and preferences, and takes into account the cultural and social needs of the patient and family.

What Is Shared Decision Making?

All people involved in decision-making do not have to agree with the decision but should feel that they have had appropriate input into the decision and their views are respected. [9] The physician's discussion with the patient and family, especially when presenting the bad news of ESRD and dialysis/no dialysis should include techniques that have been proven to help in the breaking of bad news. This way of discussing and reaching a decision regarding no dialysis plus conservative care versus dialytic intervention is called shared decision-making.

In this model, the physician and the patient reach a consensus on the treatment plan, which also could include a time trial of dialysis. This is excellently discussed in the RPA Clinical Practice Guidelines. [9]

RPA Guidelines

The RPA Clinical Practice Guideline, *Shared Decision Making in the Appropriate Initiation of and Withdrawal from Dialysis,* describes the current best model in helping patients and families to decide autonomously whether to initiate dialysis at all (withhold) or to remove the patient from dialysis (withdraw). These guidelines were developed by a Renal Physicians Association working group and address the making of shared decisions to withdraw or to withhold dialysis in patients with acute kidney injury and end-stage renal disease. [9]

If dialysis is not appropriate, a decision about whether to initiate or discontinue therapy must be made. Occasionally conflict arises; this is a very sensitive experience for families and patients. Physician support and guidance here is crucial. Once consensus has been reached, palliative care can be initiated.

When Care will not Make a Difference

International data show that there is very high mortality in older patients who choose to have dialytic intervention, especially in the United States and in Australia/New Zealand. One of the reasons for the high mortality in this group of elderly dialysis patients is the presence of multiple severe comorbidities. Poor six-month survival is common, and data indicate, multifactorial. For example, some are already in the dying process and should not be dialyzed because the procedure will not alter the inevitable course of illness to the death of the patient. Also, either the dialytic procedure itself or issues involving the vascular access may lead causally to the death of the patient via adverse effects on the heart, infections in the access (particularly in catheter accesses) and accelerated loss of residual kidney function, often seen after initiating hemodialysis. Unfortunately, those patients who reside in long-term care facilities at the time of beginning dialytic intervention have a very poor outcome including both poor survival and poor quality of life. [10]

O'Hare et al. [11] have shown that older patients with CKD may more slowly progress to Stage 5 CKD and are considerably more likely to die(without receiving dialysis) of their other comorbidities and never come to the uremic state. It may well be that elderly CKD patients should best be managed with an individualized plan of care which achieves each patient's goals and at the same time assures relief of suffering, preservation of underlying renal function and striving to achieve maximum quality of life. [10] The outcomes of this approach reveal that older patients managed conservatively may actually live as long (or even longer) and certainly live "better" not having to go to regular dialysis and doctor visits. [10,12,13]

Prognosis and Suitability

Medical ethics, law and professionalism require that the physician promote the patient's ability to make informed decisions regarding the initiation of or withdrawal from interventions, including dialysis. [14] Health care professionals are ethically obliged, under the Principle of Informed Consent (autonomy), to discuss in depth and in terms that the patient can understand just what dialytic interventions are possible.

It is also ethically required, via the principles of Beneficence and Nonmaleficence, that the physician ensure that all reversible factors constituting the patient's illness be addressed and treated so that a decision to forgo dialysis is not negatively influenced by the presence of reversible factors. These principles demand that we explore if there are unmet needs (physical or spiritual pain, depression) affecting the decision to forgo therapy and that we address them before abandoning dialytic intervention.

Adequately informing patients or their representatives and their families requires being able to assess the potential prognosis. It the prognosis is poor, the risks of dialysis outweigh its benefits. This is also true for those in whom the access will create a significant risk and/or cause an unacceptable quality of life. Severe psychiatric or behavior disorders that prevent adherence to dialysis treatments may also be good reasons for dialysis to be withheld or withdrawn. It is also reasonable to consider withdrawal for a patient who has a terminal illness or whose medical condition precludes the technical process of dialysis. [9]

When appropriate, and the answer to the "surprise" question is: I will not be surprised if this patient dies six months from now, the patient can transition, if he chooses, to hospice care. [15] Other tools, such as the Charlson Comorbidity Index and the Karnofsky Score are readily assessable from the Renal Physician's Association [9] or Touchcalc. [16]

Making the Decision to Forgo Dialysis

The appropriate time for patients who are fully informed to voluntarily choose to require dialysis or request that it be discontinued is when they still have decision-making capacity. Ideally, they should also make contingency plans that would become effective if their medical condition worsened. At that point, a "legal agent" should be designated to fulfill their wishes in the event they are incapacitated. Appointing a surrogate legal agent in advance can reduce the potential for confusion, guilt and conflict. If the patient is already receiving dialysis therapy, the interdisciplinary team should meet with the family and important caregivers and assist them in making these decisions.

Patients who have the capacity to make their own decisions, after being fully informed (which respects autonomy) may, ethically, voluntarily refuse dialysis or request that the therapy be discontinued. If, however, a patient no longer possesses decision-making capacity but had let others know, when he had capacity, that he did not desire to be dialyzed, dialysis may be withheld or withdrawn.

Patients without capacity who have a legally appointed surrogate decision maker may be removed from dialysis by the surrogate acting in the best interest of the patient. [9,14,17,18] Those with profound neurological impairment incapable of thought, sensation, purposeful movement and self-awareness most certainly may have dialytic intervention withheld or withdrawn. [9,10]

If a patient no longer possesses capacity but had previously indicated that he would refuse dialysis, it may be withheld, but it is optimal that this be documented, and part of the patient's medical record. The legal agent has the power to make the decision to withdraw dialysis given no previous documentation.

The responsibilities that burden the physician who is trying to act ethically and morally towards a patient requiring dialysis are heavy. Circumstances all too often arise where there is no legal agent or prior authorization. This is particularly true in the emergency room or critical care setting. Patients who are neurologically profoundly impaired, lacking signs of thought, sensation, purposeful behavior and awareness, may have dialysis withheld or withdrawn at the discretion of their physician. [9] When a situation arises in which the physician thinks that offering/providing dialysis will burden the patient unnecessarily, the physician is not obligated to provide the service.

Even in situations in which cultural issues are preventing patients and families from refusing to withhold or to withdraw dialysis, the demands for treatment must be addressed in light of what is in the patient's best interest and consistent with his values and preferences, often a very difficult balance to achieve. [10]

Appropriate palliative care needs to be assured as part of the very fabric of the patient's total care. [10,12] The patient's preference regarding withholding or withdrawing dialytic intervention must be evaluated against the possibility that the burdens of the treatment outweigh any foreseeable benefits. The physician is not obliged to provide dialytic intervention in cases in which the burden outweighs any probable benefit. [6]

Conflict Resolution

Forgoing dialysis will, in due time, result in the death of in some but not all patients. Because of this fact, end-of-life patient management skills become important for physicians to develop, including an appreciation of the cultural differences at end-of-life and palliative care and hospice benefits for patients and their families. The physician's role as a facilitator is paramount. Meeting the needs of the patient is by nature in the context of care that is multifaceted, and often met with difficulty. Unfortunately, data exist suggesting that factors such as age, cognitive impairment, prior mental health and financial concerns may play a role in physicians' decisions on offering dialytic therapies. [10,13]

Conflict may arise in cases where there is not consensus between factions of the family, or between care givers and the health team. Most often, this conflict results from miscommunication or interpersonal relationships. In these circumstances it is often prudent to offer a time-limited trial of therapy. This trial is most often useful when the benefits of therapy are not clearly known. The trial must be offered with the understanding that if predefined expectations are not met, therapy can be withdrawn.

Sometimes, there is conflict about what therapy should be offered to the dialysis patients. This is particularly true in a critical care setting. This conflict can arise, not only among care givers, but also among different participants on the health team. The RPA Guidelines suggest that a systemic due process approach should be established. Physicians should understand the views, particularly of the patient/legal agent, provide data to support recommendations and correct misunderstandings. When immediate dialysis is necessary, and has been requested by the patient or legal agent, it should be initiated while the conflict is being resolved.

Meeting Cultural Needs

People of different cultures may well approach the discussions regarding withholding or withdrawing dialysis in different ways than prevailing culture. The principle of respect for patient autonomy is still very much present for all patients regardless of their cultural approaches to end of life. For many cultures, the patient right to self-determination is more family centered or community centered and thus the patient may defer to family or community for decisions regarding dialysis, even if the patient is competent to make the decision. Cultural approaches to illness can also serve to affect how medical decisions are made, how much information is shared with family or community as opposed to with the patient himself. This allows the family/community to share the information necessary for decision making in a way that they think correct. Health care providers need to appreciate that this may be appropriate in some contexts and that they must determine how the patient wishes to make the decisions. [10] Other factors that greatly affect decision-making include religious philosophies related to end-of-life and family dynamics, which can be critical in their effect on decision-making, especially if the patient lacks decision-making capacity and the adult child is the surrogate decision maker. Another important issue in decision-making to withhold or to withdraw dialysis therapy is the belief of the nephrologist regarding the issue. Beliefs of the nephrologist can color how the discussions with the patient proceeds and may be an important reason why, in the United States, initiation of dialysis in patients with a poor prognosis is the norm. The ESRD population in the USA has one of the highest withdrawal rates and end of life costs and lower hospice use worldwide. [19] It is likely that initiating dialysis in elderly patients will actually result in more rapid loss of residual kidney function than if the patient had continued with conservative medical management of his CKD. [11,12]

Principle of Pain Management

Physicians have an obligation to relieve pain and suffering and to respect the dignity of the dying patient. [6] One of the under-recognized symptoms interfering with HRQOL is pain, a symptom fraught with concern and fear. Hard data are few but studies have shown that moderate to severe chronic pain is common in Stage 5 CKD requiring dialysis. [20]

Painful syndromes that may be experienced in ESRD, and are unique to ESRD include calciphylaxis, renal osteodystrophy and neuropathy. Polycystic kidney disease, osteomyelitis, discitis, ischemic limbs, and muscle cramping are also painful afflictions seen in patients with ESRD. Musculoskeletal pain appears to be the most common and equal in severity to neuropathic pain. [20]

Since the population of ESRD patients is so much older now and has comorbidities and polypharmacy, pain management is complicated and unsatisfactory. Despite the availability of effective agents for pain control, there are barriers that we fail to notice or overcome. Patients themselves can be barriers. They fail to seek help with pain control until they are in severe pain, partly because they and their physicians fear "becoming addicted". Sometimes the adverse effects associated with opioids, such as nausea, vomiting and constipation, as well as lethargy, are taken as signs of allergic reactions and patients then discontinue the medications with bad recurrence of severe pain [20] which can affect their decisions regarding initiating or continuing dialysis.

Doctors and nurses often have inadequate training in pain management, often resulting in poor recognition of the extent and severity physical and emotional pain in the ESRD patient. There is increased risk of toxicity and adverse effects with pain medications (opioids) due to altered pharmacokinetics and pharmacodynamics of pain medications in CKD patients. These are distinct barriers in the CKD population to receiving safe and adequate pain management [6] and may also color their decisions regarding forgoing ongoing dialysis or of withholding it altogether.

Sometimes, the symptom burdens of the patient with ESRD contribute to the decision to forgo dialysis. Some common and both physically and emotionally distressing symptoms include pain (physical and existential), depression, anorexia, fatigue, anxiety and significant cognitive impairment. All of these may well interfere with the patient's ability to cope and therefore impact negatively on the patient's quality of life and his tendency to forgo dialytic intervention. These issues are often under-recognized and definitely undertreated. It is important that physicians become better able to recognize and treat especially the pain and depression that are rampant in this population. [6,10] Healthcare providers need to proactively identify patients with these comorbidities and, as patients decline, be able to have discussions including forgoing dialysis, so that their care is consistent with their stated preferences, either personally or through their surrogates. Since "intractable" pain may be a proper reason to consider forgoing dialysis, it should not be so considered until all reasonable attempts to control pain have been made. Recall that patients may have more than one kind of pain and it needs to be assessed in its site, character, intensity, extent, temporal relationship and what, if any, factors relieve and/or aggravate it. It may not be necessary to completely alleviate the pain, only to control it to a level acceptable to the patient. Non-pharmaceutical methods can be very helpful, such as physical therapy, therapeutic massage and pet therapy. Pain may be increased by various psychosocial factors such as nutrition, mood, anxiety, and depression. Any unmet needs of the patient, such as spiritual or financial concerns, may add to the inability to control pain. This is the concept of "total pain". [20] It may be greatly lessened with the addition of spiritual counseling and/or psychological intervention. Therefore, if total pain is controlled, the patient is more comfortable, then decisions regarding withholding or withdrawing of dialysis can be more freely made.

Time Limited Trial

It has been suggested in the RPA guideline [9] considering a time-limited trial of dialysis for patients for whom dialysis therapy may be a poor choice, not benefitting the patient medically or in terms of quality of life. If such a trial is undertaken, clear parameters need to be discussed in advance so it will be possible to determine the next steps (continue or withdraw) at the end of the trial. If after 2 months the patient has shown no improvement in HRQOL or deteriorating functional status dialysis would be discontinued. It is really only appropriate when it is expected that there will be benefit and the patient's individual goals can be met.

Palliation

The ethical principles of beneficence and nonmaleficence demand that we health care professionals provide those interventions that give a reasonable expectation of benefit without a larger expectation of harm. [14] Therefore, dialysis, ethically, should be provided only if there is reasonable likelihood that the therapy will help the patient achieve his medical and emotional/spiritual goals. If the goals are likely to be unmet, then a more palliative course of therapy should be offered, focusing on treating symptoms and preserving mental and physical function as well as possible. [9]

Management of patients who choose to forgo dialytic therapy should include palliative care, best provided by a palliative care team. Issues including pain (physical and existential) management, spirituality, family dynamics and psychosocial factors are addressed thoroughly by the team that can include physician, nurse practitioner, social worker, case manager, chaplain and nurse. Although palliative care is no longer focused prolonging life, it focuses heavily on preserving the quality of life. This includes amelioration of pain, maintaining mental alertness for as long as possible, and maximizing time with loved ones and family.

Conclusion

In summary, the answer to the question *Is dialysis ever inappropriate therapy?* the answer is "Yes, of course!" We have reviewed some of the principles that can guide physicians helping their patients make appropriate decisions about dialysis care, particularly when the benefits to the patient are minimal. It is important that physicians embrace the philosophy that in the appropriate setting, forgoing dialysis, accompanied by intensive and compassionate medical therapy is a perfectly acceptable alternative to the provision of or maintenance of dialysis.

Important reasons to dialyze should include prolonging life of good quality and providing good symptom control. Similar goals can be achieved in appropriate patients who forgo dialysis and, in some, may provide longer quality of life and symptom control than if they had chosen a dialytic option.

With the approach to non-dialytic care of the patient, quality of life (and also length of life in many cases) is maximized. Pain is controlled. Family is involved and informed, and when the patient does die, has an excellent probability of dying with dignity.

Table 1. Is Dialysis ever an inappropriate Therapy?

NEVER DIALYSE	GRAY ZONE	OF COURSE, DIALYZE
Severe dementia	Moderate dementia	Cognitively intact
Informed refusal	Timed trial of dialysis	Patient or surrogate choice if medically appropriate
Persistent vegetative state	Cultural factors	Benefit outweighs risk
Risk outweighs benefit		
Technically unstable		
No survival benefit		

References

[1] National Health Expenditure Data. Baltimore: Centers for Medicare & Medicaid Services; 2011 [cited 14 Aug 2011]. Available from: http://www.cms.gov /NationalHealthExpendData/.

[2] Geithner TF, Solis HL, Sebelius K, Blahous CP III, Reischauer RD. Social Security Administration Annual Report 2011. [cited 13 Aug 2011]. Available from: http://www.ssa.gov/oact/trsum/index.html.

[3] Gawande A. Letting Go - What should medicine do when it can't save your life? New Yorker. 2010 Aug 2;1-15.

[4] Medicare Improvements for Patients and Providers Act of 2008 (MIPPA) Public Law 110-275.

[5] U.S. Renal Data System, USRDS Annual Data Report 2010. [cited 23 Nov 2011]. Available from: http://www.usrds.org/adr.aspx.

[6] Deciding to Forgo Life-Sustaining Treatment: A Report on the Ethical, Medical and Legal Issues in Treatment Decisions. President's Commission for the Study of Ethical Problems in Medicine and Biomedical and Behavioral Research. Washington, D.C. 1987.

[7] VanScuy L. "DNR" Real Stories of Life, Death and Somewhere Inbetween. Perkasie, Pa: Pitkow Associates; 2011.

[8] Im K, Belle SH, Schulz R, Mendelsohn AB, Chelluri L. Prevalence and outcomes of caregiving after prolonged (> or =48 hours) mechanical ventilation in the ICU. Chest. 2004 Feb;125(2):597-606.

[9] Renal Physicians Association. Shared Decision Making in the Appropriate Initiation of and Withdrawal From Dialysis. 2nd Ed. Rockville, MD: RPA. 2010.

[10] Germain MJ, Davison SN, Moss AH. When enough is enough: the nephrologist's responsibility in ordering dialysis treatments. Am J Kidney Dis. 2011 Jul;58(1):135-43.

[11] O'Hare AM, Choi AI, Bertenthal D, Bacchetti P, Garg AX, Kaufman JS, et al. Age affects outcomes in chronic kidney disease. J Am Soc Nephrol. 2007 Oct;18(10):2758-65.

[12] Schell JO, Germain MJ, Finkelstein FO, Tulsky JA, Cohen LM. An integrative approach to advanced kidney disease in the elderly. Adv Chronic Kidney Dis. 2010 Jul;17(4):368-77.

[13] Murtagh FE, Marsh JE, Donohoe P, Ekbal NJ, Sheerin NS, Harris FE. Dialysis or not? A comparative survival study of patients over 75 years with chronic kidney disease stage 5. Nephrol Dial Transplant. 2007 Jul;22(7):1955-62.

[14] Beauchamp TL, Childress JF. Principles of Biomedical Ethics 5ed. Oxford: Oxford University Press; 2011.

[15] Meier D, Isaacs S, Hughes R. Palliative Care – Transforming the Care of Serious Illness. Hoboken, NJ: Jossey-Bass; 2010.

[16] Fadem S. Predictors of morbidity and mortality in CKD. Houston: nephron.com; 2011 [cited 13 Aug 2011]. Available from: http://touchcalc.com/predictors.

[17] Wittmann-Price R, Celia LM. Exploring perceptions of "do not resuscitate" and "allowing natural death" among physicians and nurses. Holist Nurs Pract. 2010 Nov-Dec;24(6):333-7.

[18] Guidelines on the Termination of Life-Sustaining Treatment and the Care of the Dying: A Report by the Hastings Center. Briarcliff, NY 1987.

[19] Robinson BM, Port FK. Caring for dialysis patients: international insights from the Dialysis Outcomes and Practice Patterns Study (DOPPS). Identifying best practices and outcomes in the DOPPS. Semin Dial. 2010 Jan-Feb;23(1):4-6.

[20] Davison SN. Chronic pain in end-stage renal disease. Adv Chronic Kidney Dis. 2005 Jul;12(3):326-34.

In: Issues in Dialysis
Editor: Stephen Z. Fadem

ISBN: 978-1-62417-576-3
© 2013 Nova Science Publishers, Inc.

Chapter IX

The Pre-Eminent Role for Control of Extra-Cellular Volume in Dialysis Therapy

Richard J. Glassock [*]
Geffen School of Medicine at UCLA, Laguna Niguel, California, US

Abstract

Patients with end-stage renal disease (ESRD) treated by dialysis continue to experience and unacceptably high mortality and morbidity, especially in the United States. Undoubtedly this is due to many factors, including pre-treatment co-morbidity, advancing age and poor control of elements contributing to risk by the treatment itself. This Chapter will consider inadequate control of chronically expanded extra-cellular fluid volume (ECFV) during and between treatments as having a pre-eminent role in determining outcomes of dialysis therapy for ESRD. Such dysvolemia contributes to poor outcomes by fostering left ventricular hypertrophy and fibrosis and encouraging the development of hypertension, congestive heart failure and sudden (arrythmogenic) cardiac death. Efforts to improve control of ECFV in dialysis treated ESRD patients critically depend on development of better, simpler, more accurate and reliable methods and tools to assess the status of ECFV on an ongoing basis, both during the intra-dialytic and inter-dialytic intervals. Excessive ultra-filtration and administration of NaCl (covertly or overtly) during dialysis can be harmful. More prolonged (slower) dialysis can be beneficial. Excessive inter-dialytic weight gain is hazardous to health and NaCl restriction between dialysis treatments is essential. Rigorous attempts to achieve near euvolemia will likely be rewarded by lower blood pressure (without drugs), better rehabilitation, fewer hospitalizations and re-hospitalizations and more prolonged survival accompanied by an improved quality of life.

---

[*] Address Correspondence To: Richard J. Glassock, MD, MACP; 8 Bethany, Laguna Niguel, CA, 92677; glassock@cox.net.

Introduction

The continued health of the human organism is dependent on its ability to maintain relative constancy of the internal milieu, also known as homeostasis, despite wide fluctuations in the environment and dietary intake. [1] Failure of the excretory function of the kidneys impairs these homeostatic functions, imposing limits on adaptations to change in the environment or diet, also called "homeostenosis". [2] The extreme of this pathological situation is represented by end-stage renal disease (ESRD) where the filtration and excretory capacity of the kidney has been reduced to 10% or less of normal. Treatment of ESRD by dialysis can partially restore the imbalances in the *milieu interiore* but only on an imprecise and temporary basis. The fine-tuning of homeostasis requires the interaction of a complex set of neuro-humoral pathways and well-functioning kidneys--- it is incapable of being duplicated artificially by a machine or a procedure, at least at the present time.

Maintenance of a normal status of the extra-cellular volume (ECFV) and its composition are two of the paramount tasks of homeostasis, and it thus is not surprising that in ESRD and dialysis patients this regulation is severely disturbed. [3] Specifically, consumption of dietary sodium chloride (NaCl) in amounts that would be readily excreted by the kidneys in a normal individual are partially retained (with water) and lead to expansion of the ECFV. Thirst is a main driving force in water addition commensurate with the retained NaCl. While dialysis with ultra-filtration does remove some of the retained NaCl and water, the benefits are only temporary unless dialysis is provided continuously over an extended period of time. Thus, under most dialysis treatment situations, the ECFV fluctuates to an extent much greater than seen in normal subjects and very often some degree of chronic ECFV expansion persists between dialysis treatment sessions. These fluctuations exact a toll, principally upon the heart and cardio-vascular system and they contribute to the morbidity and mortality observed in ESRD therapy. [4,5] To some extent, these adverse consequences of dysregulation of ECFV can be mitigated by restricting access to NaCl, increasing its elimination by non-renal routes, and by enhancing NaCl and water removal by the dialysis procedure (principally by osmotic or hydraulically driven ultra-filtration in peritoneal and hemodialysis respectively) commensurate with the perceived status of the ECFV. [6,7] This essay will deal with this topic, emphasizing the crucial role of ECFV volume control in the determination of outcomes of dialysis therapy. It is the opinion of this author that the issue of such volume control in dialysis therapy for ESRD is a neglected area of therapeutics that is "ripe" for development of clinical performance measures (CPM) if methods for accurate, reliable and simple assessment of the status of the ECFV can be developed and validated in "real-life" circumstances.

Normal Control of ECFV

An in-depth survey of the mechanisms by which constancy of the ECFV is maintained in normal subjects is beyond the scope of this essay- only a brief overview will be provided. [1,8,9]

In a normal 70 kg man, the ECFV is about 14-15 Liters (although this may vary according to the degree of adiposity) containing 2250 mol of Na+, 1500 mmol of Cl- and 60 mmol of K+. The ECFV is divided into intra-vascular (IVFV) and interstitial (ISFV) compartments of about 2.8 Liters and 11,2 Liters respectively. [8,9] In addition, the ECFV contains about 300 grams of protein (60% albumin), 2/3 of which is in the interstitial-vascular compartment. [8,9] The distribution of ECFV between the intra-vascular and interstitial compartments is determined by the Starling forces (hydraulic and oncotic) in the capillaries and the capacity of return of interstitial fluid to the vascular compartment by the lymphatics. [9] The capillary permeability to protein (albumin), is normally constant, but may vary in disease. The distribution of fluid between the ECFV and intra-cellular compartment (ICFV; about 30 Liters in a 70 kg man) is determined largely by osmotic forces generated by the Na+ gradients produced by cellular metabolism and energetics. Regulation of the ECFW about rather narrow set-points is accomplished by a network of interacting factors involving sensors (in the atria, ventricles, pulmonary veins, carotid and aortic arch, liver, central nervous system and the kidney). These sensors monitor the status of the central and peripheral vascular (venous and arterial) volume. Effectors systems regulate NaCl and water excretion by the kidney and involve an equally complex array of neuro-humoral factors (Sympathetic nervous system outflow, vasopressin, renin-angiotensin-aldosterone, norepinephrine, natriuretic peptides, prostaglandins, nitric oxide, endothelin). [8] In normal subjects, any increase in ECFV is perceived by the sensor system and results in increased renal NaCl and water excretion, thus restoring homeostatic balance. Of course, in ESRD this sequence of events is perturbed, and despite the sensor activation when ECFV is expanded beyond critical limits, the ability of the kidneys to respond appropriately is impaired (*homeostenosis*), both in terms of speed and magnitude of the response. [2] This leads to ECFV expansion—a new steady state is acquired at the cost of a chronically expanded ECFV, the magnitude of which is determined by the imbalance of NaCl intake and maximal renal excretory capacity.

Very recently a new twist on the extra-renal control of ECFV has been added: Exogenous NaCl, once distributed in the ECFV, can be osmotically inactivated by interactions with charged glycosoaminoglycans (GAG) in the skin. [10,11] Thus Na+ and Cl- can accumulate without an isosmotic equivalent of water in tissues. The water-free NaCl storage in tissues promotes a macrophage dependent secretion of VEGF Factor C, which in turn can impact lymphatic generation and nitric oxide production, thus influencing blood pressure (BP) independent of ECFV changes. Such processes effectively blunt the impact of egress of NaCl on the ECFV. [10,11] Anything that impairs this osmotic inactivation of NaCl would be expected, therefore, to augment the effect of any given NaCl load on the ECFV and BP. Both Na+ and its attendant anion, Cl-, are involved in this process. This may be one possible explanation for the lesser effects of NaHCO3 administration on ECFV compared to NaCl administration at equimolar amounts of Na+. [12] Whether these observations have relevance to ECFV control in ESRD is not well-understood but, theoretically, if "uremia" impairs osmotic inactivation of NaCl then they may have great significance.

The Expansion of ECFV Has an Impact on the Cardio-vascular System in CKD and ESRD

Not surprisingly, there is substantial evidence that the ECFV in patients with CKD and ESRD is chronically expanded. [13,14] Whether this expansion will lead to overt edema depends on its magnitude and the forces that govern the distribution between the IVFV and the ISFV (Starling forces, intravascular oncotic pressure. lymphatic re-circulation) often determined by concomitant disease, such as congestive heart failure, nephrotic syndrome or hepatic cirrhosis. In the absence of these organ-based disorders, patients with CKD, and even ESRD, can be free of detectable edema or ascites despite expansion of the ECVF. [15,16] However, an expanded ECFV in CKD and ERSD often leads to an increase in the systemic arterial blood pressure (BP), frequently in the presence of an incomplete suppression of the renin-angiotensin-aldosterone system (RAAS). [16,17] The relationship of ECFV to BP in ESRD is governed by a quite complex pathophysiology. [17] Intrinsic renal disease (such as glomerulonephritis or polycystic kidney disease) and perhaps activation of the sympathetic nervous system may be responsible for the failure of the RAAS to suppress, despite expansion of the ECFV. [17] Accumulation of ouabain-like substances (marinobufagenins) can also inhibit ATP-ase and lead to an increase in intra-cellular Ca++ concentration thus augmenting vasoconstriction, [18,19] and also promote intra-myocardial fibrosis (see below). [20] Nevertheless, hypertension in ESRD is very responsive to reduction in ECFV, even though many factors undoubtedly contribute to elevations of BP in patients with chronic progressive renal disease Paradoxically, a chronically expanded ECFV can result in "intra-dialytic" hypertension when fluid is removed by dialysis too rapidly. The "volume dependent" hypertension associated with ESRD can lead to disturbances in cardiac anatomy and function (Left ventricular hypertrophy [LVH] or dilated cardiomyopathy and congestive heart failure [CHF]) as well as to aggravation of atherosclerotic disease, include coronary artery disease (CAD) peripheral arterial disease (PAD) and strokes. [21] However, experimental studies in animals have also shown that NaCl retention and ECVF expansion can induce LVH (and intra-myocardial fibrosis) independently of changes in systemic arterial BP. [22-24] Experimental studies in surgically induced CKD in mice have also elegantly shown that LVH is independent of changes in BP and may involve activation of mammalian target of rapamycin (mTOR) perhaps within the heart itself. [25]

Thus, it is not surprising that LVH is a very common accompaniment of CKD and ESRD, almost inevitable by current management standards, even though BP may not be greatly elevated. [26-28] Hypertrophy of the left ventricle in states of ECFV expansion is often asymmetric (similar to that found in high output states with augmented pre-load like severe anemia) while that associated with increased after-load (systolic blood pressure) or impedance (aortic compliance) is frequently concentric. [26,29] Very importantly, the LVH associated with ECFV expansion in CKD and ESRD can also be complicated by intra-myocardial fibrosis, itself due to pro-fibrotic forces elaborated endogenously by NaCl excess. [18-20,22,24,29,30] Such intra-myocardial fibrosis can predispose to arrythmogenic, electrical remodeling of cardiac tissue. [26,30-32] Sudden cardiac death due to ventricular arrhythmias must be regarded as a possible lethal complication of chronic ECFV excess in CKD and ESRD in addition to dilated cardiomyopathy and CHF. [31,32] Biochemical and physical features of an expanded ECFV are common in CKD and ESRD, including elevated NT-pro BNP and ANP levels, increased atrial volume, widened inferior vena caval diameter and expanded fluid volumes by bio-electrical impedance. [33-37] Rigorous NaCl restriction (or loop active diuretics) can often improve blood pressure and reduce LVH in CKD and ESRD, even when the BP is not affected. [38,39]

An Expanded ECFV Influences Outcomes in ESRD Treated by Dialysis

Many observational studies have shown a strong association between inter-dialytic weight gain (InterDWG) and mortality and morbidity in patients treated with thrice weekly hemodialysis. [40,41] In a recent extensive observational study of 34,107 hemodialysis patients, Kalantar-Zadeh and co-workers found a dramatic and association of the interDWG weight gain on mortality, even after adjustment for co-variates.(see Figure 1). [40] An interDWG of >3.0kg was associated with excess mortality. The fully adjusted relative risk for all-cause and CV mortality was increased by 28% and 25% respectively by an interDWG weight gain of >4.0 kg. Forty percent of the subjects had interDWG in excess of 3.0kg. If weight gain between dialysis reflects an increase in ECFV, as it almost certainly does, then events occurring *between* dialysis sessions and *not during* dialysis treatments (such as the dialysis dose or intra-dialytic ultrafiltration) represent an important, and potentially controllable, influence on outcome. Residual urine volume, thirst, salt-craving and the willingness and ability of patients to comply with advice regarding NaCl intake during the inter-dialytic interval are likely to be important factors in determining the interDWG.

Very clearly, ECFV can be reduced by hydraulic pressure gradient induced ultra-filtration in standard hemodialysis and hemodiafiltration or by the osmotic forces available in peritoneal dialysis using hyper-osmotic solute (e.g. glucose) containing solutions. In standard thrice weekly hemodialysis session of 4 hours each, the ECVF is potentially "normalized" for only a fraction of the week (about 16 hours of 168 hours or 10%), depending on how rapidly the patient regains the weight (a function of inter dialytic NaCl and water consumption and residual urine volume); and whether the dialysis procedure itself truly returned ECFV to a "normal" value for the patients anthropomorphic features (such as body weight, fat mass and lean body mass) is unlikely. More continuous dialysis procedures, like continuous ambulatory peritoneal dialysis (CAPD), likely result in a more prolonged period of ECFV control. Likewise, the use of hemodialysis regimens that are more frequent or more prolonged, such a nocturnal dialysis on a 5-6 days per week schedule, would lead to shortened inter-dialysis interval compared to standard thrice weekly hemodialysis (from 156 hours per week to about 120 hours per week). Such a shortening of the inter-dialysis interval can contribute to lower interDWG and better control of ECFV, regardless of the extent of intra-dialytic ultrafiltration. These more intensive regimens of hemodialysis have been shown to reduce the burden of LVH compared to standard thrice weekly treatment programs. [42]

The principle that better control of ECFV as associated with better outcomes was recognized very early in the history of dialysis therapy, first by Scribner, and was later exploited with great success in the Tassin unit in France. [5,13,43,44] Rigorous control of ECFV by longer dialysis and meticulous regulation of NaCl and water intake led to very superior outcomes (survival free of CV events), and satisfactory blood pressure control, without drugs in the great majority of patients despite negligible residual renal function. Indeed, substitution of BP control by drugs for adequate control of ECFV by dialysis and NaCl restriction led to inferior outcomes and failure to reverse LVH, one of the most hazardous consequences of ECFV mis-management. [26] Attempts to control ECFV by intra-dialytic ultra-filtration alone (without NaCl restriction) in standard hemodialysis are often unsuccessful and may be harmful. McIntyre and colleagues have elegantly documented the unfavorable ischemia- inducing effect on the myocardium of repeated episodes of excessive ultra-filtration. [45,46] Such "myocardial stunning" can have disastrous long-term sequelae. Every patient on standard hemodialysis deserves a rigorous effort to control BP by means of NaCl and fluid restriction and gentle, slow ultra-filtration before being maintained on antihypertensive drugs, which only compound the problem rather than alleviates it. The optimum control of hypertension in dialysis patients is by ECFV control, not drugs, with few exceptions. [5] Excessive intra-dialytic ultra-filtration can not only be harmful, as mentioned above, to the myocardium it may also stimulate thirst and NaCl craving in the post-dialysis period and contribute to rapid inter-DWG. Administration of NaCl parenterally in an attempt to treat intra-dialytic symptoms (e.g., muscle cramps), "sodium-profiling" during dialysis and use of a dialysate Na+ concentration that exceeds the patient's plasma Na+ concentration can also be additional sources of a positive Na+ balance during the dialysis treatment session. Elevation of the plasma Na+ concentration above about 139 mmol/L can cause a "stiffening" of the arterial circulation and contribute to elevations of intra-dialytic BP. [26,47] The Na+ concentration of dialysate should be aligned with the patient's serum Na+ concentration so as to avoid excessive Na+ diffusion into the patient during dialysis. [48]

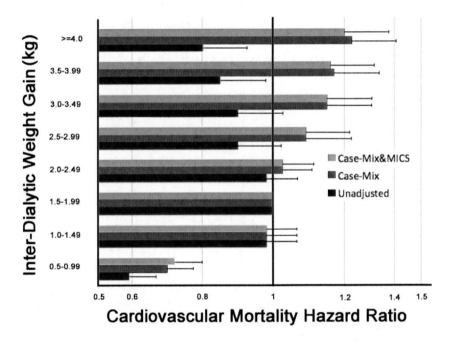

Figure 1. The association between cardiovascular mortality hazard ratio and interdialytic weight gain (in Kg) in 34,107 hemodialysis patients followed for over two years. Blue- unadjusted; Red - case-mix adjusted; Green - case-mix and malnutrition-inflammatory-cachexia adjusted. (Redrawn from Kalantar-Zadeh K, Regidor DL, Kovesdy CP [40]).

One of the most dangerous results of chronically expanded ECFV in CKD and ESRD is the development of LVH and eventually dilated cardiomyopathy and CHF. [26] An increase in LV mass with attendant intra-myocardial fibrosis can also provoke lethal arrhythmias, as mentioned above. Measures that are taken to reduce the expanded ECFV can ameliorate the LVH, even in the absence of a lower occasionally monitored BP. [37,38] Standard thrice weekly hemodialysis without meticulous attention to ECFV can permit LVH to persist or even progress, with significant adverse effects on outcome. [26] Thus, there is a direct link between ECFV control and outcome in dialysis treatment, and these effects are independent of dialysis dose (Kt/V) and anemia management.

Measurement of ECFV in Dialysis Patients: A Clinical Conundrum

Management of the ECFV in dialysis patients depends on the accuracy and reliability of assessment of its status on a regular, ongoing basis. Unfortunately beside clinical examination lacks the sensitivity and specificity required for a reliable evaluation. Edema can be lacking in dialysis patients with expanded ECFV. [15] Normal values for ECFV relative to body weight can vary according to fat mass. Central venous pressure (and atrial volume) can also be normal and influenced by cardiac function. Elevated BP is a sign of expanded ECFV but "normal" values can still be associated with subtle increases in ECFV and persistence of LVH. Indeed, it can be proposed that the presence of LVH and its magnitude can serve as a very crude estimate of the chronic status of the ECFV in a dialysis patient [26]--- a sort of a "hemoglobin A1c for ECFV". Nevertheless, other factors can contribute to the persistence of LVH in dialysis patients, independent of the expanded state of the ECFV, including severe anemia (Hemoglobin <10gms/dL), poorly controlled hypertension, hyper-phosphatemia [and elevated levels of FGF-23], the presence of an arterio-venous fistula (in hemodialysis patients only), severe hyperparathyroidism (iPTH values >500pg/ml), reduced aortic compliance due to vascular calcification, activation of the sympathetic nervous and renin-angiotensin systems and possibly reduced Vitamin D levels (see 26 for a Review). A possible role for intra-cardiac modulation of the mTOR pathway has been mentioned previously. [25]

It is impractical to directly measure ECFV (or total body exchangeable sodium content) on a regular and ongoing basis; (e.g., by isotope dilution techniques or neutron beam analysis). Therefore, a number of possible techniques to assess the status of the ECFV in dialysis patients have been advocated (see Table 1). [49-53] None of these fully meet the requirements of an ideal assay and few have undergone robust testing in clinical situations relative to "hard" outcomes such as survival or CV events. We still lack a Hemoglobin A1c-glycemia control equivalent for ECFV. Assessment of LVH by serial echocardiography may be one answer, but this has not been tested in a rigorous fashion using "gold-standard" assessment of ECFV, and might be influenced by too many non-ECFV factors to be clinically useful. [26]

"Dry Weight" (DW) is the time-honored (but seriously flawed) concept for estimation of ECFV in dialysis. [49-53] The achievement of "dry weight" has been variously defined. A recent definition is: "the lowest tolerated post-dialysis body weight at which there are minimal signs or symptoms of either hypovolemia or hypervolemia (as achieved by a gradual rather than abrupt decrease in post-dialysis body weight)". [54] As such DW is not a constant value in an individual patient and will be influenced by concomitant changes in lean body or adipose tissue mass. Total body weight (as assessed by BMI) is complex admixture of lean body mass, adipose tissue mass and fluid volume (including ECFV)—each of these can vary independently of each other.

Table 1. Possible Approaches to Assessment of Extra-Cellular (and Intra-Vascular) Fluid Volumes in Dialysis Patients

- Clinical Examination (edema. blood pressure, venous pressure)
- Right Atrial Volume (by Ultrasound)
- Inferior Vena Caval Diameter and Collapsibility (by Ultrasound)
- Relative Blood Volume Changes (ΔRBF by in-line hematocrit monitoring)
- Body or Calf Water and Electrolyte content (By multifrequency bioelectrical impedance spectroscopy)
- Serum Levels of Biomarkers (Atrial Natriuretic peptide. NT-pro-brain natriuretic peptides levels)
- Left Ventricular Hypertrophy (by Ultrasound or Magnetic Resonance Imaging without contrast)

In order to probe DW it is often necessary to provoke symptoms (dizziness, nausea, cramps, hypotension) which can lead to non-compliance and may lead to temporary interruption of dialysis treatment, excessive administration of Na+ salts, and even promote clotting of vascular access sites. Another definition of DW is also useful--- DW being "that body weight at the end of dialysis at which the patient can remain normotensive until the next dialysis session despite retention of salt and water, ideally without the use of anti-hypertensive agents". [55] I prefer this latter definition as it emphasized the importance of the inter-dialytic interval.

In any case, probing DW can be aided by non-invasive "on-line" measurement of changes in relative plasma volume (ΔRPV) by the "Crit-Line" instrument. [49,53] A flat slope of the ΔRPV over time on dialysis (<1.33% per hour) is indicative of a non-DW status, due to plasma volume refilling from an expanded interstitial space. A steeper curve for the ΔRPV (>1.33% per hour) indicates that DW has been achieved. [53] Among hypertensive dialysis patients the DRIP study found that ΔRPV slopes predicted subsequent reductions in ambulatory BP, a feature indicating better control, of ECFV. [56,57] However, the reproducibility of ΔRBV can be poor. The redistribution of fluid from hematocrit-poor compartments can influence ΔRBV and may not always predict the changes in intra-dialytic ECFV or BP. [58] The use of bio-electrical whole body impedance analysis (BIA)is another way to assess ECFV (and nutritional status as well). [59-64] By this test at least 25-30% of dialysis patients have a chronically expanded ECFV and about ½ of these is hypertensive as well. Serial multi-frequency BIA of calf muscle (using the patient as his/her own control) can give reasonably reliable values for the status of total body water and ECFV and aid in the achievement of "true" DW status without aggravation of symptoms, but such devices are not yet approved for use by the FDA in the USA. Interestingly, control of ECFV by means of routine BIA to achieve ideal control of time- averaged fluid overload (TAFO) can reduce LVH, despite no change in DW or BMI.(Velasco N, Chamney P, Wabel P, et al. Abstract, World Congress of Nephrology- Vancouver, BC, 2010 and Personal Communication) The process of serial BIA shows great promise in managing ECFV in dialysis patients, but needs further evaluation. [64,65] Widening of the inferior vena cava, and its collapse with ultra filtration, with abdominal ultrasound is another objective way to assess ECFV and DW. [66-68] This test is very observer dependent and may be difficult to perform in very obese subjects. It also requires a delay in measurement for equilibration for optimal use. The introduction of hand held (mobile) ultrasound devices may be an appealing way of bringing this test to the bedside in a cost-effective manner, but this procedure has not been tested rigorously for its long-term benefits in ECFV control. Measurement of circulating NT-pro-BNP and ANP can add to the assessment of ECVF expansion but the values are influenced by LVH and by concomitant CHF and may lack specificity required for an ideal ECFV method. [69,70] At the present time the use of serial calf multifrequency BIA appears to be the most promising objective way of monitoring of the status of the ECFV, but its superiority over other methods has not yet been rigorously shown. [65-71]

Obstacles to the Achievement of Normal ECFV in Dialysis

Numerous barriers attenuate the ability to achieve a normal ECFW in a dialysis treated population of ESRD patients. Among these include the formidable issue of non-compliance with dietary prescription for NaCl and water intake in the inter-dialytic interval. Such strict measures, often requiring NaCl intakes of <1.0gram per day on a temporary basis, can impair the pleasure of food and thus impede calorie intake and are difficult to maintain over long periods of time. If an oral resin exchanging Calcium for Sodium or a Na+ binding GAG was available it might allow for greater variation in dietary intake of NaCl with lower GI absorption of Na+. Very short hemodialysis treatment sessions (<4 hours) make it difficult to achieve normal ECFV without an unacceptable and possibly risky rate of ultrafiltration (>10ml/hour/kg). Excess Na+ administration from too high a dialysate Na+ concentration (e.g. greater than the patients plasma Na+ concentration at the start of dialysis of >139mmol/L), use of hypertonic saline during dialysis sessions and employment of "sodium profiling" in standard hemodialysis also impede greatly the ability to achieve normal ECFV. For many reasons, CAPD or more prolonged hemodialysis (such as used in Tassin) or the two together may be a preferable way to approach "normality" of the ECFV in ESRD.

Suggested Ways to Manage ECFV in ESRD Patients

First and foremost, education of patient and his/her family members on the importance of NaCl combined with water restriction (depending on the residual urinary volume) by aggressive and repetitive counseling and dietary advice is crucial to help control the tendency for excessive interDWG. Fluid restriction alone, without curtailment of NaCl intake, will not be beneficial. The average patient (without overt CHF) should be started on a 2-3gram/d NaCl diet and about 1000-ml/d of fluid from all sources (depending on residual urine volume). This can be adjusted according to the response to treatment. Patients with CHF may require more rigorous NaCl restriction temporarily. InterDWG consistently exceeding 2.5-3.0 kg should be a "red-flag" for triggering more aggressive counseling and lowering of NaCl and water intake. Loop acting diuretics can be employed if the eGFR is >10ml/min/Kg. All sources of excess NaCl in the dialysis treatment session itself should be scrupulously avoided. Blood pressure control should be achieved by slow and gradual ultra-filtration without the aid of anti-hypertensive agents whenever possible. Long-duration or more frequent hemodialysis session should encouraged and CAPD used whenever feasible. Dry weight should be probed, preferably aided by RPV changes (or BIA or IVC collapse) whichever is available and in which the unit has experience and comfort with the reliability of the assessments. The overall efficacy of ECFV control could also be monitored by periodic assessment of LV ventricular mass index (with echocardiography or cardiac magnetic resonance imaging without contrast).

It is hoped that these measures would lead to better outcomes over standard dialysis with limited attention to ECFV status (better survival, avoidance of hospitalizations and improved rehabilitation). A suitably designed long-term randomized controlled trial would be needed to prove this hypothesis, but I believe that the preponderance of evidence available today indicates that the pathway suggested by this essay is the correct one for the great majority of patients with ESRD requiring regular dialysis treatment. It is no longer appropriate to consider as "standard" therapy for the average patient with ESRD a regimen of thrice weekly sessions of <4 hours each, using a dialysate Na+ concentration of >139mmol/L, sodium modeling and an ultrafiltration rate of >10ml/hr/kg without some objective measure of ECFV. The lack of attention to Na+ and fluid intake during the inter-dialytic period and excessive use of anti-hypertensive agents to control BP is to be deplored. Inevitably patients managed in this less than ideal manner will experience adverse outcomes, included death, disability and unnecessary hospitalization. Surely our patients deserve better.

Acknowledgments

The Author is indebted to Drs. Thomas Parker III and Nathan Levin who provided many helpful and constructive suggestions during the preparation of the manuscript. The author also is grateful for the excellent secretarial and reference service provided by Mark Glassock, BS, MPH.

References

[1] Kleeman C. Volume Composition. In: Massry S, Glassock R, editors. Textbook of Nephrology. Philadelphia: Lippincott, Williams and Wilkins; 2001. p. 233-235.
[2] Schreiner GE. Management of end-state nephritis: biochemical alterations. Bull N Y Acad Med. 1970 Oct;46(10):838-849.
[3] Fishbane S, Natke E, Maesaka JK. Role of volume overload in dialysis-refractory hypertension. Am J Kidney Dis. 1996 Aug;28(2):257-261.
[4] Diroll A. Blood volume monitoring a crucial step in reducing mortality. Nephrol News Issues. 2011 Feb;25(2):32-34.
[5] Charra B, Chazot C. Volume control, blood pressure and cardiovascular function. Lessons from hemodialysis treatment. Nephron Physiol. 2003;93(4):p94-101.
[6] Daugirdas J. Handbook of dialysis. 4th ed. Philadelphia: Lippincott Williams & Wilkins; 2007.

[7] Khannā R. Nolph and Gokal's textbook of peritoneal dialysis. 3rd ed. New York: Springer; 2009.

[8] Elhassan E, Schrier R. Disorders of Extracellular Volume. In: Floege J, Johnson R, Feehally J, editors. Comprehensive Clinical Nephrology. Philadelphia: Elsevier; 2010. p. 85-99.

[9] Joles J, Koomans H. Transcapillary Fluid Exchange in Normal and Pathologic States. In: Massry S, Glassock R, editors. Textbook of Nephrology. Philadelphia: Lippincott Williams & Wilkins; 2001. p. 235-238.

[10] Carroll HJ, Gotterer R, Altshuler B. Exchangeable sodium, body potassium, and body water in previously edematous cardiac patients: evidence for osmotic inactivation of cation. Circ. 1965;32:185-192.

[11] Titze J, Machnik A. Sodium sensing in the interstitium and relationship to hypertension. Curr Opin Nephrol Hypertens. 2010 Jul;19(4):385-392.

[12] Ziomber A, Machnik A, Dahlmann A, Dietsch P, Beck F-X, Wagner H, et al. Sodium-, potassium-, chloride-, and bicarbonate-related effects on blood pressure and electrolyte homeostasis in deoxycorticosterone acetate-treated rats. Am J Physiol Renal Physiol. 2008 Jun;295(6):F1752-F1763.

[13] Blumberg A, Nelp WB, Hegstrom RM, Scribner BH. Extracellular volume in patients with chronic renal disease treated for hypertension by sodium restriction. Lancet. 1967 Jul 8;2(7506):69-73.

[14] Agarwal R, Light RP. Intradialytic hypertension is a marker of volume excess. Nephrol Dial Transplant. 2010 Oct;25(10):3355-3361.

[15] Agarwal R, Andersen MJ, Pratt JH. On the importance of pedal edema in hemodialysis patients. Clin J Am Soc Nephrol. 2008 Jan;3(1):153-158.

[16] Sinha AD, Agarwal R. Can chronic volume overload be recognized and prevented in hemodialysis patients? The pitfalls of the clinical examination in assessing volume status. Semin Dial. 2009 Oct;22(5):480-482.

[17] Luik AJ, Kooman JP, Leunissen KM. Hypertension in haemodialysis patients: is it only hypervolaemia? Nephrol Dial Transplant. 1997 Aug;12(8):1557-1560.

[18] Titze J, Ritz E. Salt and its effect on blood pressure and target organ damage: new pieces in an old puzzle. J Nephrol. 2009 Apr;22(2):177-189.

[19] Bagrov AY, Shapiro JI. Endogenous digitalis: pathophysiologic roles and therapeutic applications. Nat Clin Pract Nephrol. 2008;4:378-382.

[20] Elkaeh J, Perlyasamy SM, Shidyak A, Vetteth S, Schroder J, Raju V, Hariri IM, El-Okdi N, Gupta S, Fedorova L, Liu J, Kahaleh MB, Xie Z, Malhotra D, Watson DK, Bagrov AY, Shapiro JI. Marinobufagenin induces increases in pro-collagen expression in a process involving protein kinase C and Fli-1: implications or uremic cardiomyopathy. Am J Physiol Renal Physiol. 2009;296:F1219-F1226.

[21] Penne EL, Levin NW, Kotanko P. Improving Volume Status by Comprehensive Dietary and Dialytic Sodium Management in Chronic Hemodialysis Patients. Blood Purif. 2010;30(1):71-78.

[22] Yu HC, Burrell LM, Black MJ, Wu LL, Dilley RJ, Cooper ME, et al. Salt induces myocardial and renal fibrosis in normotensive and hypertensive rats. Circ. 1998 Dec 8;98(23):2621-2628.

[23] Frohlich ED, Varagic J. The role of sodium in hypertension is more complex than simply elevating arterial pressure. Nat Clin Pract Cardiovasc Med. 2004 Nov;1(1):24-30.

[24] Varagic J, Frohlich ED, Díez J, Susic D, Ahn J, González A, et al. Myocardial fibrosis, impaired coronary hemodynamics, and biventricular dysfunction in salt-loaded SHR. Am J Physiol Heart Cir Physio. 2006 Apr;290(4):H1503-1509.

[25] Siedlecki AM, Jin X, Muslin AJ. Uremic cardiac hypertrophy is reversed by rapamycin but not by lowering of blood pressure. Kidney Int. 2009 Apr;75(8):800-808.

[26] Glassock RJ, Pecoits-Filho R, Barberato SH. Left Ventricular Mass in Chronic Kidney Disease and ESRD. Clin J Am Soc Nephrol. 2009 Dec;4(Supplement 1):S79-S91.

[27] Paoletti E, Bellino D, Cassottana P, Rolla D, Cannella G. Left ventricular hypertrophy in nondiabetic predialysis CKD. Am. J. Kidney Dis. 2005 Aug;46(2):320-327.

[28] McMahon LP, Roger SD, Levin A. Development, prevention, and potential reversal of left ventricular hypertrophy in chronic kidney disease. J Am Soc Nephrol. 2004 Jun;15(6):1640-1647.

[29] Ritz E. Left ventricular hypertrophy in renal disease: beyond preload and afterload. Kidney Int. 2009 Apr;75(8):771-773.

[30] Gross ML, Ritz E. Hypertrophy and fibrosis in the cardiomyopathy of uremia--beyond coronary heart disease. Semin Dial. 2008 Aug;21(4):308-318.

[31] Bleyer AJ, Hartman J, Brannon PC, Reeves-Daniel A, Satko SG, Russell G. Characteristics of sudden death in hemodialysis patients. Kidney Int. 2006 Jun;69(12):2268-2273.

[32] Ritz E, Wanner C. The challenge of sudden death in dialysis patients. Clin J Am Soc Nephrol. 2008; 3: 920-929r

[33] Wang AY-M, Lai K-N. Use of cardiac biomarkers in end-stage renal disease. J Am Soc Nephrol. 2008 Sep;19(9):1643-1652.

[34] Ortega O, Rodriguez I, Gracia C, Sanchez M, Lentisco C, Mon C, et al. Strict volume control and longitudinal changes in cardiac biomarker levels in hemodialysis patients. Nephron Clin Pract. 2009;113(2):c96-103.

[35] Satyan S, Light RP, Agarwal R. Relationships of N-terminal pro-B-natriuretic peptide and cardiac troponin T to left ventricular mass and function and mortality in asymptomatic hemodialysis patients. Am J Kidney Dis. 2007 Dec;50(6):1009-1019.

[36] Zhu F, Kotanko P, Handelman GJ, Raimann JG, Liu L, Carter M, et al. Estimation of normal hydration in dialysis patients using whole body and calf bioimpedance analysis. Physiol Meas. 2011 Jul;32(7):887-902.

[37] Charra B, Chazot C. Extra cellular volume assessment methods in dialysis, a critical analysis . Nephrol Ther. 2007 Sep;3 Suppl 2:S112-120.

[38] Zamboli P, De Nicola L, Minutolo R, Chiodini P, Crivaro M, Tassinario S, et al. Effect of furosemide on left ventricular mass in non-dialysis chronic kidney disease patients: a randomized controlled trial. Nephrol Dial Transplant. 2011 May;26(5):1575-1583.

[39] Kayikcioglu M, Tumuklu M, Ozkahya M, Ozdogan O, Asci G, Duman S, et al. The benefit of salt restriction in the treatment of end-stage renal disease by haemodialysis. Nephrol Dial Transplant. 2009 Mar;24(3):956-962.

[40] Kalantar-Zadeh K, Regidor DL, Kovesdy CP, Van Wyck D, Bunnapradist S, Horwich TB, et al. Fluid Retention Is Associated With Cardiovascular Mortality in Patients Undergoing Long-Term Hemodialysis. Circ. 2009 Feb;119(5):671-679.

[41] Banerjee D, Ma JZ, Collins AJ, Herzog CA. Long-term survival of incident hemodialysis patients who are hospitalized for congestive heart failure, pulmonary edema, or fluid overload. Clin J Am Soc Nephrol. 2007 Nov;2(6):1186-1190.

[42] Chertow GM, Levin NW, Beck GJ, Depner TA, Eggers PW, Gassman JJ, et al. In-center hemodialysis six times per week versus three times per week. N Engl J Med. 2010 Dec 9;363(24):2287-2300.

[43] Charra B, Chazot C. The neglect of sodium restriction in dialysis patients: a short review. Hemodial Int. 2003 Oct 1;7(4):342-347.

[44] Charra B, Chazot C, Jean G, Hurot J-M, Terrat J-C, Vanel T, et al. Role of sodium in dialysis. Minerva Urol Nefrol. 2004 Sep;56(3):205-213.

[45] Jefferies HJ, Virk B, Schiller B, Moran J, McIntyre CW. Frequent Hemodialysis Schedules Are Associated with Reduced Levels of Dialysis-induced Cardiac Injury (Myocardial Stunning). Clin J Am Soc Nephrol. 2011 Jun;6(6):1326-1332.

[46] McIntyre CW. Recurrent circulatory stress: the dark side of dialysis. Semin Dial. 2010 Oct;23(5):449-451.

[47] Oberleithner H, Riethmüller C, Schillers H, MacGregor GA, de Wardener HE, Hausberg M. Plasma sodium stiffens vascular endothelium and reduces nitric oxide release. Proc Natl Acad Sci USA. 2007 Oct 9;104(41):16281-16286.

[48] de Paula FM, Peixoto AJ, Pinto LV, Dorigo D, Patricio PJM, Santos SFF. Clinical consequences of an individualized dialysate sodium prescription in hemodialysis patients. Kidney Int. 2004 Sep;66(3):1232-1238.

[49] Agarwal R, Weir MR. Dry-weight: a concept revisited in an effort to avoid medication-directed approaches for blood pressure control in hemodialysis patients. Clin J Am Soc Nephrol. 2010 Jul;5(7):1255-1260.

[50] Charra B. "Dry weight" in dialysis: the history of a concept. Nephrol Dial Transplant. 1998 Jul;13(7):1882-1885.

[51] Raimann J, Liu L, Tyagi S, Levin NW, Kotanko P. A fresh look at dry weight. Hemodial Int. 2008 Oct;12(4):395-405.

[52] Chazot C, Charra B, Vo Van C, Jean G, Vanel T, Calemard E, et al. The Janus-faced aspect of "dry weight." Nephrol Dial Transplant. 1999 Jan;14(1):121-124.

[53] Agarwal R, Bouldin JM, Light RP, Garg A. Probing dry-weight improves left ventricular mass index. Am J Nephrol. 2011;33(4):373-380.

[54] Sinha AD, Agarwal R. Can chronic volume overload be recognized and prevented in hemodialysis patients? The pitfalls of the clinical examination in assessing volume status. Semin Dial. 2009 Oct;22(5):480-482.

[55] Charra B, Laurent G, Chazot C, Calemard E, Terrat JC, Vanel T, et al. Clinical assessment of dry weight. Nephrol Dial Transplant. 1996;11 Suppl 2:16-19.

[56] Agarwal R, Alborzi P, Satyan S, Light RP. Dry-weight reduction in hypertensive hemodialysis patients (DRIP): a randomized, controlled trial. Hypertension. 2009 Mar;53(3):500-507.

[57] Agarwal R. Volume-associated ambulatory blood pressure patterns in hemodialysis patients. Hypertension. 2009 Aug;54(2):241-247.

[58] Booth J, Pinney J, Davenport A. Do changes in relative blood volume monitoring correlate to hemodialysis-associated hypotension? Nephron Clin Pract. 2011;117(3):c179-183.

[59] Voroneanu L, Cusai C, Hogas S, Ardeleanu S, Onofriescu M, Nistor I, et al. The relationship between chronic volume overload and elevated blood pressure in hemodialysis patients: use of bioimpedance provides a different perspective from echocardiography and biomarker methodologies. Int Urol Nephrol. 2010 Sep;42(3):789-797.

[60] Goldfarb-Rumyantzev AS, Chelamcharla M, Bray BE, Leypoldt JK, Lavasani I, Nelson N, et al. Volume indicators and left ventricular mass during aggressive volume management in patients on thrice-weekly hemodialysis. Nephron Clin Pract. 2009;113(4):c270-280.

[61] Kotanko P, Levin NW, Zhu F. Current state of bioimpedance technologies in dialysis. Nephrol Dial Transplant. 2007 Oct;23(3):808-812.

[62] Piccoli A. Bioelectric impedance measurement for fluid status assessment. Contrib Nephrol. 2010;164:143-152.

[63] Kuhlmann MK, Zhu F, Seibert E, Levin NW. Bioimpedance, dry weight and blood pressure control: new methods and consequences. Curr Opin Nephrol Hypertens. 2005 Nov;14(6):543-549.

[64] Onofriescu M, Mardare NG, Segall L, Voroneanu L, Cuşai C, Hogaş S, et al. Randomized trial of bioelectrical impedance analysis versus clinical criteria for guiding ultrafiltration in hemodialysis patients: effects on blood pressure, hydration status, and arterial stiffness. Int Urol Nephrol [Internet]. 2011 Jun 19. [cited 22 Jul 2011]. Available from: http://www.ncbi.nlm.nih.gov/pubmed/21688195.

[65] Passauer J, Petrov H, Schlesser A, Leicht J, Pucalka K. Evaluation of clinical dry weight assessment in hemodialysis patients using bioimpedance spectroscopy: a cross sectional study. Nephrol Dial Transplant. 2010; 25: 545-551.

[66] Guiotto G, Masarone M, Paladino F, Ruggiero E, Scott S, Verde S, et al. Inferior vena cava collapsibility to guide fluid removal in slow continuous ultrafiltration: a pilot study. Intensive Care Med. 2010 Apr;36(4):692-696.

[67] Agarwal R, Kelley K, Light RP. Diagnostic utility of blood volume monitoring in hemodialysis patients. Am. J. Kidney Dis. 2008 Feb;51(2):242-254.

[68] Agarwal R, Bouldin JM, Light RP, Garg A. Inferior vena cava diameter and left atrial diameter measure volume but not dry weight. Clin J Am Soc Nephrol. 2011 May;6(5):1066-1072.

[69] Booth J, Pinney J, Davenport A. N-terminal proBNP--marker of cardiac dysfunction, fluid overload, or malnutrition in hemodialysis patients? Clin J Am Soc Nephrol. 2010 Jun;5(6):1036-1040.

[70] Zhou Y-L, Liu J, Sun F, Ma L-J, Han B, Shen Y, et al. Calf bioimpedance ratio improves dry weight assessment and blood pressure control in hemodialysis patients. Am J Nephrol. 2010;32(2):109-116.

[71] Zhu F, Kuhlmann MK, Kotanko P, Seibert E, Leonard EF, Levin NW. A method for the estimation of hydration state during hemodialysis using a calf bioimpedance technique. Physiol Meas. 2008 Jun;29(6):S503-516.

In: Issues in Dialysis
Editor: Stephen Z. Fadem

ISBN: 978-1-62417-576-3
© 2013 Nova Science Publishers, Inc.

Chapter X

Mechanisms Causing Muscle Wasting in Kidney Disease and Other Catabolic Conditions

William E. Mitch[*]
Nephrology Division, Baylor College of Medicine, Houston, Texas, US

Abstract

The ubiquitin-proteasome system (UPS) includes 3 enzymes that conjugate ubiquitin to intracellular proteins that are then recognized and degraded by the proteasome. The process participates in the regulation of cell metabolism. In the kidney, the UPS participates in the regulation of the turnover of transporters and signaling proteins. In chronic kidney disease (CKD), muscle wasting occurs because complications of CKD including acidosis, insulin resistance, inflammation, and increased angiotensin II levels stimulate the UPS to degrade muscle proteins. This response also includes caspase-3 which acts to cleave muscle proteins providing substrates for the UPS. For example, caspase-3 degrades actomyosin, leaving a 14kD fragment of actin in muscle. The 14 kD actin fragment is increased in muscle of patient with kidney disease, burn injury and surgery. In addition, acidosis, insulin resistance, inflammation and angiotensin II stimulate glucocorticoid production. Glucocorticoids are also required for the muscle wasting that occurs in CKD. Thus, the UPS participates in highly organized responses that degrade muscle protein in response to loss of kidney function.

Keywords: Ubiquitin-proteasome system (UPS), muscle wasting, protein degradation, chronic kidney disease (CKD), 14kD actin fragment, caspase-3

---

[*] Correspondence to: William E. Mitch, M.D. Nephrology Division M/S: BCM 285; Baylor College of Medicine; One Baylor Plaza, Alkek N-520; Houston, TX 77030. Telephone: 713-798-8350; Fax: 713-798-5010; Email: mitch@bcm.edu

Introduction

Chronic kidney disease (CKD) is associated with an excessive risk of mortality and morbidity. [1,2] Several mechanisms have been advanced to explain this association but none is universally accepted. For example, in patients with other chronic diseases (e.g., cancer), the risks of morbidity and mortality increase when there is depletion of protein stores, a condition known as cachexia. [3] In CKD patients, however, hypoalbuminemia is the principal evidence for subnormal protein stores leading to the conclusion that CKD patients have "protein malnutrition". [4-6] This conclusion was supported by the report that some patients with advancing CKD spontaneously restrict their protein intake. [7] Attributing the metabolic problems of CKD patients to protein malnutrition is erroneous because malnutrition is defined as abnormalities related to an insufficient amount of food in the diet or to an imbalance among dietary nutrients. There at least two reasons that the morbidity and mortality associated with CKD is rarely caused by malnutrition. [5,8,9] First, if protein malnutrition were the cause of defects in protein stores, then the abnormalities should be corrected by simply altering the diet. This hypothesis has been examined and found to be wanting: Ikizler and colleagues measured rates of protein synthesis and degradation in fasting hemodialysis patients using standard techniques of labeled amino acid turnover. [10] Protein metabolism was measured before, during and finally, at 2 hours after completing the dialysis treatment. At every stage, protein degradation exceeded protein synthesis indicating significant loss of body protein stores. Subsequently, the group changed their protocol and tested the influence of adding intravenous parenteral nutrition (IDPN) during the hemodialysis procedure. [11] The same measurements were made. The IDPN supplement did improve both protein synthesis and degradation measured during dialysis but there still was a persistent increase in protein degradation lasting through the two hours after completing dialysis. Thus, abnormalities in protein metabolism were not eliminated by simply increasing the intake of protein and calories during dialysis. Pupim et al. repeated their protocol a third time but in this case, they compared the influences of (IDPN) with those of an oral nutritional supplement; both were given during the dialysis. As before, protein balance improved with both supplements but at two hours after completing dialysis, protein balance was still negative. [12] These carefully collected results not only provide new information about dialysis and protein metabolism they also demonstrate that increasing protein in the diet al.one will not be sufficient to eliminate CKD-stimulated protein losses. Others report similar conclusions: a randomized, controlled trial of responses to IDPN compared to those obtained without a dietary supplement was carried out in hemodialysis patients. [13] After two years, the supplement had not improved mortality, body mass index, laboratory markers of nutritional status or the rate of hospitalization. In summary, the excessive morbidity and mortality occurring in patients with CKD cannot be corrected simply by changing the diet. Therefore, hypoalbuminemia in CKD patients should not be attributed to malnutrition. [5,8] Obviously, it is critical to plan the diet of CKD patients in order to ensure they receive an adequate amount of protein and calories. It is also necessary to avoid an excess of dietary protein because accumulation of waste products will contribute to complications of CKD. [14]

The Taxonomy of Protein Wasting

These considerations have prompted the use of different terms to identify CKD patients with protein wasting. A task force of the International Society of Renal Nutrition and Metabolism (ISRNM) concluded that malnutrition is inadequate to serve as a description of the problems of CKD patients. [9] They recommended obtaining several measurements to classify protein stores, including serum albumin or prealbumin and cholesterol plus measurements of body mass and anthropometry. The group also suggested that protein-energy wasting or (PEW) be the descriptive term for CKD patients who have evidence of abnormal protein stores. This term was chosen to avoid the implication that changing the diet will correct lost protein stores (see above). Use of the term sarcopenia was ruled out because it is generally used to describe patients with aging-induced muscle wasting. Labeling these patients as cachetic was not recommended because it implies there is a more severe state of protein depletion and a dire prognosis. PEW on the other hand, describes CKD patients with a milder form of metabolic depletion not suffering from other catabolic conditions.

In 2006, another group of scientists and clinicians concluded that cachexia identifies a complex metabolic syndrome that is associated with catabolic conditions and is characterized by prominent loss of muscle and fat mass. [3] It was emphasized that a major stumbling block in identifying stages of cachexia is the absence of a reliable measure of protein stores or muscle mass. To diagnose cachexia, it was recommended that the following be present: loss of edema free body weight within 12 months; anthropometry abnormalities; plus evidence of inflammation and hypoalbuminemia. A summary of these deliberations is presented to emphasize that there is a problem with imprecision of the measurements and hence, confusion arises when diagnosing protein wasting. Importantly, these shortcomings will interfere with the evaluation of treatment strategies directed at blocking the development of protein wasting.

CKD-Induced Stimuli of Protein Wasting

A major focus of clinical studies of CKD has been to evaluate the consequences of hypoalbuminemia and other complications. For example, it is documented that circulating levels of cytokines are frequently increased in patients with CKD suggesting that inflammation is the cause of hypoalbuminemia. [6,15,16] In a study of hemodialysis patients receiving long term, standardized treatments, monthly measurements of circulating levels of α-1 acid glycoprotein and ceruloplasmin (representing markers of inflammation) and serum albumin were collected. Analysis of these measurements indicated that higher levels of inflammatory markers measured in one month predicted that serum albumin will be lower in the succeeding month. [16] In contrast, dietary factors exerted minimal influence on the serum albumin concentration. It was concluded that inflammation is a key cause of hypoalbuminemia. This is relevant because changing the diet will not cure inflammation.

Another complication of CKD, metabolic acidosis, also causes hypoalbuminemia. When normal adults were given NH_4Cl to induce acidosis, their ability to synthesize albumin was significantly decreased. [17] Using an interventional protocol, Movilli et al. gave hemodialysis patients $NaHCO_3$ supplements for 3 months, producing significant improvements in serum albumin and HCO_3 as well as arterial blood pH. [18] These responses were independent of the protein in the diet or the intensity of dialysis. [19] The conclusion is that at least two complications of CKD do cause hypoalbuminemia, responses that are minimally influenced by dietary factors. In fact, the diet can play a negative role because raising the amount of protein in the diet of CKD patients can increase the degree of metabolic acidosis which will stimulate the degradation of protein in muscle jeopardizing the maintenance of protein stores (see below).

Catabolic Pathways Affecting Protein Stores

All intracellular and extracellular proteins are continually "turning over", being degraded to amino acids and replaced by synthesis of new proteins. Specific proteins in the nucleus, cytoplasm, endoplasmic reticulum or mitochondria are degraded at widely different rates varying from minutes for some regulatory enzymes or transcription factors, to days or weeks for proteins like actin and myosin in skeletal muscle and months for hemoglobin in red blood cells. This distribution in protein half-lives is possible because their degradation is highly regulated. If this were not true, uncoordinated proteolysis would cause disastrous changes in cellular functions and protein stores in muscle and other organs. The need for precise regulation of protein metabolism is underscored by two facts: first, the daily rates of protein turnover (3.7 to 4.7 g/kg/day) are enormous so that even a small, sustained decrease in synthesis or acceleration of protein degradation, would cause a marked loss of protein stores. [20] Secondly, the minute to minute regulation of transcriptional events or metabolic pathways requires adjusting the levels of specific proteins precisely. Therefore, it is somewhat surprising that the same proteolytic system (the ATP-dependent, ubiquitin-proteasome system (UPS)) is responsible for the degradation of the majority of intracellular proteins in all tissues. [20]

The Ubiquitin-Proteasome System

The UPS initiates two major functions when degrading proteins (Figure 1). First, it "tags" proteins destined for degradation by conjugating them with ubiquitin (Ub); and secondly, the tagged protein is degraded by the 26S proteasome. [20,21] Ub-conjugation begins with the activation of UB by a single E1 isoform (Ub-activating enzyme) which interacts with one of the 20-40 isoforms of the E2 Ub-carrier proteins. These initial steps are ATP dependent. They also provide a degree of specificity to the breakdown of proteins because a single E2 Ub-carrier protein can interact with only a limited variety of substrate proteins and a specific group of E3 ubiquitin ligases. These latter enzymes are the key to determining the specificity of proteolysis. There are more than 1000 of these enzymes and each recognizes only a specific protein substrate (or possibly a class of proteins). The specific E3 ligase activated in this process has two functions: it recognizes the protein to be degraded and then transfers ubiquitin to lysines in the substrate protein or to lysines in Ub. The transfer of activated Ub's continues until a chain of 4-5 Ub's is attached to the protein. This chain can then be recognized by the 26S proteasome, a very large organelle consisting of >60 proteins organized into two particles, a 20S, barrel-shaped particle and 19S regulatory particles present at either or both ends of the 20S particle. The 19S particles recognize the polyubiquitin chain and in the presence of ATP, cleaves the Ub chain from the substrate protein. The 19S particle then unfolds the protein and translocates it into the 20S particle where it is degraded to peptides. The peptides are converted to amino acids by cytosolic peptidases. [22] The importance of these reactions is underscored by the 2004 Nobel Prize in Chemistry awarded to Avram Hershko, Aaron Ciechanover and Irwin Rose (http://nobelprize.org/chemistry/laureates/2004/) for their discovery of Ub and its biochemistry.

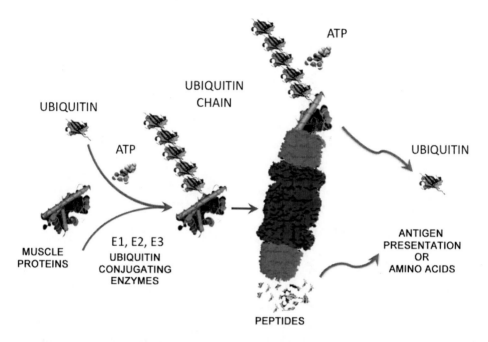

Figure 1. The ubiquitin-proteasome system (UPS) degrades muscle proteins efficiently with remarkable specificity. Substrate proteins to be degraded are first conjugated with a chain of ubiquitins, proteins of the heat-shock family that are present in the cytoplasm and nuclei of all cells. The conjugation process requires ATP and is mediated by two enzymes (E1 and E3) and a ubiquitin-carrier protein, E2. In muscle, the specificity is mainly achieved by two E3-ubiquitin conjugases, Atrogin-1 and MuRF-1, enzymes that recognize specific lysines in protein substrates of muscle and transfer the activated ubiquitin to these lysines. When a chain of 4-5 ubiquitins has been conjugated to the doomed muscle protein, it is recognized by the proteasome, a large structure which uses ATP to unfold the protein, removes the ubiquitins for recycling and injects the protein substrate into the central cavity of the proteasome. Inside the proteasome, the protein is degraded to peptides that are rapidly removed by peptidases in the cytoplasm of muscle cells. Alternatively, the peptides can be used in antigen presentation.

Both the conjugation of Ub to substrate proteins and degradation of the protein are accelerated in muscle wasting conditions. Considering the complexity of Ub conjugation to a substrate protein, it is not surprising that the expression of key contributors to this process, Ub, subunits of the 26S proteasomes, and two E3 Ub-ligases, Atrogin-1 (also known as MAFbx) and MuRF-1, increase in muscle. These E3 Ub-ligases are critical for the breakdown of muscle proteins and their expression increases dramatically (8-20 fold) in rodent models of muscle wasting conditions. [23-27] In cultured muscle cells, the content of atrogin-1 mRNA correlates closely with rates of protein breakdown. [26] Consequently, understanding how these E3 Ub-conjugating enzymes are activated has been extensively studied. Two factors have been identified: the forkhead transcription factors (FoxO); and the inflammatory transcription factor, NFκB. FoxO and NFκB activate the promoters for Atrogin-1/MAFbx and MuRF-1 respectively to increase expression of the E3 Ub ligases and ultimately, muscle wasting. [24,28,29]

In response to progressive loss of kidney function, muscle protein synthesis may decrease somewhat, but the more prominent response is an increase in rates of protein degradation. [30-32] Specifically, CKD accelerates proteolysis by initiating a coordinated, multistep process. First, there is activation of the UPS and caspase-3. The latter performs an initial cleavage of the complex structure of actomyosin and myofibrils to produce substrates for the UPS. Second, there are higher levels of mRNAs encoding certain components of the UPS. Notably, accelerated muscle wasting in CKD involves cellular mechanisms that are very similar to those causing muscle wasting in other catabolic conditions, such as cancer cachexia, starvation, insulin deficiency or resistance and or sepsis. [20,21] In fact, there are changes in the expression of about 100 atrophy-related genes called atrogenes in catabolic conditions. [32,33,33-35] These results indicate that there is a common transcriptional program with multiple transcriptional factors which change in a coordinated fashion to cause loss of muscle mass. [33,36]

Caspase-3 Interacts with the UPS to Produce Muscle Atrophy

Catabolic conditions stimulate a specific loss of contractile proteins which comprise about 2/3 of the protein in muscle. Loss of these proteins is largely responsible for the disability of patients who experience muscle wasting. [37] The UPS readily degrades the individual proteins, actin, myosin, troponin or tropomyosin but it exhibits only limited proteolytic activity for these same proteins when they are in complexes. This means that other proteases must initially cleave muscle proteins in complexes yielding substrates for the UPS. [38] We have found that caspase-3 performs this task and that this protease is activated by certain catabolic conditions (e.g., high circulating TNFα levels or resistance to insulin or IGF-1). [15,39,40] The role of caspase-3 was uncovered in cultured muscle cells when it was found that activated caspase-3 cleaves actomyosin to produce protein fragments that are rapidly degraded by the UPS. However, this proteolytic action of caspase-3 also leaves a "footprint", a 14 kD C-terminal fragment of actin which is most easily detected in the insoluble fraction of muscle; it is rarely found in the soluble fraction presumably because of rapid degradation by the UPS. [40] The conditions that activate caspase-3 in muscles include complications of CKD such as acidosis, diabetes, and angiotensin II. [24,40,41,41] These findings are not limited to mouse models. In muscle biopsies of patients with CKD, the level of the 14 kD actin fragment in muscle biopsies is increased and it responds to therapy: the 14 kD actin fragment decreases in patients who complete a prolonged exercise program directed at increasing the patient's endurance. [42] Moreover, in patients undergoing hip surgery to treat osteoarthritis, the level of the14 kD actin fragment in muscle was highly correlated (r = 0.78) with the measured rate of protein degradation. Finally, the level of the fragment was high in uninjured muscles of patients who had suffered a major burn injury. The finding that the 14 kD actin fragment is increased in muscle suggests that it might serve as a biomarker of accelerated muscle protein degradation. More extensive data are needed to address this possibility.

Recently, caspase-3 was found to exert another property which stimulates muscle proteolysis: activation of caspase-3 actually stimulates the proteolytic activity of the proteasome. Caspase-3's influence on proteasome activity was discovered when proteolytic activity of the proteasome was measured using a short peptide containing a fluorescent tag (i.e., there was no requirement for an initial cleavage of a protein by caspase-3). Subsequent experiments revealed that the increase in proteolysis was due to caspase-3-mediated cleavage of specific subunits of the 19S particle of the proteasome. [43] This response apparently opens the entrance to the 20S proteasome permitting substrate proteins to enter the proteasome where they are degraded. In summary, in rodent models and in patients responding to catabolic conditions, caspase-3 exerts two functions that increase muscle protein degradation: 1) it performs an initial cleavage of complexes of muscle proteins, providing substrates for degradation by the UPS; and 2) it stimulates proteolytic activity of the proteasome. These properties exert a "feed-forward" stimulation of muscle proteins when caspase-3 is activated.

The calpains have also been suggested as another protease that initially cleaves myofibrillar proteins in catabolic conditions. Calpains are calcium-dependent, cysteine proteases that are active in muscular dystrophy or sepsis-induced muscle wasting. [44,45] Their role in breaking down muscle proteins in other conditions is unclear since the muscle wasting induced by uremia or impaired insulin/IGF-1 signaling is unaffected by inhibition of calpain activity. [32;40]

Muscle Proteolytic Activities Present in Patients

In humans, evidence that catabolic conditions stimulate the activation of the UPS in muscle has been mainly examined by evaluating changes in the mRNAs encoding Ub and proteasome subunits. In muscles of patients with trauma, cancer, CKD and sepsis, the level of these mRNAs is increased. [46-49] For example, CKD patients being treated by chronic ambulatory peritoneal dialysis (CAPD), were examined repeatedly during a year long, randomized trial to determine the influence of correcting metabolic acidosis. [50] Not only was there an increase in serum bicarbonate values, there also was an increase in body weight and muscle mass and fewer hospitalizations. [46] Using a similar protocol that lasted for 4 weeks, we found that correction of even mild metabolic acidosis led to decreased levels of Ub mRNA in muscles. These reports indicate that catabolic conditions activate the UPS in muscle of CKD patients. As noted earlier, there also is evidence that caspase-3 is activated in muscles of patients with accelerated protein degradation due to CKD, severe burns injury or surgery for osteoarthritis. [42]

Factors Triggering Muscle Wasting in CKD and other Catabolic States

Certain complications of CKD are well documented stimuli of muscle wasting. The complications include metabolic acidosis, decreased responsiveness to insulin or IGF-1, increased angiotensin II levels, and/or inflammation. [32,34,51,52] The complexity of these mechanisms is illustrated by examining the role of glucocorticoids. For example, metabolic acidosis stimulates muscle protein breakdown but only when there is a physiologic increase in glucocorticoid production plus impairment in the intracellular signaling processes of insulin or IGF-1. [24,41,53,54] Likewise, an increase in glucocorticoids is also required in the muscle protein degradation that occurs in models of diabetes, high levels of angiotensin II or sepsis. [35,51,55]

Why are glucocorticoids required to stimulate muscle wasting in catabolic conditions? The mechanism depends on decreased responses to insulin or IGF-1. The latter decreases activation of the phosphatidylinositol 3-kinase/Akt (PI3K/Akt) signaling pathway, resulting in reduced production of phosphadidylinositol-3,4,5 phosphate (the active product of PI3K) and a decrease in the phosphorylation and activity of the serine/threonine kinase, Akt. [24,56] A lower p-Akt in turn, decreases the phosphorylation of downstream kinases, mTOR and S6kinase to suppress protein synthesis. It also stimulates protein degradation in muscle. This mechanism depends on a decrease in p-Akt because the lower level reduces the phosphorylation of the forkhead family of transcription factors [FoxO1, 3,4] This allows FoxOs to migrate into the nucleus where they stimulate transcription of the muscle-specific E3 Ub ligases, Atrogin-1 and MuRF-1. The increase in these enzymes enhances muscle protein degradation. [24,28,57] Impairment in insulin/IGF-1-PI3K/Akt signaling also activates caspase-3. In this case, the pro-apoptotic factor, Bax, is activated and it migrates to mitochondria causing a release of cytochrome C which increases caspase-3 activity. [24]

Glucocorticoids exert two responses that change the regulation of muscle protein turnover. One response is to a physiologic level of glucocorticoids; it acts when there is decreased signaling from insulin or IGF-1 by a mechanism that is independent of gene transcription (i.e., non-genomic). The second mechanism is a response to pharmacologic doses of glucocorticoids causing a change gene expression. In both cases, the increase in protein degradation is related to stimulation of Atrogin-1 and the UPS. [26,58,59] The response to a physiologic level of glucocorticoids was discovered in studies of adrenalectomized rodents. When they were treated with NH_4Cl to induce metabolic acidosis or made insulin-deficient with streptozotocin or starved (to reduce circulating insulin levels), muscle protein degradation did not increase unless the animals were also given a physiological dose of glucocorticoids. [35,54,60] This requirement for glucocorticoids is also present in models of muscle wasting induced by angiotensin II or sepsis. [51,61] These responses act to suppress the level of p-Akt, leading to transcription and expression of Atrogin-1 with activation of caspase-3 and the UPS. In response to large doses of glucocorticoids, there also is increased transcription of Atrogin-1 and activation of the UPS but the mechanism for these responses is unknown because the promoter of Atrogin-1 does not respond to glucocorticoids.

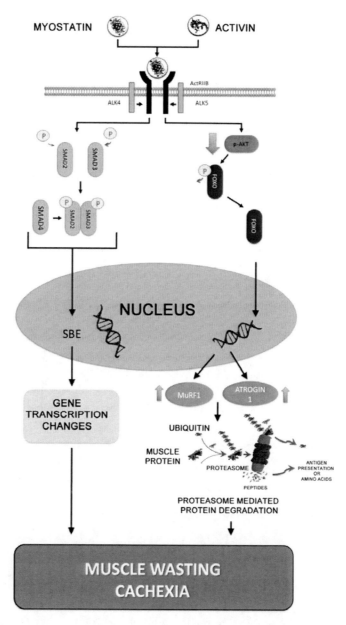

Figure 2. Myostatin is released from the complex in response to proteolysis (or to free radicals or decreased pH). The liberated myostatin can then bind to a high-affinity, type-2 activin receptor (ActRIIB) which is present on muscle membranes. This leads to recruitment and activation of the type I activin receptor transmembrane kinases ALK4 or ALK5. Subsequently, there is phosphorylation of the transcription factors, Smad2 and Smad3, and recruitment of Smad4 to form a Smad complex of the Smad-binding element, SBE. This complex can enter the nucleus to stimulate transcriptional changes in downstream genes, resulting in muscle protein degradation and loss of muscle mass. Notably, myostatin/activin binding to ActRIIB receptor also reduces Akt activity, leading to diminished FoxO phosphorylation. This response is pertinent because dephosphorylated FoxO will enter the nucleus to activate transcription of atrophy-specific E3 ligases, MuRF1 and Atrogin1. These ligases are responsible for the specificity of the ubiquitination of muscle proteins and their degradation by the proteasome. When myostatin activity is inhibited, muscle protein degradation and the consequences of a low p-Akt are eliminated.

Recent results have identified another contributor to muscle wasting in CKD, namely, abnormal responses of satellite cells. These function as muscle "stem" cells and in quiescent states, they are located under the basal lamina of myofibrils. When stimulated by muscle injury or when muscle mass is low, satellite cells proliferate and differentiate into myofibrils. [62] IGF-1 regulates the responses of satellite cells and CKD impairs IGF-1 intracellular signaling. Therefore, it is not surprising that CKD impairs responses of satellite cells, including their proliferation and differentiation. [25,63]

Therapeutic Rationale for Interfering with Myostatin

Myostatin Signaling

Myostatin is a member of the transforming growth factor-β (TGF-β) family of secreted proteins but unlike TGF-β, myostatin is predominantly expressed in skeletal muscle although low levels of myostatin are present in cardiac muscle and adipose tissue. In skeletal muscle, the precursor of myostatin. Prepromyostatin, is cleaved yielding promyostatin, consisting of a propeptide and myostatin. This propeptide functions to bind myostatin producing an inactive, "latent complex". Myostatin is released from the complex in response to proteolysis (or to free radicals or decreased pH). The liberated myostatin can then bind to a high-affinity, type-2 activin receptor (ActRIIB) which is present on muscle membranes. [64] Activation of this receptor initiates signals that lead to phosphorylation of SMAD transcription factors to regulate gene transcription. Notably, TGF-b family members (e.g., activin A) also can bind to ActRIIB and stimulate the same intracellular signaling pathway. (Figure 2).

Genetic Evidence for Myostatin Responses

There is conclusive genetic evidence that myostatin plays a pivotal role in regulating skeletal muscle mass and function. For example, deletion of the myostatin gene in mice produces a phenotype with a dramatic increase in the sizes and number of skeletal muscle fibers. [65] Other models include transgenic mice that overexpress a dominant-negative myostatin receptor or the propeptide (see above) or proteins that can sequester myostatin yield animals that exhibit a dramatic increase in muscle mass. In addition to the mouse phenotypes, cattle, sheep, dogs and a human with a loss-of-function myostatin mutation exhibit an enormous increase in muscle mass. [66-68] There also is evidence that these myostatin mutations influence athletic performance, whippet dogs bearing a single copy of the myostatin mutation are among the fastest dogs in competitive racing. [67] But, whippets bearing two copies of the same mutation produce such an increase in muscle that they win no races. Likewise, myostatin polymorphism in elite thoroughbred horses suggests that these horses have a decided advantage due to the loss of the myostatin allele. [69] Since myostatin deficiency leads to muscle hypertrophy and improved physical performance, manipulating myostatin could be the basis for a therapeutic strategy that blocks muscle wasting.

Myostatin Pathway Activation in Catabolic Condition

Myostatin protein and the myostatin-activin signaling pathway are increased in catabolic conditions that are characterized by muscle wasting. In aging subjects or in response to prolonged bed rest, there are increased muscle levels of myostatin a. [70] Myostatin is also increased in muscles of patients with AIDS [71], renal failure, [72,73] or heart failure. [74] Likewise models of cancer cachexia, [64] glucocorticoid administration, [75] mechanical unloading and space flight [76,77] also have high levels of myostatin in muscle. Muscle activin A which can interact with the myostatin receptor is increased in cancer [64] and heart failure. [78] Experimentally, mice given either myostatin or activin A experienced an almost 30% decrease in muscle mass. [64,79] These responses document that both myostatin and activin A influence muscle size. Could their function be blocked by a treatment strategy based on antibodies, including a peptibody, or administration of the myostatin propeptide, follistatin or soluble ActRIIB receptors? The tentative answer is yes because this strategy blocks the muscle wasting induced by different forms of cancer or CKD. [64,73]

Beneficial Responses from Blocking Myostatin Pathway in Cancer Models

Cancer is a "poster child" of muscle wasting since as many as 80% of patients with advanced cancers develop muscle wasting and 25% of cancer-related deaths are ascribed to cachexia. The main mechanism causing loss of muscle mass is acceleration of protein degradation by the UPS, initiated by hormones or cytokines that impair p-Akt signaling. The response to a low p-Akt activates the UPS and caspase-3 to increase muscle protein breakdown (see above). Blocking this pathway can produce remarkable responses. For example, administration of an ActRIIB decoy receptor, blocked both myostatin and **activin A** activity and protected mice from the muscle wasting that is induced by different cancers. Zhou et al. administered an ActRIIB decoy receptor to cancer-bearing mice including CDF1 mice implanted with colon-26 carcinoma, nude mice transplanted with human TOV-21G ovarian carcinoma or human G361 melanoma and inhibin-deficient mice that spontaneously develop gonadal tumors. [64] In each case, muscle wasting was prevented and there was a significant increase in survival. In mice bearing the colon-26 carcinoma, muscle wasting was prevented even though the tumor continued to grow. Secondly, the treatment increased muscle levels of p-Akt and p-FoxO3a, which decreased the transcription of Atrogin-1/MAFbx and MuRF1 (see above). Thirdly, there were improved functions of satellite cells, including an increase in their proliferation. These responses contribute to the rapid reversal of cancer-induced muscle atrophy when ActRIIB signaling is inhibited. Finally, reversal of muscle losses occurred even though circulating levels of TNF-a, IL-1b and IL-6 in the colon-26 were not suppressed. [64] These results suggest that inflammation alone would not interfere with the ability of the ActRIIB decoy receptor to block activin/myostatin actions in muscle.

Beneficial Responses to Blocking Myostatin in Chronic Kidney Disease

CKD exhibits properties that are present in other disorders (e.g., diabetes, starvation and some forms of cancer): there is an increase in circulating markers of inflammation, an increase in glucocorticoid production, impaired insulin/IGF-1signaling and muscle protein wasting. These same catabolic disorders are associated with similar patterns of gene expression in muscles (see above) plus reduced levels of p-Akt and increased expression of Atrogin-1/MAFbx. The result is accelerated muscle proteolysis (see above). Since the muscle level of myostatin is increased by CKD, its contribution to muscle wasting was studied. [72,73] Zhang et al. evaluated a mouse model of CKD (subtotal nephrectomy plus a high protein diet). [73] Mice with BUN values >80 mg/dL were paired for BUN and weight and pair-fed for 4 weeks. In each pair, one mouse with CKD received subcutaneous injections every other day of an anti-myostatin peptibody (a genetically engineered myostatin-neutralizing peptide fused to Fc). The paired mouse was injected with the diluent. Treatment with the peptibody suppressed myostatin in muscle and reversed the loss of body weight while increasing the weights of individual muscles. The mechanisms that prevented muscle atrophy included an increase in the rate of protein synthesis and a decrease in protein degradation. There also were improvements in satellite cell function.

Myostatin inhibition in CKD mice also decreased the circulating levels of inflammatory cytokines and especially, IL-6, unlike the results found in cancer-bearing mice treated with the decoy ActRIIB receptor. The decrease in IL-6 is especially interesting because earlier results indicated that inflammation increased the circulating levels of IL-6 and serum amyloid A. [80] The increase in inflammatory mediators impaired intracellular IGF-1 signaling and decreased muscle levels of p-Akt leading to accelerated protein degradation in muscle. Treatment with the peptibody, therefore, corrected these responses and blocked muscle catabolism.

To understand you myostatin was linked to IL-6, cultured muscle cells were initially treated with TNF-α which initiated a response that raised myostatin production in muscle cells. But, when muscle cells were treated with myostatin, more IL-6 was produced. Therefore, when myostatin was blocked, there was suppression of IL-6 and hence, improved IGF-1 intracellular signaling. This led to an increased level of p-Akt and improved muscle metabolism.

Conclusion

Cancer and catabolic disorders characterized by inflammation, impaired insulin/IGF-1 signaling, increased glucocorticoid production and muscle protein wasting are associated with an increased risk of morbidity and mortality. The physiologic and indeed, the molecular mechanisms that cause muscle protein wasting are being uncovered. Despite these advances, there are no reliable therapies that prevent or reverse the muscle atrophy which contributes to the excessive morbidity and mortality of these disorders. Recent reports suggest we are entering a new era in which blocking myostatin signaling in muscle might prevent a loss of muscle mass and improve survival from catabolic conditions. It is especially exciting that blocking myostatin does not require a genetic manipulation. Instead, myostatin signaling in muscle can be blocked pharmacologically. Although much information about pathophysiology and pharmacology is needed before using such therapy in patients, we are no longer stuck at devising new definitions for the degree of muscle wasting.

References

[1] Division of Kidney UaHDNN. USRDS 2009 Annual data report: atlas of end-stage renal disease in the United States. Bethesda: NIH; 2003.

[2] Go AS, Chertow GM, Fan D, McCulloch CE, Hsu CY. Chronic kidney disease and the risks of death, cardiovascular events, and hospitalization. N Engl J Med 2004 Sep 23;351(13):1296-305.

[3] Evans WJ, Morley JE, Argiles J, Bales C, Baracos V, Guttridge D, et al. Cachexia: a new definition. Clin Nutr 2008 Dec;27(6):793-9.

[4] Lowrie EG, Lew NL. Death risk in hemodialysis patients: The predictive value of commonly measured variables and an evaluation of the death rate differences among facilities. Am J Kid Dis 1990;15:458-82.

[5] Stenvinkel P, Heimburger O, Lindholm B. Wasting, but not malnutrition, predicts cardiovascular mortality in end-stage renal disease. Nephrol Dial Transpl 2004;19:2181-3.

[6] Carrero JJ, Chmielewski M, Axelsson J, Snaedal S, Heimburger O, Barany P, et al. Muscle atrophy, inflammation and clinical outcome in incident and prevalent dialysis patients. Clin Nutr 2008 Aug;27(4):557-64.

[7] Hakim RM, Lazarus JM. Initiation of dialysis. J Am Soc Nephrol 1995;6:1319-20.

[8] Mitch WE. Malnutrition: a frequent misdiagnosis for hemodialysis patients. J Clin Invest 2002;110:437-9.

[9] Fouque D, Kalantar-Zadeh K, Kopple JD, Cano N, Chauveau P, Cuppari L, et al. A proposed nomenclature and diagnostic criteria for protein–energy wasting in acute and chronic kidney disease. Kidney Int 2008 May 9;73:391-8.

[10] Ikizler TA, Pupim LB, Brouillette JR, Levenhagen DK, Farmer K, Hakim RM, et al. Hemodialysis stimulates muscle and whole body protein loss and alters substrate oxidation. Amer J Physiol 2002;282:E107-E116.

[11] Pupim LB, Flakoll PJ, Brouillette JR, Levenhagen DK, Hakim RM, Ikizler TA. Intradialytic parenteral nutrition improves protein and energy homeostasis in chronic hemodialysis patients. J Clin Invest 2002;110:483-92.

[12] Pupim LB, Majchrzak KM, Flakoll PJ, Ikizler TA. Intradialytic oral nutrition improves protein homeostasis in chronic hemodialysis patients with deranged nutritional status. J Am Soc Nephrol 2006 Nov;17(11):3149-57.

[13] Baumeister W, Walz J, Zuhl F, Seemuller E. The proteasome: paradigm of a self-comparmentalizing protease. Cell 1998;92:367-80.

[14] Masud T, Mitch WE. Requirements for protein, calories and fat in the predialysis patient. In: Mitch WE, Ikizler TA, editors. Handbook of Nutrition and the Kidney. 6 ed. Philadelphia: Lippincott-Williams & Wilkins; 2010. p. 92-108.

[15] Kimmel PL, Phillips TM, Simmens SJ, Peterson RA, Weihs KL, Alleyne S, et al. Immunologic function and survival in hemodialysis patients. Kidney Int 1998;54:236-44.

[16] Kaysen GA, Dubin JA, Muller H-G, Rosales L, Levin NW, Mitch WE. Inflammation and reduced albumin synthesis associated with stable decline in serum albumin in hemodialysis patients. Kidney Int 2004;65:1408-15.

[17] Ballmer PE, McNurlan MA, Hulter HN, Anderson SE, Garlick PJ, Krapf R. Chronic metabolic acidosis decreases albumin synthesis and induces negative nitrogen balance in humans. J Clin Invest 1995;95:39-45.

[18] Flier JS, Lowell BB. Obesity research springs a proton leak. Nat Genet 1997;15:223-4.

[19] Movilli E, Zani R, Carli O, Sangalli L, Pola A, Camerini C, et al. Direct effect of the correction of acidosis on plasma parathyroid hormone concentrations, calcium and phosphate in hemodialysis patients: a prospective study. Nephron 2001;87:257-62.

[20] Mitch WE, Goldberg AL. Mechanisms of muscle wasting: The role of the ubiquitin-proteasome system. N Engl J Med 1996;335:1897-905.

[21] Lecker SH, Goldberg AL, Mitch WE. Protein degradation by the ubiquitin-proteasome pathway in normal and disease states. J Am Soc Nephrol 2006;17:1807-19.

[22] Lecker SH, Mitch WE. Proteolysis by the ubiquitin-proteasome system and kidney disease. J Am Soc Nephrol 2011 May;22(5):821-4.

[23] Bodine SC, Latres E, Baumhueter S, Lai VK, Nunez L, Clark BA, et al. Identification of ubiquitin ligases required for skeletal muscle atrophy. Sci 2001;294:1704-8.

[24] Lee SW, Dai G, Hu Z, Wang X, Du J, Mitch WE. Regulation of muscle protein degradation: coordinated control of apoptotic and ubiquitin-proteasome systems by phosphatidylinositol 3 kinase. J Am Soc Nephrol 2004;15:1537-45.

[25] Bailey JL, Price SR, Zheng B, Hu Z, Mitch WE. Chronic kidney disease causes defects in signaling through the insulin receptor substrate/phosphatidylinositol 3-kinase/Akt pathway: implications for muscle atrophy. J Am Soc Nephrol 2006;17:1388-94.

[26] Sacheck JM, Ohtsuka A, McLary SC, Goldberg AL. IGF-1 stimulates muscle growth by suppressing protein breakdown and expression of atrophy-related ubiquitin ligases, atrogin-1 and MuRF1. Am J Physiol 2004;287:E591-E601.

[27] Hu Z, Wang H, Lee IH, Du J, Mitch WE. Endogenous glucocorticoids and impaired insulin signaling are both required to stimulate muscle wasting under pathophysiological conditions in mice. J Clin Invest 2009;119:7650-9.

[28] Sandri M, Sandri C, Gilbert A, Skuck C, Calabria E, Picard A, et al. FoxO transcription factors induce the atrophy-related ubiquitin ligase atrogin-1 and cause skeletal muscle atrophy. Cell 2004;117:399-412.

[29] Cai D, Frantz JD, Tawa NE, Melendez PA, Oh BC, Lidov HG, et al. IKKbeta/NF-kappaB activation causes severe muscle wasting in mice. Cell 2004;119:285-98.

[30] Goodship THJ, Mitch WE, Hoerr RA, Wagner DA, Steinman TI, Young VR. Adaptation to low-protein diets in renal failure: Leucine turnover and nitrogen balance. J Am Soc Nephrol 1990;1:66-75.

[31] May RC, Kelly RA, Mitch WE. Mechanisms for defects in muscle protein metabolism in rats with chronic uremia: The influence of metabolic acidosis. J Clin Invest 1987;79:1099-103.

[32] Bailey JL, Wang X, England BK, Price SR, Ding X, Mitch WE. The acidosis of chronic renal failure activates muscle proteolysis in rats by augmenting transcription of genes encoding proteins of the ATP-dependent, ubiquitin-proteasome pathway. J Clin Invest 1996;97:1447-53.

[33] Lecker SH, Jagoe RT, Gomes M, Baracos V, Bailey JL, Price SR, et al. Multiple types of skeletal muscle atrophy involve a common program of changes in gene expression. FASEB J 2004;18:39-51.

[34] Price SR, Bailey JL, Wang X, Jurkovitz C, England BK, Ding X, et al. Muscle wasting in insulinopenic rats results from activation of the ATP-dependent, ubiquitin-proteasome pathway by a mechanism including gene transcription. J Clin Invest 1996;98:1703-8.

[35] Mitch WE, Bailey JL, Wang X, Jurkovitz C, Newby D, Price SR. Evaluation of signals activating ubiquitin-proteasome proteolysis in a model of muscle wasting. Am J Physiol 1999;276:C1132-C1138.

[36] Sacheck JM, Hyatt JP, Raffaello A, Jagoe RT, Roy RR, Edgerton VR, et al. Rapid disuse and denervation atrophy involve transcriptional changes similar to those of muscle wasting during systemic diseases. FASEB J 2007 Jan;21(1):140-55.

[37] Clarke BA, Drujan D, Willis MS, Murphy LO, Corpina RA, Burova E, et al. The E3 Ligase MuRF1 degrades myosin heavy chain protein in dexamethasone-treated skeletal muscle. Cell Metab 2007 Nov;6(5):376-85.

[38] Solomon V, Goldberg AL. Importance of the ATP-ubiquitin-proteasome pathway in degradation of soluble and myofibrillar proteins in rabbit muscle extracts. J Biol Chem 1996;271:26690-7.

[39] Hotamisligil GS, Peraldi P, Budavari A, Ellis R, White MF, Spielgelman BM. IRS-1-mediated inhibition of insulin receptor tyrosine kinase activity in TNF-a- and obesity-induced insulin resistance. Sci 1996;271:665-8.

[40] Du J, Wang X, Meireles CL, Bailey JL, Debigare R, Zheng B, et al. Activation of caspase 3 is an initial step triggering muscle proteolysis in catabolic conditions. J Clin Invest 2004;113:115-23.

[41] Wang XH, Hu Z, Hu JP, Du J, Mitch WE. Insulin resistance accelerates muscle protein degradation: activation of the ubiquitin-proteasome pathway by defects in muscle cell signaling. Endocrin 2006;147:4160-8.

[42] Workeneh B, Rondon-Berrios H, Zhang L, Hu Z, Ayehu G, Ferrando A, et al. Development of a diagnostic method for detecting increased muscle protein degradation in patients with catabolic conditions. J Am Soc Nephrol 2006;17:3233-9.

[43] Wang XH, Zhang L, Mitch WE, LeDoux JM, Hu J, Du J. Caspase-3 cleaves specific proteasome subunits in skeletal muscle stimulating proteasome activity. J Biol Chem 2010;285:3527-32.

[44] Wei W, Fareed MU, Evenson A, Menconi MJ, Yang H, Petkova V, et al. Sepsis stimulates calpain activity in skeletal muscle by decreasing calpastatin activity but does not activate caspase-3. Am J Physiol Regul Integr Comp Physiol 2005 Mar;288(3):R580-R590.

[45] Tidball JG, Spencer MJ. Expression of a calpastatin transgene slows muscle wasting and obviates changes in myosin isoform expression during murine muscle disuse. J Physiol 2002;545:819-28.

[46] Pickering WP, Price SR, Bircher G, Marinovic AC, Mitch WE, Walls J. Nutrition in CAPD: Serum bicarbonate and the ubiquitin-proteasome system in muscle. Kidney Int 2002;61:1286-92.

[47] Mansoor O, Beaufrere Y, Boirie Y, Ralliere C, Taillandier D, Aurousseau E, et al. Increased mRNA levels for components of the lysosomal, Ca++-activated and ATP-ubiquitin-dependent proteolytic pathways in skeletal muscle from head trauma patients. Proc Natl Acad Sci USA 1996;93:2714-8.

[48] Tiao G, Hobler S, Wang JJ, Meyer TA, Luchette FA, Fischer JE, et al. Sepsis is associated with increased mRNAs of the ubiquitin-proteasome proteolytic pathway in human skeletal muscle. J Clin Invest 1997;99:163-8.

[49] Williams AB, Sun X, Fischer JE, Hasselgren P-O. The expression of genes in the ubiquitin-proteasome proteolytic pathway is increased in skeletal muscle from patients with cancer. Surgery 1999;126:744-9.

[50] Stein A, Moorhouse J, Iles-Smith H, Baker R, Johnstone J, James G, et al. Role of an improvement in acid-base status and nutrition in CAPD patients. Kidney Int 1997;52:1089-95.

[51] Song Y-H, Li Y, Du J, Mitch WE, Rosenthal N, Delafontaine P. Muscle-specific expression of insulin-like growth factor-1 blocks angiotensin II-induced skeletal muscle wasting. J Clin Invest 2005;115:451-8.

[52] Stenvinkel P, Heimburger O, Paultre F, Diczfalusy U, Wang T, Berglund L, et al. Strong association between malnutrition, inflammation and atherosclerosis in chronic kidney failure. Kidney Int 1999;55:1899-911.

[53] May RC, Kelly RA, Mitch WE. Metabolic acidosis stimulates protein degradation in rat muscle by a glucocorticoid-dependent mechanism. J Clin Invest 1986;77:614-21.

[54] Price SR, England BK, Bailey JL, Van Vreede K, Mitch WE. Acidosis and glucocorticoids concomitantly increase ubiquitin and proteasome subunit mRNAs in rat muscle. Am J Physiol 1994;267:C955-C960.

[55] Tiao G, Fagan J, Roegner V, Lieberman M, Wang J-J, Fischer JE, et al. Energy-ubiquitin-dependent muscle proteolysis during sepsis in rats is regulated by glucocorticoids. J Clin Invest 1996;97:339-48.

[56] Bodine SC, Stitt TN, Gonzalez M, Kline WO, Stover GL, Bauerlein R, et al. Akt/mTOR pathway is a crucial regulator of skeletal muscle hypertrophy and can prevent muscle atrophy in vivo. Nat Cell Biol 2001;3:1014-9.

[57] Stitt TN, Drujan D, Clarke BA, Panaro F, Timofeyva Y, Klinenber JR, et al. The IGF-1/PI3K/Akt pathway prevents expression of muscle atrophy-induced ubiquitin ligases by inhibiting FOXO transcription factors. Mol Cell 2004;14:395-403.

[58] Tran H, Brunet A, Griffith EC, Greenberg ME. The many forks in FOXO's road. Sci STKE 2003 Mar 4;2003(172):RE5.

[59] Dardevet DD, Sornet C, Taillandier D, Savary I, Attaix D, Grizard J. Sensitivity and protein turnover response to glucocorticoids are different in skeletal muscle from adult and old rats: Lack of regulation of the ubiquitin-proteasome proteolytic pathway in aging. J Clin Invest 1995;96:2113-9.

[60] Wing SS, Goldberg AL. Glucocorticoids activate the ATP-ubiquitin-dependent proteolytic system in skeletal muscle during fasting. Am J Physiol 1993;264:E668-E676.

[61] Hall-Angeras M, Angeras U, Zamir O, Hasselgren P-O, Fischer JE. Effect of the glucocorticoid receptor antagonist RU 38486 on muscle protein breakdown in sepsis. Surgery 1991;109:468-73.

[62] Tedesco FS, Dellavalle A, az-Manera J, Messina G, Cossu G. Repairing skeletal muscle: regenerative potential of skeletal muscle stem cells. J Clin Invest 2010 Jan;120(1):11-9.

[63] Zhang L, Wang XH, Wang H, Hu Z, Du J, Mitch WE. Satellite cell dysfunction and impaired IGF-1 signaling contribute to muscle atrophy in chronic kidney disease. J Am Soc Nephrol 2010;21:419-27.

[64] Zhou X, Wang JL, Lu J, Song Y, Kwak KS, Jiao Q, et al. Reversal of Cancer Cachexia and Muscle Wasting by ActRIIB Antagonism Leads to Prolonged Survival. Cell 2010 Aug 20;142(4):531-43.

[65] Mahajan A, Simoni J, Sheather SJ, Broglio KR, Rajab MH, Wesson DE. Daily oral sodium bicarbonate preserves glomerular filtration rate by slowing its decline in early hypertensive nephropathy. Kidney Int 2010 Aug;78(3):303-9.

[66] McPherron AC, Lee SJ. Double muscling in cattle due to mutations in the myostatin gene. Proc Natl Acad Sci U S A 1997 Nov 11;94(23):12457-61.

[67] Mosher DS, Quignon P, Bustamante CD, Sutter NB, Mellersh CS, Parker HG, et al. A mutation in the myostatin gene increases muscle mass and enhances racing performance in heterozygote dogs. PLoS Genet 2007 May 25;3(5):e79.

[68] Schuelke M, Wagner KR, Stolz LE, Hubner C, Riebel T, Komen W, et al. Myostatin mutation associated with gross muscle hypertrophy in a child. N Engl J Med 2004 Jun 24;350(26):2682-8.

[69] Binns MM, Boehler DA, Lambert DH. Identification of the myostatin locus (MSTN) as having a major effect on optimum racing distance in the Thoroughbred horse in the USA. Anim Genet 2010 Dec;41 Suppl 2:154-8.

[70] Reardon KA, Davis J, Kapsa RM, Choong P, Byrne E. Myostatin, insulin-like growth factor-1, and leukemia inhibitory factor mRNAs are upregulated in chronic human disuse muscle atrophy. Muscle Nerve 2001 Jul;24(7):893-9.

[71] Gonzalez-Cadavid NF, Taylor WE, Yarasheski K, Sinha-Hikim I, Ma K, Ezzat S, et al. Organization of the human myostatin gene and expression in healthy men and HIV-infected men with muscle wasting. Proc Natl Acad Sci U S A 1998 Dec 8;95(25):14938-43.

[72] Verzola D, Procopio V, Sofia A, Villaggio B, Tarroni A, Bonanni A, et al. Apoptosis and myostatin mRNA are upregulated in the skeletal muscle of patients with chronic kidney disease. Kidney Int 2011 Apr;79(7):773-82.

[73] Zhang L, Rajan V, Lin E, Hu Z, Han HQ, Zhou X, et al. Pharmacological inhibition of myostatin suppresses systemic inflammation and muscle atrophy in mice with chronic kidney disease. FASEB J 2011 May;25(5):1653-63.

[74] Breitbart A, uger-Messier M, Molkentin JD, Heineke J. Myostatin from the heart: local and systemic actions in cardiac failure and muscle wasting. Am J Physiol Heart Circ Physiol 2011 Jun;300(6):H1973-H1982.

[75] Ma K, Mallidis C, Bhasin S, Mahabadi V, Artaza J, Gonzalez-Cadavid N, et al. Glucocorticoid-induced skeletal muscle atrophy is associated with upregulation of myostatin gene expression. Am J Physiol 2003;285:E363-E371.

[76] Carlson CJ, Booth FW, Gordon SE. Skeletal muscle myostatin mRNA expression is fiber-type specific and increases during hind limb unloading. Am J Physiol 1999 Aug;277(2 Pt 2):R601-R606.

[77] Lalani R, Bhasin S, Byhower F, Tarnuzzer R, Grant M, Shen R, et al. Myostatin and insulin-like growth factor-I and -II expression in the muscle of rats exposed to the microgravity environment of the NeuroLab space shuttle flight. J Endocrinol 2000 Dec;167(3):417-28.

[78] Yndestad A, Ueland T, Oie E, Florholmen G, Halvorsen B, Attramadal H, et al. Elevated levels of activin A in heart failure: potential role in myocardial remodeling. Circ 2004 Mar 23;109(11):1379-85.

[79] Zimmers TA, Davies MV, Koniaris LG, Haynes P, Esquela AF, Tomkinson KN, et al. Induction of cachexia in mice by systemically administered myostatin. Sci 2002;296:1486-8.

[80] Zhang L, Du J, Hu Z, Han G, Delafontaine P, Garcia G, et al. IL-6 and serum amyloid A synergy mediates angiotensin II-induced muscle wasting. J Am Soc Nephrol 2009 Mar;20(3):604-12.

In: Issues in Dialysis
Editor: Stephen Z. Fadem

ISBN: 978-1-62417-576-3
© 2013 Nova Science Publishers, Inc.

Chapter XI

The Dysregulated Immune System of Patients on Dialysis

Alexander Grabner, Hermann Pavenstädt,
Detlef Lang and Stefan Reuter[*]
Department of Medicine D, University of Münster, Münster, Germany

Abstract

Patients on dialysis present with diseases directly related to a dysfunctional immune system, a high infectious morbidity, enhanced carcinoma incidence, impaired wound healing, and reduced effect of vaccination. Yet, an activation of the immune system accompanied by elevated systemic inflammatory markers is observed early in renal insufficiency, and increases with progressive chronic kidney disease (CKD). Hence, it is not surprising that the presence of chronic inflammation predicts poor outcome in CKD patients.

In the following, uremia- and dialysis-related factors and mechanisms impacting on different cell types of the immune system (with a focus on monocytes/macrophages) are discussed.

Keywords: immune system, dialysis, end stage renal disease, uremia

Introduction

In consequence of risk factors clustering, morbidity and mortality rates are clearly higher in patients with chronic kidney disease (CKD). CKD is associated with a complex disorder of both the adaptive and innate immune system. CKD-related immune dysfunction is characterized by a coexistence of immune activation (e.g., resulting in low-grade

---

[*] Correspondence to: Stefan Reuter, MedizinischeKlinik und Poliklinik D, 48149 Münster, Germany. Phone: +49-251-83-56983; fax: +49-251-83-56973; E-mail: sreuter@uni-muenster. de

inflammation associated with cardiovascular diseases) as well as immune suppression (e.g., contributing to the high prevalence of infections among these patients). In a large study including 252,516 Canadian outpatients, James et al. showed that the risks of hospitalization and death after pneumonia were increased in patients with CKD and increased significantly with decreasing glomerular filtration rate (eGFR). [1] Especially patients on hemodialysis (HD) present with a high infectious morbidity, enhanced carcinoma incidence, impaired wound healing and poor response to vaccination - disease entities directly related to immunodeficiency. [2-6] Thus, it was not surprising that dialysis was identified in an Australian study including approximately 23,000 cardiac surgical procedures as an independent risk factor for deep sternal wound infections. [7] On the other hand, hypercytokinemia-related immune activation plays a decisive role. Elevated systemic inflammatory markers such as C-reactive protein (CRP) and interleukin-6 (IL-6) can already be observed in acute renal insufficiency and at early stages of chronic renal insufficiency further increasing with progression of CKD. [8-11] Even in end stage renal disease (ESRD) inflammatory serum markers still correlate to residual kidney function (as assessed in patients on peritoneal dialysis. [12-14]) as well as to the length of the HD session (as assessed in patients on chronic HD. [15,16] However, it remains controversial whether ESRD or HD-related elevation of CRP directly translates into increased mortality. [17-19] One contributing factor might be that CRP is in fact excreted in low amounts with the urine. Correspondingly, excretion of pro-inflammatory urinary soluble IL-6 receptor declines with kidney function. [20,21] Interestingly, basal IL-6 synthesis from monocytes equals in CKD and healthy subjects. [22] Nevertheless, due to decreased renal elimination mainly pro-inflammatory cytokines accumulate. Thus, decreasing kidney function per se might be individually more or less responsible for hypercytokinemia.

Despite a controversial debate about the adequate biomarkers and factors involved, it is widely accepted that high CKD mortality is associated with persistent systemic inflammation.

CKD patients experience a chronic activation of the acute phase response usually related to an activated immune state. To sum up, the immune system is on one hand handicapped while on the other hand alert.

Not surprisingly, malfunction of leukocytes is an attribute of patients on dialysis. [23,24] Nearly all types of leukocytes have been characterized to suffer in these patients as it is evident e.g., by reduced phagocytosis and intracellular killing capability of granulocytes and macrophages, decreased anti-apoptotic potential of monocytes, shortened lymphocyte survival, and inhibition of plasma cell and suppressor T-cell activity. Since monocytes/macrophages (Mphi) are major effectors of the immune system with widespread microbicidal and tumoricidal functions that are altered in uremia we herein focus on Mphi. [24-28]

Roughly divided, factors impairing the host defence in patients on dialysis are related to 1) patients' underlying renal disease, 2) uremia, 3) oxidative stress 4) medication 5) catabolism and malnutrition, and 6) HD-related factors. Except for renal diseases, these factors and mechanisms impacting on different cell types of the immune system are discussed in the following.

Immune System

The immune system consists of two major components, the innate (non-specific) and the adaptive (specific) immune system. While the innate immune system builds up the initial defense against pathogenic invaders (rapid response), the adaptive immune system acts as a second line of defense (slow response). Moreover, working as an immunological memory it provides protection in cases of re-exposure. Both systems rely on cellular, humoral, and in case of the innate immune system, anatomical effectors which are necessary for appropriate immunocompetence. Although both parts of the immune system have defined functions, they act synergistically driven by interactions and cross-talks through e. g. cytokines, chemokines and antibodies, between each other.

Uremic Stress

Uremia-derived immune dysfunction is characterized by a coexistence of hypercytokinemia-related immune activation as well as immune suppression. On the one hand uremic toxins, oxidative stress, volume overload, and comorbidities correspond to an increased monokine generation. [29,30] On the other hand, the uremic milieu and its toxins impact directly or via bone marrow toxicity on immunocompetent cells. This is described in the following.

Innate Immune System

In HD patients, cells of the innate immune system, e. g., granulocytes, mast cells, Mphi, and natural killer cells, present decreased chemotactic, phagocytotic, and bactericidal activities. [31] Under uremic conditions granulocytes respond to a phagocytotic challenge with reduced production of reactive oxygen species (ROS). [32] and tend to higher rates of spontaneous cell death. [33] In contrast, a dysbalance between apoptosis and necrosis of neutrophils is observed when uremia delays apoptosis execution. Thereby, neutrophils are driven into (secondary) necrosis, a promoter of inflammation. [34] However, if the net effect of neutrophil death in the uremic milieu is calculated, one can observe that the overall apoptosis rate of normal neutrophils in uremic plasma is accelerated. [33] Among uremic solutes mainly middle weight proteins have been identified to affect granulocyte function. For instance, granulocyte inhibiting protein GIP I and GIP II inhibit granulocyte glucose uptake thereby suppressing respiratory burst activity. [35] In addition, Mphi are those immune cells which are mostly affected by uremia. Recently, Lim et al. have shown that uremia impairs endocytosis and maturation of monocytes, whereas IL-12 production and consecutive allogeneic T-cell proliferation increase. [36] Moreover, inducible nitric oxide synthase, an effector molecule of macrophages` cytotoxicity, is directly inhibited by urea. [37]

Heat shock protein (HSP) expression is an important cytoprotective, anti-apoptotic mechanism of Mphi against stress. We and others have demonstrated that the HSP72 stress response of monocytes from patients on HD as well as from uremic rats is impaired, therefore, possibly contributing to immune dysfunction. [24,38] However, the dysfunction of innate immunity is not only characterized by suppression but also by a complex mechanism of activation. On non-cellular level, mannose-binding lectin, an activator of the complement cascade, is significantly increased in the serum of uremic patients. [39] Furthermore, expression of endocytic pattern recognition receptors such as macrophage scavenger receptor and scavenge receptor CD36, both known to play pivotal roles in atherogenesis and foam cell formation, is increased in ESRD patients resulting in an accelerated atherosclerosis development. [40,41] Mphi play a key role in promoting low-grade inflammation. Typically, monocytes in HD patients are "preactivated" and release cytokines such as of IL1-ß, IL-6, IL-12, and TNF-α. [42] Among the various uremic toxins, advanced glycosylation endproducts (AGEs) have been identified to preactivate monocytes. For instance, AGE-modified ß2-microglobulin promotes monocytic migration and cytokine secretion. [43], whereas guanidino compounds stimulate TNF-α production. [44] Other AGEs such as carboxyethyllysine and carboxymethyllysine increase the production of free radicals by monocytic cells. [45]

Hyperhomocysteinemia is a common feature of CKD. In macrophages, homocysteine activates nuclear factor-kappaB (NF- B) resulting in sustained superoxide anion production and consecutive oxidative stress. [46] On the other hand, p-cresol, a phenolic compound retained in uremia, suppresses leukocyte activity. Interestingly, when used as a serum marker, higher concentrations of free p-cresol are independently associated with increased mortality in HD patients. [47] Interestingly, recent studies revealed that most of the p-cresol produced by intestine cells conjugates to p-cresylglucuronide and p-cresylsulfate, which on the contrary have been shown to activate free radical production of leukocytes. [48] Nevertheless, in earlier studies p-cresol level and p-cresylsulfate serum level correlated. Thus, serum p-cresol concentration might still serve as a valid clinical outcome parameter. [49,50]

IL-10 is a potent deactivator of monocytes playing a key role for inflammation limitation and preactivation. When produced by monocytes it decreases the secretion of other cytokines, thereby forming a negative feedback mechanism. [51] In HD patients, the number of regulatory monocytes (i.e. monocytes producing IL-10 and not IL-6) is low. [52] Nevertheless, data regarding the sheer amount of IL-10 produced by monocytes from HD patients is controversial. [52,53] Interestingly, interindividual differences in IL-10 production seem to translate into clinical consequences. Patients with low IL-10 levels present with higher levels of pro-inflammatory cytokines. It is these patients in particular, who develop more artherosclerosis than individuals with high IL-10 serum level. [54] Since there is a genetic determination for IL-10 production (cytokine promotor polymorphisms leading to low or high production), genetic factors affecting the immune system and clinical outcome from HD patients might be involved, too. [55]

Adaptive Immune System

The adaptive immune system consists of B- and T-lymphocytes comprising a highly specified system with the ability to recognize and remember pathogens and therefore providing an effective immune response to known pathogens. It is well-known that ESRD patients' susceptibility to infection is increased, while their response to vaccination is decreased. This indicates an impairment of the adaptive immunity population. Current data suggest that mainly T-lymphocytes and antigen presenting cells (APC) are affected. Despite an often observed mild lymphopenia, the leukocyte number is usually normal in HD patients. In vitro, a uremic milieu decreases T-cell proliferation and increases the susceptibility of B-cells to apoptosis. [56,57] However, serum antibody levels of ESRD patients are not reduced in principle, indicating in fact that the humoral immunity primarily seems to be intact. [58] In contrast, T-cell function and differentiation is severely disturbed. T helper (Th) cells play a decisive role in controlling the immune response. Th1 cells, for instance, produce pro-inflammatory cytokines like TNF-α, IL-12, and IFN-γ, thereby activating macrophages and neutrophils. Th2 lymphocytes promote the humoral immunity mainly via IL-4 and IL-5 release. [59] In ESRD patients an increased Th1/Th2 ratio due to significantly elevated Th1 levels is assessed. [60] This dysbalance favors especially an impairment of B-cell function after immunization by means of reduced antibody production contributing to the clinically often disappointing response to vaccination. [61,62] Moreover, the increased Th1 level enhances monocyte preactivation which promotes low grade inflammation and artherosclerosis. [29] The increase in Th1/Th2 ratio is probably linked to IL-12 overproduction by macrophages. [63] IL-12 activates INF-γ and inhibits IL-4 production of T-cells. [64], thereby driving their differentiation towards Th1 type and polarizing the complex interacting disturbances of innate and adaptive immunity. An extensive review focusing on the disturbance of the adaptive immune system has recently been published by Eleftheriadis et al. [65]

Toll-like Receptors

Toll-like receptors (TLRs) belong to the group of cellular signaling pattern-recognition receptors of the innate immune system. They recognize various pathogens by binding to LPS or viral DNA resulting in phagocytosis, activation of complement, or mediation of cytokine production (e. g., of IL-1ß, IL-6, and TNF-α) of the hosting cell. [66] Being involved in dendritic cell maturation and in presentation of antigens to lymphocytes, TLRs link the innate and the adaptive immune system. Toll-like receptor 4 (TLR4) recognizing bacterial LPS is probably the most widely studied member of the TLR family. Since one can observe a decreased antigen presentation capability of dendritic cells in uremia, a reduced expression or an impaired function of TLRs can be assumed. Indeed, in monocytes of predialysis patients TLR4 expression is reduced along with cytokine production in response to LPS challenge. [67] Consistently, TLR2 expression is decreased in monocytes of patients on peritoneal dialysis. [68] Its suppressed expression was linked to uremic stress and chronic stimulation with endotoxins. [68]

HSP70 proteins are potent immune adjuvants (released e. g. upon tissue damage) regulating the immune-response. HSP70 also increases the expression of TLR4. [69,70] Because HSP expression response of monocytes is impaired in a uremic milieu, a reduced HSP72 response to stress might cause less effective recognition of harmful antigens and less activation of TLR4-dependent pathways. [24]

Table 1. Dysregulation of the immune system in uremia

Activation on cellular level		
Cellular type	Mechanism	Reference
Monocytes	Release of IL.1-β, IL.-6, IL.12, TNF-α	[42]
	AGE-modified B2-microglobulin promotes migration	[43]
	Guanidino compounds stimulate TNF-α production	[44]
	Hyperhomocysteinemia activates NF-κB	[46]
	Carboxyethyllysine and carboxymethyllysine increase free radical production	[45]
	P-cresylglucuronide and P-cresylsulfate activate free radical production	[48]
	Upregulation of macrophage scavenger receptor and CD36	[40,41]
	AOPPs stimulate TNF-α production	[75]
	Advanced LDL oxidation induces chemotaxis	[43]
	Elevated intracellular iron activates NF-κB	[76]
B-Lymphocytes	Increased Autoantibodies	[77-79]
	Advanced LDL oxidation induces synthesis of autoantibodies	[80]
T-Lymphocytes	Th1 cell elevation due to high IL12 increases Inf-γ production	[64,65]
Suppression on cellular level		
Granulocytes	Reduced chemotaxis, phagocytosis, production of ROS	[31,32]
	Increased apoptosis	[33]
	GIP I & II inhibit respiratory burst activity	[35]
	Downregulation of opsonin receptors via ROS	[81]
	Iron overload reduces phagocytosis and myeloperoxidaes activity	[82]
Monocytes	Impaired endocytosis and maturation	[36]
	Decreased iNOS synthesis	[37]
	Iron overload inhibits iNOS synthesis	[83]
	Decreased HSP72 synthesis	[24,38]
	P-cresol inhibits activity	[47]
	TLR4 & 2 expression decreased	[67,68]
B-Lymphocytes	Increased apoptosis	[56,57]
	Poor antibody response to vaccines	[61,62]
T-Lymphocytes	Th2 cell suppression leads to decreased IL4 and 5 production	[59]

Moreover, TLRs are important regulators of costimulatory molecules such as CD80 or CD86 of dendritic cells or macrophages. [71] Hence, this could serve as a reasonable explanation why the antigen presenting capabilities of these cells with related impaired T-lymphocyte function is affected. However, not only suppression but also activation of TLRs is present in uremia. TLR4 has recently been reported to recognize dietary saturated fatty acids. [72] Moreover, several endogenous ligands (e. g. liberated in ischemia by necrotic cells, heat-shock proteins, and extracellular matrix breakdown products) are able to mediate TLR-induced expression of inflammatory genes and trigger dendritic cell maturation. [73] As if that were not enough factors involved, potentially several uremic toxins could serve as TLR-activating ligands, too. [74]

Table 1 provides a brief summary of the dysregulation of the innate and adaptive immunity on cellular level.

Oxidative Stress

Oxidative stress can be defined as an imbalance of prooxidants and antioxidants within cells, tissues or the whole organism towards oxidation. On the one hand, ROS and reactive nitrogen species (RNS) are elevated by increased production via NAPDH oxidases and myeloperoxidases due to uremia-associated metabolic abnormalities, HD per se, and drugs (iron and erythropoietins). [84,85] On the other hand, important antioxidants such as tocopherol, carotenoids, ascorbic acid, selenium, and others are reduced because of loss during HD and reduced intake due to imposed dietary restriction. This prooxidative constellation leads to increased lipoprotein oxidation, carbamylation, and advanced oxidation protein products (AOPPs). In vitro, AOPPs retain the capacity to activate monocyte respiratory burst and TNF production, thus indicating that AOPPs may themselves act as pro-inflammatory mediators. [75] Advanced LDL oxidation provokes antigenicity, thereby initiating synthesis of antibodies against oxidized LDL. These play a pathogenic role in the development of artherosclerosis by means of Mphi activation, formation of foam cells, and proliferation of vascular smooth muscle cells. [80] This induces monocyte chemotaxis and increases secretion of inflammatory cytokines by macrophages. [43] Furthermore, progressive lipoprotein oxidation reduces the amount of intact, yet not that of oxidized lipoproteins. These have been demonstrated to protect against inflammation by binding to and neutralizing circulating LPS. [86] As already mentioned, elevated LPS bioactivity leads to a pro-inflammatory cytokine activation cascade. Further, increased generation of ROS and chlorinated oxidants via NADPH oxidases and myeloperoxidases leads to down regulation of opsonin receptors of neutrophils, resulting in impaired chemotaxis, adhesion, migration, phagocytosis, and bactericidal activities. [81]

Iron Load

Anemia is an almost universal complication of CKD usually worsening with initiation of HD. In the preerythropoetin era periodic blood transfusions and regular iron substitution were necessary for consequent treatment, both affecting immunity. The immunosuppressive effect of blood transfusions initially observed by improving graft survival after kidney transplantation in the precyclosporine era was confirmed by the suppression of delayed type hypersensitivity skin tests. [87] as well as by impaired lymphocyte function in vitro. For instance, lymphocytes from multitransfused patients exhibited a significant lower MLC (mixed lymphocyte culture) reactivity. [88] Although the precise mechanisms still remain unclear, there is evidence that blood transfusions impact on immunity via induction of regulatory CD4+ T-cells which recognize allopeptides. These affect the activated T-cells directly or indirectly by their modulatory effect on dendritic cells. [89] Another common complication of frequent blood transfusion is iron overload. At present, iron overload may complicate parenteral iron therapy which is recommended in iron-depleted HD patients receiving recombinant erythropoietins (erythropoiesis stimulating agents, ESA) Iron overload is associated with elevated susceptibility to bacterial infections affecting both innate and adaptive immunity. [90] Iron effects on the innate anti-microbial defense have been studied recently. It is well known that iron is conducive to bacterial growth, but also inhibits the expression of inducible nitric oxide synthase (iNOS). [83] On the other hand, elevated intracellular iron promotes the activation of the key immune response regulator NF- B. [76] Further, HIF-1α, a transcription factor regulating the expression of inflammatory cytokines and anti-microbial peptides produced by macrophages, is iron-regulated. Here, low intracellular iron concentrations (e. g. iron deprivation in HD patients is common due to lower intestinal iron absorption, greater iron losses, and require a larger iron turnover to maintain the ESA-driven red cell mass than do healthy individuals. [91]) lead to HIF-1α induced gene expression by preventing the degradation of the transcription factor. [92] Thus, iron within Mphi is critically involved in their defense armory against pathogens as iron catalyzes the formation of toxic hydroxyl radicals, modifies the binding affinity of transcription factors and affects cellular metabolism via modifying the activity of citric acid cycle enzymes and oxidative phosphorylation. Notably, inflammation-related iron retention within macrophages is a key mechanism for the development of anemia in chronic diseases. The role of iron metabolism of Mphi in inflammation has been recently reviewed by Weiss. [93]

Neutrophils and lymphocytes functions are negatively affected by iron overload as seen by functional impairment, e. g., reduced phagocytosis and myeloperoxidase activity. [82] In patients with hereditary hemochromatosis iron overload decreases the level of circulating CD8+ lymphocytes [94], whereas in experimental rodent settings the lymphocyte numbers do not seem to be affected. However, it was proposed that proliferative and cytokine responses are reduced. [95] At least, in patients on HD, data about iron load and its related impact on acquired immunity needs further clarification.

Erythropoiesis Stimulating Agents

ESA help to avoid complications of blood transfusions. However, ESA themselves impact on the immune system as demonstrated by the fact that administration of ESA is associated with an increased immune response to hepatitis B virus (HBV) vaccination (higher antibody titer). Interestingly, alterations of CD4+ and CD8+ T-lymphocytes as well as B-lymphocytes of patients receiving ESA have been detected. It was shown that ESA lead to increased CD8+ T-cell apoptosis via TNF-α stimulation. This promotes a favorable

CD4+/CD8+ ratio positively correlating with anti-HBs antibody titer. [96] Further, CD4+ cells treated with ESA exhibit increased proliferation, differentiation to Th1 Lymphocytes, and production of IL-2 and IL-12. [97] Consistently, monocyte preactivation in cell culture is decreased, because cells responded to phytohemagglutinin stimulation with only low IL-6 and TNF-α level. [98] Further, treatment with ESA induces the expression of HSP70, a strong anti-apoptotic and cytoprotective chaperone, in heart and kidney. [99,100] Taken together several clinical and experimental studies confirm a positive modulatory effect of ESA on the immune system of HD patients.

Vitamin D Metabolism

Vitamin D and its analogs (widely used in ESRD patients for treatment of secondary hyperparathyreoidism) impact on the innate and adaptive immunity, too. For instance, when exposed to Vitamin D macrophages develop enhanced chemotactic and phagocytic activity. [101] as well as an upregulated production of anti-microbial proteins such as cathelicidin. [102] It is of note that cholecalciferol therapy reduced circulating levels of inflammatory cytokines including IL-8, IL-6, and TNF in patients on HD. [103] Broken down to the level of APC and T-cells, a complex modulation of the adaptive immunity is observed. For instance, Vitamin D inhibits the production of Th1 cytokines while it stimulates the production of Th2 ones. Although Vitamin D-related alteration of T-cell response inevitably affects the B-cell line, too, one can observe additional direct effects of Vitamin D like inhibition of B-cell proliferation, plasma cell differentiation, and production of immunoglobulins. [104] A comprehensive review on the complex mechanisms of Vitamin D modulation of the immune system has been recently published. [105] Nevertheless, the effect of Vitamin D administration on the acquired immunity needs further elucidation. [65]

Further Medication

Apart from reducing blood pressure, angiotensin converting enzyme inhibitors (ACEI) treatment modulates the immunity of ESRD patients as well. For instance, in CAPD patients, total and subset lymphocyte counts changed under ACEI treatment. [106] Further impacts on T-cells and Mphi have been discussed. In experimental autoimmune encephalomyelitis, a blockade of ACE induced potent regulatory T-cells modulating Th1 cell-mediated autoimmunity. [107] Correspondingly, on the one hand ACEI therapy in chronic heart failure patients is associated with a reduction of IL-6 and TNF-α, on the other hand T helper cells were affected since Th1/Th2 cytokine ratios decrease. [108] Angiotensin II receptor blocker affect lymphocyte proliferation and production of interferon-γ as well, thereby suppressing Th1 and Th2 immune response. [109,110] Moreover, ACE inhibition seems somehow anti-inflammatory because macrophages release less IL-6 after coronary artery graft surgery in patients treated with ACE inhibitors. [111] In accordance, a reduction of serum TNF-α as well as CRP was observed in advanced CKD patients treated with ACEI. [112] Further, ACEI lead to a reduction of soluble (inflammatory) cell adhesion molecules like sVCAM-1 and sICAM-1, which in ESRD patients are independent predictors of all cause and cardiovascular death. [113] This was confirmed in cell culture models as well. [114] However, a detailed review on angiotensin II modulation of inflammation and immunity has recently been published elsewhere. [115]

In the following, we briefly discuss a few additional drugs widely used in patients on HD. Several of these drugs seem to modulate the immune system as suggested by treatment studies analyzing serum cytokines. However, detailed data on their mechanism on cellular level in patients on HD is still missing.

Sevelamer, a frequently used phosphate binding drug, may have immunomodulatory side effects. There is few data showing a sevelamer-related decrease in serum CRP and an increase in fetuin-A levels. [116,117] This could be due to endotoxin/LPS binding which in turn reduces pro-inflammatory stimuli and cytokine levels. [118,119] Pleiotropic effects of statins are widely discussed in the literature. It was stated that statins not only inhibit cholesterol synthesis but exert anti-inflammatory and anti-oxidative properties in HD patients. [120,121] However, as this did not translate into an effect on survival (e. g. 4D study), further studies are needed for a final evaluation. [122] Interestingly, acetylsalicylic acid decreases serum IL-6, IL-8, and TNF-α levels in HD patients. [123] Further, Vitamin E and N-acetylcysteine, two antioxidants potentially inhibiting cytokine release. [124,125], have been shown to reduce cardiovascular events in HD patients. [126,127] Moreover, low molecular heparin seems to reduce oxidative stress and inflammation in HD patients. [128]

Finally, it remains self-evident that patients on HD necessitating immunosuppressive therapy exhibit an altered immune system by means of treatment.

Catabolism and Malnutrition

Protein-energy-malnutrition and wasting (referred to as kidney disease wasting) are frequently present in ESRD patients. In the HD collective, between 23% to 76% of patients are reported to be malnourished. [129] Malnutrition in ESRD patients is usually the consequence of a various number of catabolic mechanisms stimulated by renal insufficiency. Apart from poor food intake (i.e. true malnutrition), uremia is associated with anorexia, nausea, vomiting, and loss of appetite. This is due to uremic toxicity which causes delayed gastric emptying (neuropathy) and hormonal derangements. Especially insulin resistance in diabetics and inadequate control of acidosis lead to a hypercatabolic state with hypoalbuminemia and a consecutive loss of lean body mass. However, even when uremia and acidosis are treated with dialysis, wasting occurs. This is related to dialysis treatment per se (e. g. HD alters protein turnover and amino acid transport kinetics) and to chronic inflammation playing a decisive role in the development of wasting. Since wasting and inflammation act hand in hand most likely in an equicausal status, malnutrition-inflammation complex syndrome (MICS) or malnutrition, inflammation, and atherosclerosis (MIA) syndrome are appropriate terms referring to their underlying complex mechanisms. Generally, nutrient deficiencies are associated with impaired immune responses. In particular, lymphopenia is very common and is considered as a malnutrition marker that indicates very poor prognosis in HD patients. [130] In addition, lymphocyte transformation correlates directly with blood urea nitrogen, creatinine, and albumin as well as with midarm muscle circumference, suggesting that nutritional status also may influence lymphocyte function in uremic patients. For instance, McMurray et al. have shown that malnutrition leads to an impaired blastogenic response of peripheral blood lymphocytes. [131]

In critically ill, a low plasma glutamine level impairs monocyte function leading to substantial immunosuppression. [132,133] Glutamine deprivation increases Mphi' susceptibility to stress and apoptosis, as well as it reduces their responsiveness to stimuli. [133] Glutamine starving reduces thermoresistance (to fever) of Mphi that is, according to Pollheimer et al., caused by impaired HSP70 response. [132] Thus, one can assume that glutamine depletion contributes to the reduced HSP72-heat shock response and favors apoptosis as demonstrated in patients' Mphi. [24] Further, weight loss may also be associated with reduced skeletal muscle oxidative metabolism, leading to a mitigated anti-oxidant defense. [134] Because MICS leads to a low body mass index, hypocholesterolemia, hypocreatininemia, and hypohomocysteinemia, a "reverse epidemiology" of cardiovascular risks can occur in dialysis patients, also known as „obesity paradox", indicating that obesity, hypercholesterolemia, and increased blood levels of creatinine and homocysteine appear to be protective and paradoxically associated with a better outcome. [135] Possible causes of this phenomenon include a) time-discrepancies between the competing risks for adverse events that are associated with overnutrition and undernutrition or MICS, respectively, b) sequestration/storage of uremic toxins in fat tissue, c) selection of a gene pool favorable to longer survival in dialysis patients during the course of CKD progression, which eliminates over 95% of the CKD population before they commence dialysis therapy, d) a more stable hemodynamic status, e) alterations in circulating cytokines, f) unique neurohormonal constellations, and g) endotoxin–lipoprotein interactions (higher concentrations of total cholesterol (lipoproteins) are beneficial for HD patients, since a richer pool of lipoproteins can actively bind to and remove circulating endotoxins). Therefore, the increased pool of lipoproteins may attenuate the harmful effects of endotoxins which cause inflammation and subsequence atherosclerosis if unbound. [136]

Immune Dysfunction in Chronic Kidney Disease

Causes of immune dysfunction in CKD patients and potential links between immunosuppression and immunoactivation. An immunosuppressed state leads to chronic/recurrent or subclinical infection whereas chronic inflammation is associated with increased artherosclerosis and cardiovascular disease, both leading to increased mortality. AMC: arterial media calcification

Dialysis-Related Factors

Infections

It is not only the immune defect contributing to the infectious burden of HD patients but also the accumulation of risk factors in this population which frequently leads to microbial challenges. For instance, HD induces systemic circulatory stress and recurrent regional intestinal ischemia. This may increase endotoxin translocation from the gut. [137] Resultant endotoxemia is associated with systemic inflammation, oxidative stress, markers of malnutrition, cardiac injury, and reduced survival. Besides, blood born virus infections occur. Since infections impact on the immune system e. g., by activation or alteration of leukocyte functions or induction of apoptosis, some common ones are briefly discussed. [25,138]

Staphylococcus aureus

Staphylococcus aureus carriage (with the anterior nares being the locus of choice to test) can play a key role in the pathogenesis of staphylococcal infections such as bacteremia. [139] While in the general population a prevalence rate of approximately 35% for S. aureus nasal carriage can be assessed, subgroups of patients with increased rates include those with insulin-dependent diabetes mellitus, those on intravenous drugs, chronic ambulatory peritoneal dialysis or HD. [140,141] A clearly higher carriage rate in the nose and on the skin has been reported for such patients. [142,143] Therefore, it is not surprising that S. aureus is a major cause of bacteremia among HD patients. One contributing factor is the requirement for intermittent vascular access for prolonged time periods including repeated vascular access punctures, prosthetic arteriovenous grafts, and significant higher prevalence rates of vascular catheters. Vascular access increases the risk for bacteremia, hospitalization, and mortality. [143-145] Complications include a disease pattern such as sepsis, endocarditis, osteomyelitis, septic arthritis, peritonitis, and metastatic abscesses. Thus, the immune system of HD patients is chronically activated, as it is frequently confronted with bacteremia. In this context antimicrobial therapy is often commenced. This increases the risk of bacterial resistances and the spread of nosocomial infections to other patients.

Hepatitis

The prevalence of hepatitis in maintenance hemodialysis patients substantially exceeds that in the general population and transmission among patients undergoing hemodialysis has frequently been documented. [146,147] Risk factors are the immune defect, the high prevalence of hepatitis B virus (HBV) and HCV infections in dialysis centers, blood transfusions, long-term dialysis treatment (contamination of equipment or of the hands of the staff members), frequent changes of HD units, and previous renal transplants. [147] In addition to reduced vaccination response (HBV), anti-HBs levels decline faster after immunization in HD patients compared with healthy individuals, such that in approximately 40% of responsive patients the levels are undetectable at one or three years, respectively. [147] Treatment (viral eradication or persistent suppression of viral replication) remains challenging because of altered pharmacokinetics and the increased risk of drug-related toxicity. HCV-RNA-positive patients showed lowest albumin and highest CRP levels and ESA requirements in a study of 111 HD patients. [148] Moreover, alloantigen presentation by monocytes from HCV-infected patients results in lower production of IL-17 by CD4+ T-cells. It was therefore concluded by Chung et al. that chronic stimulation of APCs with HCV core protein is associated with hyporesponsiveness in TLR-mediated innate immunity. [149] On the other hand, overexpression of TLR2 and TLR4 in addition to increased cytokine production of monocytes (TNF-α, IL-6, IL-8) after TLR challenge was assessed in chronic HCV patients as compared with controls. Despite a higher number of Tregs, T-cell exhaustion related to chronic HBV/HCV infections might also contribute. [150,151]

Human Immunodeficiency Virus (HIV)

The prevalence of HIV/AIDS is significantly higher in patients on HD than in the general population. [152] 2002 national surveillance data of dialysis-associated diseases in the United States showed that nearly 2% of HD patients were HIV positive. Since HIV mainly affects CD4+ T helper cells patients suffer more often from (opportunistic) infections and malignancy.

Cytomegalovirus

CMV diseases predominantly occur as opportunistic infections in patients with severe immunosuppression, such as renal failure patients. Among others, risk factors for CMV infection are blood transfusion and HD. [153,154] It has been suggested that latent infections with CMV or other herpes viruses, which persist for lifetime in infected individuals, are the main driving force for the generation of senescent CD8+ T-lymphocytes. [155]

Membrane-related Activation and Bioincompatibility

Several factors are involved in triggering the inflammatory process including those arising from dialysis treatment itself, mainly membrane-related activation and dialysate biocompatibility.

In HD, a large artificial surface area is exposed to blood. Therefore, interactions between blood components and the dialyzer membrane influence the immune system in several ways. The exposure of blood to the artificial surface results among others in the activation of coagulation and complement cascade. [156] Complement activation has been linked to the release of cytokines like IL-1ß and TNF-α by Mphi which get activated either due to contact with the dialyzer membrane or by compliment. Shear stress is one factor altering mononuclear cells so that they respond stronger to subsequent exposure to endotoxin. [157] An increase of these circulating cytokine levels can be assessed early after onset of HD. [158] Inconsistent results have been published regarding acute effects of HD session on up- or downregulation of apoptotic genes in leukocytes. According to Friedrich et al., the mRNA expression of pro-apoptotic genes like death receptor CD95/Fas, the death receptor 5 (DR5), and caspase 8 increases in leukocytes during HD. [159] Nevertheless, Andreoli et al. could not find an impact of dialyzer biocompatibility on spontaneous polymorphonuclear cells (PNM) apoptosis and function, cytokine synthesis by peripheral blood mononuclear cells (PBMC) or on their serum levels, serum levels of C3a, and terminal complement complex. [160] However, post HD serum levels of complement correlated negatively with PMN phagocytosis and peroxide production, and positively with PMN apoptosis and cytokine production by PBMC. In monocytes, we could neither detect dialysis session-dependent HSP72 induction (stimulation of this major anti-stress and anti-apoptotic HSP70 family member protein) nor find elevated baseline HSP72 in patients or rats with renal insufficiency. [24] One explanation for these different results can be the different reuse practices of dialyzers. Rao et al. found that the reuse process of polysulphone-based dialyzers can influence the oxidative response of PMN, whereas the type of bleach–germicide combination during reuse was associated with the phagocytosis index. However, in this study, PMN from patients dialyzed with polysulphone or cuprophane membranes showed higher respiratory burst activity compared to with those exposed to substituted cellulose (cellulose acetate or cellulose triacetate) membranes, regardless of dialyzer reuse. [161]

In contrast, Carracedo et al. criticized that cellulosic membranes in particularly affect mononuclear cells and lead to an induction of cell activation markers such as: increased production of pro-inflammatory cytokines, adhesion molecules, CD14 receptor, and phosphorylation of surface molecules. Moreover, cellulosic HD membranes may induce spontaneous apoptosis in normal mononuclear cells and mononuclear cells from HD patients while repeated in vivo stimulation during HD induces a process of replicative senescence. [162]

Another finding by Soriano et al. was that lymphocyte apoptosis is influenced not only by the biocompatibility, but also by the permeability of the dialysis membrane. [163]

One additional underestimated problem might be related to dialyzer membrane-caused complement-mediated cell sequestration (into dialyzer and lungs) which was extensively elucidated in neutrophils and monocytes. [164-168] For instance, within 20 minutes of HD, the numbers of circulating monocytes decreased in a study by Girndt et al. by two third. The remaining monocytes responded significantly weaker to LPS and surface marker studies revealed that mainly mature monocytes were removed. Thus, maybe fully differentiated cells capable of cytokine production and antigen presentation are removed whereas relatively immature cells remain in circulation. [168]

Another factor contributing to chronic inflammation may be the exposure of blood to impure dialysis fluid. Dialysate purity has rightly been a concern since the beginning of dialysis treatment because samples have frequently been demonstrated to be contaminated with bacterial-originated DNA fragments. Bacterial DNA fragments can be assessed in the blood of HD patients, and if detected they are associated with increased CRP and IL-6 levels in these individuals. [169,170] Interestingly, when the effects of non-sterile (mean endotoxin content SEM 97 $\pm$ 22 EU/ml) and ultrapure bicarbonate dialysate on cytokine serum level and PNM and Mphi activation markers (sterile and pyrogen-free, obtained by ultrafiltration through polyamide) were compared no difference was measured. [171] The authors conclude that complement cleavage products play the major role in HD-related leukocyte activation. In contrast, when Guo et al. compared conventional dialysate and high purity dialysate they detected increased monocyte apoptosis and cell inflammation when cells were incubated with conventional dialysate. Notably, conventional dialysate contained nearly tenfold more bacteria than high purity dialysate while there was no difference in endotoxin levels. [172] In this context it might be relevant that high flux dialyzers may promote backdiffusion rather than backfiltration thereby enhancing endotoxin transport through the membrane into the patient. [173]

However, if membranes- or dialysate-related activation (of pro-apoptotic pathways) is relevant in general, or is related to different types of PNM remains unclear. Despite this discussion, Sardenberg et al. stated that the higher apoptosis rate from PMN from pre-dialysis ESRD patients can be corrected by dialysis (CAPD or HD), because these patients displayed PMN apoptosis rates similar to controls. [174] One should also keep in mind that a large collective of HD patients do not exhibit significant activation of the inflammatory response, although all patients are exposed to dialysis membranes and dialysates. Thus, Kaysen suggested that patient-specific processes, such as the type of vascular access, unrecognized infections, or variable responses to the dialyzer used, may be of importance. [175]

Conclusion

It is out of question that the immune system of CKD and especially of HD-patients is dysregulated. It features signs of overactivation (chronic microinflammation, MICS, and MIA) as well as signs of malfunction (impairing the host defence against infections, enhanced carcinoma incidence, impaired wound healing, and reduced effect of vaccination) The cause of immune dysfunction is likely to be multifactorial. Effects sharing in are most likely mediated by uremic toxins, persistent endotoxin and microbial challenge, artificial surface (dialyzer)-related leukocyte activation and sequestration, shear stress, changes in serum protein structure, function, composition, and metabolism, alterations in endothelial function, nutrition and multiple medications. Therapeutic manipulation of immune balance under uremic conditions is thus a major challenge harboring potential beneficial effects on life quality and prognosis of patients on HD.

References

[1] James MT, Quan H, Tonelli M, Manns BJ, Faris P, Laupland KB, et al. CKD and risk of hospitalization and death with pneumonia. Am J Kidney Dis. 2009 Jul;54(1):24-32.

[2] Barraclough KA, Wiggins KJ, Hawley CM, van Eps CL, Mudge DW, Johnson DW, et al. Intradermal versus intramuscular hepatitis B vaccination in hemodialysis patients: a prospective open-label randomized controlled trial in nonresponders to primary vaccination. Am J Kidney Dis. 2009 Jul;54(1):95-103.

[3] Mandayam S, Shahinian VB. Are chronic dialysis patients at increased risk for cancer? J Nephrol. 2008 Mar;21(2):166-74.

[4] Vajdic CM, McDonald SP, McCredie MR, van Leeuwen MT, Stewart JH, Law M, et al. Cancer incidence before and after kidney transplantation. JAMA. 2006 Dec 20;296(23):2823-31.

[5] Cheung AH, Wong LM. Surgical infections in patients with chronic renal failure. Infect Dis Clin North Am. 2001 Sep;15(3):775-96.

[6] Powe NR, Jaar B, Furth SL, Hermann J, Briggs W. Septicemia in dialysis patients: incidence, risk factors, and prognosis. Kidney Int. 1999 Mar;55(3):1081-90.

[7] Robinson PJ, Billah B, Leder K, Reid CM. Factors associated with deep sternal wound infection and haemorrhage following cardiac surgery in Victoria. Interact Cardiovasc Thorac Surg. 2007 Apr;6(2):167-71.

[8] Gueret G, Lion F, Guriec N, Arvieux J, Dovergne A, Guennegan C, et al. Acute renal dysfunction after cardiac surgery with cardiopulmonary bypass is associated with plasmatic IL6 increase. Cytokine. 2009 Feb;45(2):92-8.

[9] Costa E, Rocha S, Rocha-Pereira P, Nascimento H, Castro E, Miranda V, et al. Neutrophil activation and resistance to recombinant human erythropoietin therapy in hemodialysis patients. Am J Nephrol. 2008;28(6):935-40.

[10] Uzun H, Konukoglu D, Besler M, Erdenen F, Sezgin C, Muderrisoglu C. The effects of renal replacement therapy on plasma, asymmetric dimethylarginine, nitric oxide and C-reactive protein levels. Clin Invest Med. 2008;31(1):E1-E7.

[11] Lacson E Jr, Levin NW. C-reactive protein and end-stage renal disease. Semin Dial. 2004 Nov;17(6):438-48.

[12] Perez-Flores I, Coronel F, Cigarran S, Herrero JA, Calvo N. Relationship between residual renal function, inflammation, and anemia in peritoneal dialysis. Adv Perit Dial. 2007;23:140-3.

[13] Wang AY, Wang M, Woo J, Lam CW, Lui SF, Li PK, et al. Inflammation, residual kidney function, and cardiac hypertrophy are interrelated and combine adversely to enhance mortality and cardiovascular death risk of peritoneal dialysis patients. J Am Soc Nephrol. 2004 Aug;15(8):2186-94.

[14] Chung SH, Heimburger O, Stenvinkel P, Qureshi AR, Lindholm B. Association between residual renal function, inflammation and patient survival in new peritoneal dialysis patients. Nephrol Dial Transplant. 2003 Mar;18(3):590-7.

[15] Caglar K, Peng Y, Pupim LB, Flakoll PJ, Levenhagen D, Hakim RM, et al. Inflammatory signals associated with hemodialysis. Kidney Int. 2002 Oct;62(4):1408-16.

[16] Docci D, Bilancioni R, Buscaroli A, Baldrati L, Capponcini C, Mengozzi S, et al. Elevated serum levels of C-reactive protein in hemodialysis patients. Nephron. 1990;56(4):364-7.

[17] Meuwese CL, Halbesma N, Stenvinkel P, Dekker FW, Molanaei H, Qureshi AR, et al. Variations in C-reactive protein during a single haemodialysis session do not associate with mortality. Nephrol Dial Transplant. 2010 Nov;25(11):3717-23.

[18] Korevaar JC, vanManen JG, Dekker FW, de Waart DR, Boeschoten EW, Krediet RT. Effect of an increase in C-reactive protein level during a hemodialysis session on mortality. J Am Soc Nephrol. 2004 Nov;15(11):2916-22.

[19] Herselman M, Esau N, Kruger JM, Labadarios D, Moosa MR. Relationship between serum protein and mortality in adults on long-term hemodialysis: exhaustive review and meta-analysis. Nutrition. 2010 Jan;26(1):10-32.

[20] Ortiz RM, Mamalis A, Navar LG. Aldosterone Receptor Antagonism Reduces Urinary C-Reactive Protein Excretion in Angiotensin II-Infused, Hypertensive Rats. J Am Soc Hypertens. 2009 May;3(3):184-91.

[21] Motie M, Schaul KW, Potempa LA. Biodistribution and clearance of 125I-labeled C-reactive protein and 125I-labeled modified C-reactive protein in CD-1 mice. Drug Metab Dispos. 1998 Oct;26(10):977-81.

[22] Memoli B, Postiglione L, Cianciaruso B, Bisesti V, Cimmaruta C, Marzano L, et al. Role of different dialysis membranes in the release of interleukin-6-soluble receptor in uremic patients. Kidney Int. 2000 Jul;58(1):417-24.

[23] Goldblum SE, Reed WP. Host defenses and immunologic alterations associated with chronic hemodialysis. Ann Intern Med. 1980 Oct;93(4):597-613.

[24] Reuter S, Bangen P, Edemir B, Hillebrand U, Pavenstadt H, Heidenreich S, et al. The HSP72 stress response of monocytes from patients on haemodialysis is impaired. Nephrol Dial Transplant. 2009 Sep;24(9):2838-46.

[25] Reuter S, Lang D. Life span of monocytes and platelets: importance of interactions. Front Biosci. 2009;14:2432-47.

[26] Schmidt S, Westhoff TH, Krauser P, Ignatius R, Jankowski J, Jankowski V, et al. The uraemic toxin phenylacetic acid impairs macrophage function. Nephrol Dial Transplant. 2008 Nov;23(11):3485-93.

The Dysregulated Immune System of Patients on Dialysis 183

[27] Heidenreich S, Schmidt M, Bachmann J, Harrach B. Apoptosis of monocytes cultured from long-term hemodialysis patients. Kidney Int. 1996 Mar;49(3):792-9.

[28] Athlin L, Domellof L. The phagocytic process of human peritoneal macrophages in cancer or uremia. Acta Pathol Microbiol Immunol Scand C. 1986 Apr;94(2):63-8.

[29] Stenvinkel P, Ketteler M, Johnson RJ, Lindholm B, Pecoits-Filho R, Riella M, et al. IL-10, IL-6, and TNF-alpha: central factors in the altered cytokine network of uremia--the good, the bad, and the ugly. Kidney Int. 2005 Apr;67(4):1216-33.

[30] Kimmel PL, Phillips TM, Simmens SJ, Peterson RA, Weihs KL, Alleyne S, et al. Immunologic function and survival in hemodialysis patients. Kidney Int. 1998 Jul;54(1):236-44.

[31] Vanholder R, Ringoir S, Dhondt A, Hakim R. Phagocytosis in uremic and hemodialysis patients: a prospective and cross sectional study. Kidney Int. 1991 Feb;39(2):320-7.

[32] Anding K, Gross P, Rost JM, Allgaier D, Jacobs E. The influence of uraemia and haemodialysis on neutrophil phagocytosis and antimicrobial killing. Nephrol Dial Transplant. 2003 Oct;18(10):2067-73.

[33] Cendoroglo M, Jaber BL, Balakrishnan VS, Perianayagam M, King AJ, Pereira BJ. Neutrophil apoptosis and dysfunction in uremia. J Am Soc Nephrol. 1999 Jan;10(1):93-100.

[34] Glorieux G, Vanholder R, Lameire N. Uraemic retention and apoptosis: what is the balance for the inflammatory status in uraemia? Eur J Clin Invest. 2003 Aug;33(8):631-4.

[35] Cohen G, Haag-Weber M, Horl WH. Immune dysfunction in uremia. Kidney Int. Suppl 1997 Nov;62:S79-S82.

[36] Lim WH, Kireta S, Leedham E, Russ GR, Coates PT. Uremia impairs monocyte and monocyte-derived dendritic cell function in hemodialysis patients. Kidney Int. 2007 Nov;72(9):1138-48.

[37] Prabhakar SS, Zeballos GA, Montoya-Zavala M, Leonard C. Urea inhibits inducible nitric oxide synthase in macrophage cell line. Am J Physiol. 1997 Dec;273(6 Pt 1):C1882-C1888.

[38] Marzec L, Zdrojewski Z, Liberek T, Bryl E, Chmielewski M, Witkowski JM, et al. Expression of Hsp72 protein in chronic kidney disease patients. Scand J Urol Nephrol. 2009;43(5):400-8.

[39] Satomura A, Endo M, Ohi H, Sudo S, Ohsawa I, Fujita T, et al. Significant elevations in serum mannose-binding lectin levels in patients with chronic renal failure. Nephron. 2002;92(3):702-4.

[40] Chmielewski M, Bryl E, Marzec L, Aleksandrowicz E, Witkowski JM, Rutkowski B. Expression of scavenger receptor CD36 in chronic renal failure patients. Artif Organs. 2005 Aug;29(8):608-14.

[41] Ando M, Gafvels M, Bergstrom J, Lindholm B, Lundkvist I. Uremic serum enhances scavenger receptor expression and activity in the human monocytic cell line U937. Kidney Int. 1997 Mar;51(3):785-92.

[42] Girndt M, Kohler H, Schiedhelm-Weick E, Schlaak JF, Meyer zumBuschenfelde KH, Fleischer B. Production of interleukin-6, tumor necrosis factor alpha and interleukin-10 in vitro correlates with the clinical immune defect in chronic hemodialysis patients. Kidney Int. 1995 Feb;47(2):559-65.

[43] Miyata T, Inagi R, Iida Y, Sato M, Yamada N, Oda O, et al. Involvement of beta 2-microglobulin modified with advanced glycation end products in the pathogenesis of hemodialysis-associated amyloidosis. Induction of human monocyte chemotaxis and macrophage secretion of tumor necrosis factor-alpha and interleukin-1. J Clin Invest. 1994 Feb;93(2):521-8.

[44] Glorieux GL, Dhondt AW, Jacobs P, Van LJ, Lameire NH, De Deyn PP, et al. In vitro study of the potential role of guanidines in leukocyte functions related to atherogenesis and infection. Kidney Int. 2004 Jun;65(6):2184-92.

[45] Glorieux G, Helling R, Henle T, Brunet P, Deppisch R, Lameire N, et al. In vitro evidence for immune activating effect of specific AGE structures retained in uremia. Kidney Int. 2004 Nov;66(5):1873-80.

[46] Au-Yeung KK, Yip JC, Siow YL, O K. Folic acid inhibits homocysteine-induced superoxide anion production and nuclear factor kappa B activation in macrophages. Can J Physiol Pharmacol. 2006 Jan;84(1):141-7.

[47] Bammens B, Evenepoel P, Keuleers H, Verbeke K, Vanrenterghem Y. Free serum concentrations of the protein-bound retention solute p-cresol predict mortality in hemodialysis patients. Kidney Int. 2006 Mar;69(6):1081-7.

[48] Schepers E, Meert N, Glorieux G, Goeman J, Van der EJ, Vanholder R. P-cresylsulphate, the main in vivo metabolite of p-cresol, activates leucocyte free radical production. Nephrol Dial Transplant. 2007 Feb;22(2):592-6.

[49] Ketteler M. Kidney failure and the gut: p-cresol and the dangers from within. Kidney Int. 2006 Mar;69(6):952-3.

[50] Vanholder R, Van LS, Glorieux G. What is new in uremic toxicity? Pediatr Nephrol. 2008 Aug;23(8):1211-21.

[51] Brunet P, Capo C, Dellacasagrande J, Thirion X, Mege JL, Berland Y. IL-10 synthesis and secretion by peripheral blood mononuclear cells in haemodialysis patients. Nephrol Dial Transplant. 1998 Jul;13(7):1745-51.

[52] Girndt M, Sester U, Kaul H, Kohler H. Production of proinflammatory and regulatory monokines in hemodialysis patients shown at a single-cell level. J Am Soc Nephrol. 1998 Sep;9(9):1689-96.

[53] Perianayagam MC, Jaber BL, Guo D, King AJ, Pereira BJ, Balakrishnan VS. Defective interleukin-10 synthesis by peripheral blood mononuclear cells among hemodialysis patients. Blood Purif. 2002;20(6):543-50.

[54] Seyrek N, Karayaylali I, Balal M, Paydas S, Aikimbaev K, Cetiner S, et al. Is there any relationship between serum levels of interleukin-10 and atherosclerosis in hemodialysis patients? Scand J Urol Nephrol. 2005;39(5):405-9.

[55] Girndt M, Sester U, Sester M, Deman E, Ulrich C, Kaul H, et al. The interleukin-10 promoter genotype determines clinical immune function in hemodialysis patients. Kidney Int. 2001 Dec;60(6):2385-91.

[56] Stachowski J, Pollok M, Burrichter H, Spithaler C, Baldamus CA. Signalling via the TCR/CD3 antigen receptor complex in uremia is limited by the receptors number. Nephron. 1993;64(3):369-75.

[57] Fernandez-Fresnedo G, Ramos MA, Gonzalez-Pardo MC, de Francisco AL, Lopez-Hoyos M, Arias M. B lymphopenia in uremia is related to an accelerated in vitro apoptosis and dysregulation of Bcl-2. Nephrol Dial Transplant. 2000 Apr;15(4):502-10.

[58] Okasha K, Saxena A, el Bedowey MM, Shoker AS. Immunoglobulin G subclasses and susceptibility to allosensitization in humans. Clin Nephrol. 1997 Sep;48(3):165-72.

[59] Mosmann TR, Sad S. The expanding universe of T-cell subsets: Th1, Th2 and more. Immunol Today. 1996 Mar;17(3):138-46.

[60] Sester U, Sester M, Hauk M, Kaul H, Kohler H, Girndt M. T-cell activation follows Th1 rather than Th2 pattern in haemodialysis patients. Nephrol Dial Transplant. 2000 Aug;15(8):1217-23.

[61] Stevens CE, Alter HJ, Taylor PE, Zang EA, Harley EJ, Szmuness W. Hepatitis B vaccine in patients receiving hemodialysis. Immunogenicity and efficacy. N Engl J Med. 1984 Aug 23;311(8):496-501.

[62] Kohler H, Arnold W, Renschin G, Dormeyer HH, Meyer zumBuschenfelde KH. Active hepatitis B vaccination of dialysis patients and medical staff. Kidney Int. 1984 Jan;25(1):124-8.

[63] Hsieh CS, Macatonia SE, Tripp CS, Wolf SF, O'Garra A, Murphy KM. Development of TH1 CD4+ T cells through IL-12 produced by Listeria-induced macrophages. Science. 1993 Apr 23;260(5107):547-9.

[64] Seder RA, Gazzinelli R, Sher A, Paul WE. Interleukin 12 acts directly on CD4+ T cells to enhance priming for interferon gamma production and diminishes interleukin 4 inhibition of such priming. Proc Natl Acad Sci USA. 1993 Nov 1;90(21):10188-92.

[65] Eleftheriadis T, Antoniadi G, Liakopoulos V, Kartsios C, Stefanidis I. Disturbances of acquired immunity in hemodialysis patients. Semin Dial. 2007 Sep;20(5):440-51.

[66] Pasare C, Medzhitov R. Toll-like receptors: linking innate and adaptive immunity. Microbes Infect. 2004 Dec;6(15):1382-7.

[67] Ando M, Shibuya A, Tsuchiya K, Akiba T, Nitta K. Reduced expression of Toll-like receptor 4 contributes to impaired cytokine response of monocytes in uremic patients. Kidney Int. 2006 Jul;70(2):358-62.

[68] Kuroki Y, Tsuchida K, Go I, Aoyama M, Naganuma T, Takemoto Y, et al. A study of innate immunity in patients with end-stage renal disease: special reference to toll-like receptor-2 and -4 expression in peripheral blood monocytes of hemodialysis patients. Int J Mol Med. 2007 May;19(5):783-90.

[69] Bangen JM, Schade FU, Flohe SB. Diverse regulatory activity of human heat shock proteins 60 and 70 on endotoxin-induced inflammation. BiochemBiophys Res Commun. 2007 Aug 3;359(3):709-15.

[70] Schmitt E, Gehrmann M, Brunet M, Multhoff G, Garrido C. Intracellular and extracellular functions of heat shock proteins: repercussions in cancer therapy. J Leukoc Biol. 2007 Jan;81(1):15-27.

[71] Girndt M, Sester M, Sester U, Kaul H, Kohler H. Defective expression of B7-2 (CD86. on monocytes of dialysis patients correlates to the uremia-associated immune defect. Kidney Int. 2001 Apr;59(4):1382-9.

[72] Tschop M, Thomas G. Fat fuels insulin resistance through Toll-like receptors. Nat Med. 2006 Dec;12(12):1359-61.

[73] Beg AA. Endogenous ligands of Toll-like receptors: implications for regulating inflammatory and immune responses. Trends Immunol. 2002 Nov;23(11):509-12.

[74] Hauser AB, Stinghen AE, Kato S, Bucharles S, Aita C, Yuzawa Y, et al. Characteristics and causes of immune dysfunction related to uremia and dialysis. Perit Dial Int. 2008 Jun;28 Suppl 3:S183-S187.

[75] Witko-Sarsat V, Friedlander M, Nguyen KT, Capeillere-Blandin C, Nguyen AT, Canteloup S, et al. Advanced oxidation protein products as novel mediators of inflammation and monocyte activation in chronic renal failure. J Immunol. 1998 Sep 1;161(5):2524-32.

[76] Vallabhapurapu S, Karin M. Regulation and function of NF-kappaB transcription factors in the immune system. Annu Rev Immunol. 2009;27:693-733.

[77] Nolph KD, Husted FC, Sharp GC, Siemsen AW. Antibodies to nuclear antigens in patients undergoing long-term hemodialysis. Am J Med. 1976 May 10;60(5):673-6.

[78] Fabrizi F, Sangiorgio R, Pontoriero G, Corti M, Tentori F, Troina E, et al. Antiphospholipid (aPL) antibodies in end-stage renal disease. J Nephrol. 1999 Mar;12(2):89-94.

[79] Sunder-Plassmann G, Kapiotis S, Gasche C, Klaar U. Functional characterization of cytokine autoantibodies in chronic renal failure patients. Kidney Int. 1994 May;45(5):1484-8.

[80] Maggi E, Bellazzi R, Falaschi F, Frattoni A, Perani G, Finardi G, et al. Enhanced LDL oxidation in uremic patients: an additional mechanism for accelerated atherosclerosis? Kidney Int. 1994 Mar;45(3):876-83.

[81] scamps-Latscha B, Jungers P, Witko-Sarsat V. Immune system dysregulation in uremia: role of oxidative stress. Blood Purif. 2002;20(5):481-4.

[82] Waterlot Y, Cantinieaux B, Hariga-Muller C, De Maertelaere-Laurent E, Vanherweghem JL, Fondu P. Impaired phagocytic activity of neutrophils in patients receiving haemodialysis: the critical role of iron overload. Br Med J. (Clin Res Ed. 1985 Aug 24;291(6494):501-4.

[83] Dlaska M, Weiss G. Central role of transcription factor NF-IL6 for cytokine and iron-mediated regulation of murine inducible nitric oxide synthase expression. J Immunol. 1999 May 15;162(10):6171-7.

[84] Chen HC, Tsai JC, Tsai JH, Lai YH. Recombinant human erythropoietin enhances superoxide production by FMLP-stimulated polymorphonuclear leukocytes in hemodialysis patients. Kidney Int. 1997 Nov;52(5):1390-4.

[85] Canaud B, Cristol J, Morena M, Leray-Moragues H, Bosc J, Vaussenat F. Imbalance of oxidants and antioxidants in haemodialysis patients. Blood Purif. 1999;17(2-3):99-106.

[86] Rauchhaus M, Coats AJ, Anker SD. The endotoxin-lipoprotein hypothesis. Lancet. 2000 Sep 9;356(9233):930-3.

[87] Valderrabano F, Anaya F, Perez-Garcia R, Olivas E, Vasconez F, Jofre R. Transfusion-induced anergy: skin test as an index for pretransplant transfusions. Proc Eur Dial Transplant Assoc. 1983;20:338-48.

[88] Fehrman I, Ringden O. Lymphocytes from multitransfused uremic patients have poor MLC reactivity. Tissue Antigens. 1981;17(4):386-95.

[89] Roelen D, Brand A, Claas FH. Pretransplant blood transfusions revisited: a role for CD(4+. regulatory T cells? Transplantation. 2004 Jan 15;77(1 Suppl):S26-S28.

[90] Seifert A, von HD, Schaefer K. Iron overload, but not treatment with desferrioxamine favours the development of septicemia in patients on maintenance hemodialysis. Q J Med. 1987 Dec;65(248):1015-24.

[91] Besarab A, Coyne DW. Iron supplementation to treat anemia in patients with chronic kidney disease. Nat Rev Nephrol. 2010 Dec;6(12):699-710.

The Dysregulated Immune System of Patients on Dialysis 187

[92] Nizet V, Johnson RS. Interdependence of hypoxic and innate immune responses. Nat Rev Immunol. 2009 Sep;9(9):609-17.

[93] Weiss G. Iron metabolism in the anemia of chronic disease. Biochim Biophys Acta. 2009 Jul;1790(7):682-93.

[94] Macedo MF, Porto G, Costa M, Vieira CP, Rocha B, Cruz E. Low numbers of CD8+ T lymphocytes in hereditary haemochromatosis are explained by a decrease of the most mature CD8+ effector memory T cells. Clin Exp Immunol. 2010 Mar;159(3):363-71.

[95] Mencacci A, Cenci E, Boelaert JR, Bucci P, Mosci P, Fe dC, et al. Iron overload alters innate and T helper cell responses to Candida albicans in mice. J Infect Dis. 1997 Jun;175(6):1467-76.

[96] Sennesael JJ, Van der NP, Verbeelen DL. Treatment with recombinant human erythropoietin increases antibody titers after hepatitis B vaccination in dialysis patients. Kidney Int. 1991 Jul;40(1):121-8.

[97] Bryl E, Mysliwska J, bska-Slizien A, Trzonkowski P, Rachon D, Bullo B, et al. Recombinant human erythropoietin stimulates production of interleukin 2 by whole blood cell cultures of hemodialysis patients. Artif Organs. 1999 Sep;23(9):809-16.

[98] Trzonkowski P, Mysliwska J, bska-Slizien A, Bryl E, Rachon D, Mysliwski A, et al. Long-term therapy with recombinant human erythropoietin decreases percentage of CD152(+. lymphocytes in primary glomerulonephritis haemodialysis patients. Nephrol Dial Transplant. 2002 Jun;17(6):1070-80.

[99] Xu B, Dong GH, Liu H, Wang YQ, Wu HW, Jing H. Recombinant human erythropoietin pretreatment attenuates myocardial infarct size: a possible mechanism involves heat shock Protein 70 and attenuation of nuclear factor-kappaB. Ann Clin Lab Sci. 2005;35(2):161-8.

[100] Yang CW, Li C, Jung JY, Shin SJ, Choi BS, Lim SW, et al. Preconditioning with erythropoietin protects against subsequent ischemia-reperfusion injury in rat kidney. FASEB J. 2003 Sep;17(12):1754-5.

[101] Xu H, Soruri A, Gieseler RK, Peters JH. 1,25-Dihydroxyvitamin D3 exerts opposing effects to IL-4 on MHC class-II antigen expression, accessory activity, and phagocytosis of human monocytes. Scand J Immunol. 1993 Dec;38(6):535-40.

[102] Martineau AR, Wilkinson KA, Newton SM, Floto RA, Norman AW, Skolimowska K, et al. IFN-gamma- and TNF-independent vitamin D-inducible human suppression of mycobacteria: the role of cathelicidin LL-37. J Immunol. 2007 Jun 1;178(11):7190-8.

[103] Stubbs JR, Idiculla A, Slusser J, Menard R, Quarles LD. Cholecalciferol supplementation alters calcitriol-responsive monocyte proteins and decreases inflammatory cytokines in ESRD. J Am Soc Nephrol. 2010 Feb;21(2):353-61.

[104] Chen S, Sims GP, Chen XX, Gu YY, Chen S, Lipsky PE. Modulatory effects of 1,25-dihydroxyvitamin D3 on human B cell differentiation. J Immunol. 2007 Aug 1;179(3):1634-47.

[105] Baeke F, Takiishi T, Korf H, Gysemans C, Mathieu C. Vitamin D: modulator of the immune system. Curr Opin Pharmacol. 2010 Aug;10(4):482-96.

[106] Grzegorzewska AE, Leander M. Lymphocyte subset counts in continuous ambulatory peritoneal dialysis patients in relation to administration of recombinant human erythropoietin and angiotensin-converting enzyme inhibitors. Adv Perit Dial. 2002;18:6-11.

[107] Platten M, Youssef S, Hur EM, Ho PP, Han MH, Lanz TV, et al. Blocking angiotensin-converting enzyme induces potent regulatory T cells and modulates TH1- and TH17-mediated autoimmunity. Proc Natl Acad Sci USA. 2009 Sep 1;106(35):14948-53.

[108] Gage JR, Fonarow G, Hamilton M, Widawski M, Martinez-Maza O, Vredevoe DL. Beta blocker and angiotensin-converting enzyme inhibitor therapy is associated with decreased Th1/Th2 cytokine ratios and inflammatory cytokine production in patients with chronic heart failure. Neuroimmunomodulation. 2004;11(3):173-80.

[109] Sagawa K, Nagatani K, Komagata Y, Yamamoto K. Angiotensin receptor blockers suppress antigen-specific T cell responses and ameliorate collagen-induced arthritis in mice. Arthritis Rheum. 2005 Jun;52(6):1920-8.

[110] Nataraj C, Oliverio MI, Mannon RB, Mannon PJ, Audoly LP, Amuchastegui CS, et al. Angiotensin II regulates cellular immune responses through a calcineurin-dependent pathway. J Clin Invest. 1999 Dec;104(12):1693-701.

[111] Brull DJ, Sanders J, Rumley A, Lowe GD, Humphries SE, Montgomery HE. Impact of angiotensin converting enzyme inhibition on post-coronary artery bypass interleukin 6 release. Heart. 2002 Mar;87(3):252-5.

[112] Stenvinkel P, Andersson P, Wang T, Lindholm B, Bergstrom J, Palmblad J, et al. Do ACE-inhibitors suppress tumour necrosis factor-alpha production in advanced chronic renal failure? J Intern Med. 1999 Nov;246(5):503-7.

[113] Suliman ME, Qureshi AR, Heimburger O, Lindholm B, Stenvinkel P. Soluble adhesion molecules in end-stage renal disease: a predictor of outcome. Nephrol Dial Transplant. 2006 Jun;21(6):1603-10.

[114] Soehnlein O, Schmeisser A, Cicha I, Reiss C, Ulbrich H, Lindbom L, et al. ACE inhibition lowers angiotensin-II-induced monocyte adhesion to HUVEC by reduction of p65 translocation and AT 1 expression. J Vasc Res. 2005 Sep;42(5):399-407.

[115] Benigni A, Cassis P, Remuzzi G. Angiotensin II revisited: new roles in inflammation, immunology and aging. EMBO Mol Med. 2010 Jul;2(7):247-57.

[116] Caglar K, Yilmaz MI, Saglam M, Cakir E, Acikel C, Eyileten T, et al. Short-term treatment with sevelamer increases serum fetuin-a concentration and improves endothelial dysfunction in chronic kidney disease stage 4 patients. Clin J Am SocNephrol. 2008 Jan;3(1):61-8.

[117] Stinghen AE, Goncalves SM, Bucharles S, Branco FS, Gruber B, Hauser AB, et al. Sevelamer decreases systemic inflammation in parallel to a reduction in endotoxemia. Blood Purif. 2010;29(4):352-6.

[118] Perianayagam MC, Jaber BL. Endotoxin-binding affinity of sevelamer hydrochloride. Am J Nephrol. 2008;28(5):802-7.

[119] Sun PP, Perianayagam MC, Jaber BL. Endotoxin-binding affinity of sevelamer: a potential novel anti-inflammatory mechanism. Kidney Int. Suppl 2009 Dec;(114):S20-S25.

[120] Vernaglione L, Cristofano C, Muscogiuri P, Chimienti S. Does atorvastatin influence serum C-reactive protein levels in patients on long-term hemodialysis? Am J Kidney Dis. 2004 Mar;43(3):471-8.

[121] Stenvinkel P, Rodriguez-Ayala E, Massy ZA, Qureshi AR, Barany P, Fellstrom B, et al. Statin treatment and diabetes affect myeloperoxidase activity in maintenance hemodialysis patients. Clin J Am SocNephrol. 2006 Mar;1(2):281-7.

[122] Wanner C, Krane V, Marz W, Olschewski M, Mann JF, Ruf G, et al. Atorvastatin in patients with type 2 diabetes mellitus undergoing hemodialysis. N Engl J Med. 2005 Jul 21;353(3):238-48.

[123] Goldstein SL, Leung JC, Silverstein DM. Pro- and anti-inflammatory cytokines in chronic pediatric dialysis patients: effect of aspirin. Clin J Am SocNephrol. 2006 Sep;1(5):979-86.

[124] Lappas M, Permezel M, Rice GE. N-Acetyl-cysteine inhibits phospholipid metabolism, proinflammatory cytokine release, protease activity, and nuclear factor-kappaB deoxyribonucleic acid-binding activity in human fetal membranes in vitro. J Clin Endocrinol Metab. 2003 Apr;88(4):1723-9.

[125] Jiang Q, Elson-Schwab I, Courtemanche C, Ames BN. gamma-tocopherol and its major metabolite, in contrast to alpha-tocopherol, inhibit cyclooxygenase activity in macrophages and epithelial cells. Proc Natl Acad Sci USA. 2000 Oct 10;97(21):11494-9.

[126] Tepel M, van der GM, Statz M, Jankowski J, Zidek W. The antioxidant acetylcysteine reduces cardiovascular events in patients with end-stage renal failure: a randomized, controlled trial. Circ. 2003 Feb 25;107(7):992-5.

[127] Boaz M, Smetana S, Weinstein T, Matas Z, Gafter U, Iaina A, et al. Secondary prevention with antioxidants of cardiovascular disease in endstage renal disease (SPACE): randomised placebo-controlled trial. Lancet. 2000 Oct 7;356(9237):1213-8.

[128] Poyrazoglu OK, Dogukan A, Yalniz M, Seckin D, Gunal AL. Acute effect of standard heparin versus low molecular weight heparin on oxidative stress and inflammation in hemodialysis patients. Ren Fail. 2006;28(8):723-7.

[129] Schoenfeld PY, Henry RR, Laird NM, Roxe DM. Assessment of nutritional status of the National Cooperative Dialysis Study population. Kidney Int. Suppl 1983 Apr;(13):S80-S88.

[130] Reddan DN, Klassen PS, Szczech LA, Coladonato JA, O'Shea S, Owen WF, Jr., et al. White blood cells as a novel mortality predictor in haemodialysis patients. Nephrol Dial Transplant. 2003 Jun;18(6):1167-73.

[131] McMurray DN, Loomis SA, Casazza LJ, Rey H, Miranda R. Development of impaired cell-mediated immunity in mild and moderate malnutrition. Am J Clin Nutr. 1981 Jan;34(1):68-77.

[132] Pollheimer J, Zellner M, Eliasen MM, Roth E, Oehler R. Increased susceptibility of glutamine-depleted monocytes to fever-range hyperthermia: the role of 70-kDa heat shock protein. Ann Surg. 2005 Feb;241(2):349-55.

[133] Eliasen MM, Brabec M, Gerner C, Pollheimer J, Auer H, Zellner M, et al. Reduced stress tolerance of glutamine-deprived human monocytic cells is associated with selective down-regulation of Hsp70 by decreased mRNA stability. J Mol Med. 2006 Feb;84(2):147-58.

[134] Imbeault P, Tremblay A, Simoneau JA, Joanisse DR. Weight loss-induced rise in plasma pollutant is associated with reduced skeletal muscle oxidative capacity. Am J Physiol Endocrinol Metab. 2002 Mar;282(3):E574-E579.

[135] Kalantar-Zadeh K, Kopple JD. Obesity paradox in patients on maintenance dialysis. Contrib Nephrol. 2006;151:57-69.

[136] Niebauer J, Volk HD, Kemp M, Dominguez M, Schumann RR, Rauchhaus M, et al. Endotoxin and immune activation in chronic heart failure: a prospective cohort study. Lancet. 1999 May 29;353(9167):1838-42.

[137] McIntyre CW, Harrison LE, Eldehni MT, Jefferies HJ, Szeto CC, John SG, et al. Circulating Endotoxemia: A Novel Factor in Systemic Inflammation and Cardiovascular Disease in Chronic Kidney Disease. Clin J Am SocNephrol. 2010 Sep 28.

[138] DeLeo FR. Modulation of phagocyte apoptosis by bacterial pathogens. Apoptosis. 2004 Jul;9(4):399-413.

[139] Wertheim HF, Vos MC, Ott A, van BA, Voss A, Kluytmans JA, et al. Risk and outcome of nosocomial Staphylococcus aureus bacteraemia in nasal carriers versus non-carriers. Lancet. 2004 Aug 21;364(9435):703-5.

[140] Nouwen JL, van BA, Verbrugh HA. Determinants of Staphylococcus aureus nasal carriage. Neth J Med. 2001 Sep;59(3):126-33.

[141] Kluytmans J, van BA, Verbrugh H. Nasal carriage of Staphylococcus aureus: epidemiology, underlying mechanisms, and associated risks. Clin Microbiol Rev. 1997 Jul;10(3):505-20.

[142] Kaplowitz LG, Comstock JA, Landwehr DM, Dalton HP, Mayhall CG. Prospective study of microbial colonization of the nose and skin and infection of the vascular access site in hemodialysis patients. J Clin Microbiol. 1988 Jul;26(7):1257-62.

[143] Yu VL, Goetz A, Wagener M, Smith PB, Rihs JD, Hanchett J, et al. Staphylococcus aureus nasal carriage and infection in patients on hemodialysis. Efficacy of antibiotic prophylaxis. N Engl J Med. 1986 Jul 10;315(2):91-6.

[144] Powe NR, Jaar B, Furth SL, Hermann J, Briggs W. Septicemia in dialysis patients: incidence, risk factors, and prognosis. Kidney Int. 1999 Mar;55(3):1081-90.

[145] Mokrzycki MH, Lok CE. Traditional and non-traditional strategies to optimize catheter function: go with more flow. Kidney Int. 2010 Dec;78(12):1218-31.

[146] Patel PR, Thompson ND, Kallen AJ, Arduino MJ. Epidemiology, surveillance, and prevention of hepatitis C virus infections in hemodialysis patients. Am J Kidney Dis. 2010 Aug;56(2):371-8.

[147] Edey M, Barraclough K, Johnson DW. Review article: Hepatitis B and dialysis. Nephrology. (Carlton.2010 Mar;15(2):137-45.

[148] Tutal E, Sezer S, Ibis A, Bilgic A, Ozdemir N, Aldemir D, et al. The influence of hepatitis C infection activity on oxidative stress markers and erythropoietin requirement in hemodialysis patients. Transplant Proc. 2010 Jun;42(5):1629-36.

[149] Chung H, Watanabe T, Kudo M, Chiba T. Hepatitis C virus core protein induces homotolerance and cross-tolerance to Toll-like receptor ligands by activation of Toll-like receptor 2. J Infect Dis. 2010 Sep 15;202(6):853-61.

[150] Watanabe T, Bertoletti A, Tanoto TA. PD-1/PD-L1 pathway and T-cell exhaustion in chronic hepatitis virus infection. J Viral Hepat. 2010 Jul;17(7):453-8.

[151] Wang JP, Zhang Y, Wei X, Li J, Nan XP, Yu HT, et al. Circulating Toll-like receptor (TLR. 2, TLR4, and regulatory T cells in patients with chronic hepatitis C. APMIS. 2010 Apr;118(4):261-70.

[152] Finelli L, Miller JT, Tokars JI, Alter MJ, Arduino MJ. National surveillance of dialysis-associated diseases in the United States, 2002. Semin Dial. 2005 Jan;18(1):52-61.

[153] Ikram H. Cytomegalovirus infections in hemodialysis centers. Clin Nephrol. 1981 Jan;15(1):1-4.

[154] Hardiman AE, Butter KC, Roe CJ, Cunningham J, Baker LR, Kangro HO, et al. Cytomegalovirus infection in dialysis patients. Clin Nephrol. 1985 Jan;23(1):12-7.

[155] Pawelec G, Akbar A, Caruso C, Solana R, Grubeck-Loebenstein B, Wikby A. Human immunosenescence: is it infectious? Immunol Rev. 2005 Jun;205:257-68.

[156] Pertosa G, Tarantino EA, Gesualdo L, Montinaro V, Schena FP. C5b-9 generation and cytokine production in hemodialyzed patients. Kidney Int. Suppl 1993 Jun;41:S221-S225.

[157] Pomianek MJ, Colton CK, Dinarello CA, Miller LC. Synthesis of tumor necrosis factor alpha and interleukin-1 receptor antagonist, but not interleukin-1, by human mononuclear cells is enhanced by exposure of whole blood to shear stress. ASAIO J. 1996 Jan;42(1):52-9.

[158] Singh NP, Bansal R, Thakur A, Kohli R, Bansal RC, Agarwal SK. Effect of membrane composition on cytokine production and clinical symptoms during hemodialysis: a crossover study. Ren Fail. 2003 May;25(3):419-30.

[159] Friedrich B, Janessa A, Schmieder R, Risler T, Alexander D. Acute effects of haemodialysis on pro-/anti- apoptotic genes in peripheral blood leukocytes. Cell Physiol Biochem. 2008;22(5-6):423-30.

[160] Andreoli MC, Dalboni MA, Watanabe R, Manfredi SR, Canziani ME, Kallas EG, et al. Impact of dialyzer membrane on apoptosis and function of polymorphonuclear cells and cytokine synthesis by peripheral blood mononuclear cells in hemodialysis patients. Artif Organs. 2007 Dec;31(12):887-92.

[161] Rao M, Guo D, Jaber BL, Sundaram S, Cendoroglo M, King AJ, et al. Dialyzer membrane type and reuse practice influence polymorphonuclear leukocyte function in hemodialysis patients. Kidney Int. 2004 Feb;65(2):682-91.

[162] Carracedo J, Ramirez R, Soriano S, Alvarez de Lara MA, Rodriguez M, Martin-Malo A, et al. Monocytes from dialysis patients exhibit characteristics of senescent cells: does it really mean inflammation? Contrib Nephrol. 2005;149:208-18.

[163] Soriano S, Martin-Malo A, Carracedo J, Ramirez R, Rodriguez M, Aljama P. Lymphocyte apoptosis: role of uremia and permeability of dialysis membrane. Nephron. Clin Pract 2005;100(3):c71-c77.

[164] Tabor B, Geissler B, Odell R, Schmidt B, Blumenstein M, Schindhelm K. Dialysis neutropenia: the role of the cytoskeleton. Kidney Int. 1998 Mar;53(3):783-9.

[165] Grooteman MP, Nube MJ, van Houte AJ, Schoorl M, van LJ. Granulocyte sequestration in dialysers: a comparative elution study of three different membranes. Nephrol Dial Transplant. 1995 Oct;10(10):1859-64.

[166] Sester U, Sester M, Heine G, Kaul H, Girndt M, Kohler H. Strong depletion of CD14(+. D16(+. monocytes during haemodialysis treatment. Nephrol Dial Transplant. 2001 Jul;16(7):1402-8.

[167] Nockher WA, Wiemer J, Scherberich JE. Haemodialysis monocytopenia: differential sequestration kinetics of CD14+CD16+ and CD14++ blood monocyte subsets. Clin Exp Immunol. 2001 Jan;123(1):49-55.

[168] Girndt M, Kaul H, Leitnaker CK, Sester M, Sester U, Kohler H. Selective sequestration of cytokine-producing monocytes during hemodialysis treatment. Am J Kidney Dis. 2001 May;37(5):954-63.

[169] Schindler R, Beck W, Deppisch R, Aussieker M, Wilde A, Gohl H, et al. Short bacterial DNA fragments: detection in dialysate and induction of cytokines. J Am SocNephrol. 2004 Dec;15(12):3207-14.

[170] Bossola M, Sanguinetti M, Scribano D, Zuppi C, Giungi S, Luciani G, et al. Circulating bacterial-derived DNA fragments and markers of inflammation in chronic hemodialysis patients. Clin J Am SocNephrol. 2009 Feb;4(2):379-85.

[171] Tielemans C, Husson C, Schurmans T, Gastaldello K, Madhoun P, Delville JP, et al. Effects of ultrapure and non-sterile dialysate on the inflammatory response during in vitro hemodialysis. Kidney Int. 1996 Jan;49(1):236-43.

[172] Guo LL, Pan Y, Zhu XJ, Tan LY, Xu QJ, Jin HM. Conventional, but not high-purity, dialysate-induced monocyte apoptosis is mediated by activation of PKC-{delta} and inflammatory factors release. Nephrol Dial Transplant. 2010 Oct 5.

[173] Hosoya N, Sakai K. Backdiffusion rather than backfiltration enhances endotoxin transport through highly permeable dialysis membranes. ASAIO Trans. 1990 Jul;36(3):M311-M313.

[174] Sardenberg C, Suassuna P, Andreoli MC, Watanabe R, Dalboni MA, Manfredi SR, et al. Effects of uraemia and dialysis modality on polymorphonuclear cell apoptosis and function. Nephrol Dial Transplant. 2006 Jan;21(1):160-5.

[175] Kaysen GA. The microinflammatory state in uremia: causes and potential consequences. J Am SocNephrol. 2001 Jul;12(7):1549-57.

In: Issues in Dialysis
Editor: Stephen Z. Fadem

ISBN: 978-1-62417-576-3
© 2013 Nova Science Publishers, Inc.

Chapter XII

Is Serum Albumin a Useful Marker of Nutritional Status in Chronic Kidney Disease?

Allon N. Friedman

Division of Nephrology, Indiana University School of Medicine,
Indianapolis, Indiana, US

Abstract

Serum albumin has long been accepted as a useful marker of nutritional status in the chronic kidney disease (CKD) population. Yet a more detailed examination reveals that it is in fact a poor nutritional measure. Animal and human studies using healthy and CKD models confirm that protein consumption must be negligible for serum albumin levels to be affected, and even then they are influenced only modestly. Such a severe level of protein restriction cannot explain the persistently low levels of serum albumin (e.g. 3.2 g/dl) observed in the US dialysis population, especially when obesity rates have been climbing. Moreover, the literature does not consistently support the premise that protein supplementation leads to increased serum albumin levels. In fact, serum albumin is an excellent marker of illness. Clinicians should take advantage of this fact by using serum albumin to identify and treat occult illnesses.

Introduction

The problem of malnutrition in patients with kidney disease remains of major concern to the nephrology community. Though numerous markers of nutritional status have been identified over the past few decades, one in particular—serum albumin—has established itself as the most influential, practical, and cost-effective. Nephrologists, renal dieticians, clinical investigators, large dialysis companies, and payors all use serum albumin for this purpose. But how good is serum albumin as a measure of nutrition, and what does it actually measure?

These questions have important consequences not only for patient care but also for clinicians, because nutritional quality goals may in the future affect reimbursement, and the health care system as a whole, which reimburses expensive nutritional interventions.

What Is Malnutrition?

Malnutrition can concisely be defined as "inadequate or excess intake of protein, energy, and micronutrients such as vitamins, and the frequent infections and disorders that result". [1] By this definition then, the state is malnutrition is reversible by simply providing deficient nutrients or withholding excess nutrients. This is a critical point to consider when determining whether serum albumin is a useful marker of nutrition. In nephrology patients, malnutrition has classically referred to the state in which protein and/or calories are lacking, so henceforth this is the definition that will be used in this discussion.

The Synthesis and Role of Albumin

Serum albumin is a negatively charged, water-soluble molecule of approximately 65 kD in weight. [2] It is synthesized in the liver at a rate of approximately 12-14 gm daily [2] and is normally present in the serum of adults at between 3.5 and 5.0 g/dl. The half-life of serum albumin in healthy adults humans is about 3 weeks. [3] Albumin serves two main physiologic purposes. First, it maintains osmotic pressure. Second, it acts as a carrier for metals, ions, fatty acids, amino acids, metabolites, bilirubin, enzymes, drugs, and hormones. [2,4,5]

Determinants of Serum Albumin

Serum albumin levels are influenced by the balance between liver synthesis and secretion, distribution between the intravascular and other compartments, degradation within the body, and body losses. As described below, the two most important external factors that regulate hepatic synthesis are dietary protein intake and illness/stress. [6]

Animal Models

Data from rat and perfused rat liver models describe how severely protein restricted diets or diets devoid of any protein lead to reduced hepatic albumin mRNA synthesis. [7-10] While this leads to lower serum albumin levels, the drop is ameliorated by a concomitant reduction in serum albumin degradation. Refeeding leads to a rapid reversal of the process and a normalization of serum albumin. [7,10] The degree of dietary protein depletion necessary to cause lower serum albumin levels has not been directly addressed, though the preponderance of studies that did observe a reduction in serum albumin involved diets with negligible protein content (i.e. 0.5% of total energy) or no protein altogether. [7-10] 0.5% of total energy is roughly equivalent to a 70 kg man consuming 3 gm of protein per day. Higher amounts of protein intake, even when relatively low, do not significantly reduce serum albumin. For example, consuming 3.2% protein (of total energy intake) over 6 weeks caused only a minimal reduction in plasma albumin (from 3.2 to 3.1 g/l). [9] What is clear from these animal studies is that dietary protein content must be at minimum severely restricted in order for significant reductions in serum albumin to be observed.

Studies in Healthy Humans

Data in human subjects confirm the results in the animal models. Hoffenberg et al. observed that restricting daily protein intake to 10gm for 3 to 6 weeks mildly reduced serum albumin levels from 4.2 to 3.8 gm/dl (p<0.02). [11] These findings were confirmed in a later study. [4] Intake only slightly greater had no appreciable impact on serum albumin. [11] A study of short term starvation also observed no effect on serum albumin, although dehydration and hemocontentration could have confounded the results. [12]

Another important determinant of serum albumin levels is the presence of inflammation or illness, which causes reductions in serum albumin by down regulation of hepatic mRNA synthesis, accelerated albumin catabolism, and increased vascular permeability. [13-15]

Studies in Chronic Kidney Disease

A number of human studies have established that a reduction in the glomerular filtration rate is not in itself associated with a shorter half-life of albumin or a lower albumin synthesis/catabolism ratio. [16,17] Some reports actually describe a higher synthesis rate. [18] These findings also true for pre-dialysis and dialysis patients. [16,18-20] Loss of albumin in the urine or dialysate was not found to affect albumin levels, [19] nor was intravascular volume expansion. [20] Of note, these studies did not examine the influence of conditions common to the uremic or dialysis populations such as concurrent illnesses [21] or chronic metabolic acidosis, [22] which could independently reduce albumin synthesis and increase catabolism.

Serum Albumin Levels in the U.S. Dialysis Population

Table 1 describes the trend over time of serum albumin levels in US patients initiating renal replacement therapy. The data are notable in three ways. First, excess adiposity (as estimated by the body mass index) continues to rise, making it difficult to implicate malnutrition as a widespread issue in these patients. Second, mean albumin levels have remained remarkably stable over time. Third, albumin levels are far lower than one would expect from a simple lack of dietary protein intake (as observed in experimental studies reviewed above and clinical studies below). This raises the basic questions of how serum albumin has become so entrenched as an accepted marker of nutritional status in patients with kidney disease, and its corollary, which is why is malnutrition considered so prevalent in end-stage renal disease.

**Table 1. Trends in Serum Albumin and Body Mass Index Levels in the U.S.
End-Stage Renal Disease Population: 1996-2006**

	Year										
	1996	1997	1998	1999	2000	2001	2002	2003	2004	2005	2006
Body Mass Index (kg/m^2)											
Mean ±Standard Deviation	25.5± 6.6	25.6± 6.7	26.0± 6.9	26.5± 7.0	27.0± 7.0	27.2± 7.1	27.5± 7.2	27.6± 7.2	27.8± 7.3	28.2± 7.5	28.5± 7.6
Median	24.4	24.6	24.9	25.3	25.8	25.8	26.1	26.3	26.4	26.7	27.1
25% Percentile	21.1	21.2	21.5	21.8	22.2	22.4	22.5	22.7	22.8	23.0	23.2
75% Percentile	28.7	28.9	29.4	29.8	30.5	30.6	31.0	31.2	31.4	31.9	32.3
Serum Albumin (g/dL)											
Mean± Standard Deviation	3.2± 0.7	3.2± 0.7	3.2± 0.7	3.1± 0.7	3.1± 0.7	3.1± 0.7	3.1± 0.7	3.1± 0.7	3.1± 0.7	3.1± 0.7	3.2± 0.7
Median	3.2	3.2	3.2	3.2	3.2	3.2	3.2	3.2	3.2	3.2	3.2
25% Percentile	2.8	2.8	2.8	2.7	2.7	2.7	2.7	2.7	2.6	2.7	2.7
75% Percentile	3.7	3.7	3.7	3.6	3.6	3.6	3.6	3.6	3.6	3.6	3.7

Reprinted with permission from reference. [55]
Data courtesy of the U.S. Renal Data System, USRDS 2008 Annual Data Report special data request: Atlas of End-Stage Renal Disease in the United States, National Institutes of Health, National Institute of Diabetes and Digestive and Kidney Diseases, Bethesda, MD, 2008.

The Origins of Serum Albumin as a Measure of Nutrition

The use of serum albumin to identify underlying malnutrition probably evolved from classic descriptions of kwashiorkor, a nutritional disorder especially common in children from developing nations. Kwashiorkor is a process that has been associated with the consumption of a diet adequate in calories but very deficient in protein. [23-26] In fact, the underlying pathophysiology is not well understood and could be caused by due to occult inflammatory conditions such as infections. [27-29] Kwashiorkor patients manifest edema, dermatitis, and spared subcutaneous fat stores but still remain relatively thin and underweight. They also present with hypoalbuminemia. [28-31] On the other hand, marasmus, another childhood nutritional derangement often mentioned in the same breath as kwashiorkor, originates from a prolonged lack of dietary protein and calories, so-called "protein-energy malnutrition". [23] The typical marasmic appearance is what one would expect with extreme malnutrition: a skeletal appearance and apathetic, listless behavior. Unlike kwashiorkor, however, the serum albumin levels of marasmic patients remain within the normal range. [26] This key difference highlights the fact that unlike illness or inflammation, a lack of protein and/or calories even when severe is unlikely to substantially reduce the serum albumin level.

Clinical Observations Of Serum Albumin

General Population

Anorexia nervosa is a useful model to help determine how severe malnutrition affects serum albumin levels because it is an excellent example of "pure malnutrition." That is, anorexia patients usually suffer from profound protein and energy deficits without the confounding effects of underlying inflammatory conditions, altered vascular permeability, or albumin losses. [32] If serum albumin is a sensitive nutritional marker, one would expect to see large reductions in serum albumin associated with severe malnutrition. Yet observations show that anorexia patients maintain serum albumin levels in the normal range even when their body mass index is in the teens. [32-35] Only when patient becomes moribund does the serum albumin fall. [33]

An additional source of insight into the albumin-nutrition relationship is the noted Minnesota Experiment, initiated in the 1940s by nutritional researcher Ancel Keys. [36] This study examined the effects of forced starvation in thirty two healthy young males who complied with a semistarvation diet (less than 1600 kcal/day) over a six month period. As shown in Table 2, while both lean and fat mass drastically declined over the study period, and the subjects' appearance became skeletal, mean serum albumin was only modestly affected (drop from 4.3 to 3.9g/dl). Interestingly, albumin levels either remained unchanged or rose in nearly a third of study subjects. These findings confirm the relative insensitivity of serum albumin to even profound changes in nutritional status.

Table 2. The Minnesota Experiment: Effects on Body Composition and Serum Albumin

	24 Week Semi-Starvation Diet[*] (n=32)	
	Baseline	End of Study
Body Mass Index (kg/m^2)	21.7 ± 1.7	16.4 ± 0.9
Body Composition[†] (kg) Total Weight (% of baseline) "Active" Body Mass (% of baseline) Fat Mass (% of baseline)	69.4 ± 5.9 (100) 39.9 (100) 9.8 ± 4.2 (100)	52.6 ± 4.0 (76) 29.2 (73) 3.1 ± 2.5 (32)
Serum Albumin (g/dL)	4.3 ± 0.5	3.9 ± 0.5

Reprinted with permission from reference. [55]
[*] Mean $\pm$ SD (though no SD available for "Active" body mass)
[†] "Active" body mass is total body weight less the sum of the fat, intracellular, and bone mineral weight; Fat mass was measured on the basis of specific gravity.

Table 3. Effects of Randomized Oral Nutritional Interventions on Serum Albumin Levels in Dialysis Patients

Study	N/Location/ Dialysis Modality[*]	Group Interventions[†]	Study Length (weeks)	Baseline BMI (kg/m^2)	Serum Albumin (g/dl) Baseline	End	Blinded Study?[*]	Comments
Kuhlmann [56], 1999	22/ Germany/ HD	I_1: high protein/energy diet I_2: standard diet I_3: low protein/energy diet	12	I_1:18 I_2: 22 I_3: 22	I_1: 4.14 I_2: 4.08 I_3: 4.19	I_1: 5.14 I_2: no change I_3: no change (no significant change in any group)	N	Unclear how group assignments were performed
Eustace [43], 2000	47/ USA/ HD+PD	C: matched placebo I: amino acid tablets	12	*PD* C: 23 I: 24 *HD* C: 25 I: 31	*PD* C: 3.00 I: 3.43 *HD* C: 3.47 I: 3.57	*PD* C: +0.02 I: +0.04 (p=NS) *HD* C: +0.04 I: +0.26 (p=0.02)	Y	Nonsignificant effect on combined groups (p=0.08)
Hiroshige [44], 2001	44/ Japan/ HD	C: matched placebo I: amino acid granules	52	C: 18 I: 19	C: 3.27 I: 3.31	C: no increase I: increase	Y	Mean dialysis vintage 6-7 years. Only 28 subjects randomized.
Sharma [57], 2002	40/ India/ HD	C: dietary counseling I_1: home-prepared supplement I_2: commercial supplement	4	C: 17 I_1: 18 I_2: 17	C: 3.4 I_1: 3.4 I_2: 3.4	C: +0.1 I_1: +0.6 I_2: +0.5 (p<0.001)	N	Diabetic patients excluded
Kloppenberg [58], 2004	45/ Netherlands/ HD	C: regular protein diet I: high protein diet	80	C: 25 I: 24	C: 4.77 I: 4.19	no significant change in either group	N	Intervention also included high vs. regular dialysis dose
Akpele [59], 2004	40/ USA/ HD	C: dietary counseling I: 1-2 supplement cans/day	29 (mean)	n/a	C: 3.01 I: 3.11	C: +0.03/mos I: -0.04/mos (p=0.03)	N	

Study	N/Location/ Dialysis Modality[*]	Group Interventions[†]	Study Length (weeks)	Baseline BMI (kg/m^2)	Serum Albumin (g/dl)		Blinded Study?[*]	Comments
					Baseline	End		
Gonzalez-Espinoza [60], 2005	28/ Mexico/ PD	C: usual care I: oral protein supplement	24	C: 25 I: 23	C: 2.66 I: 2.4	C: +0.14 I:+0.41 ($p<0.05$)	N	
Leon [61], 2006	180/ USA/ HD	C: usual care I: strategies to lower dialysis/nutritional barriers	52	C: 28 I: 29	C: 3.40 I: 3.40	C: +0.06 I: +0.21 ($p<0.01$)	N	Non-nutritional interventions also included
Moretti [62], 2009	49/ USA/ HD+PD	C: usual care I: oral protein supplement	52	C: 27 I: 25	C_1: 3.6 I_1: 3.5 C_2: 3.4 I_2: 3.5	$P<0.05$ only between I_2 and C_2 after 6 months	N	Overall no significant trend of improvement

Reprinted with permission in revised form from reference. [55]
[*] HD: Hemodialysis; PD: peritoneal dialysis; Y: yes; N: no.
[†] Letters indicate study arms: C=control, I=intervention.

Chronic Kidney Disease

A number of studies in the pre-dialysis kidney disease population have reported that even severe restriction of daily protein intake (e.g. 0.3 to 0.5 g/kg) does not lead to reduction in serum albumin. [37-40] Of these, the Modification of Diet in Renal Disease (MDRD) study is the most prominent. This large, randomized trial restricted daily protein consumption to as little as 0.56 g/kg over a mean of at least two years without noting any change in normal baseline serum albumin levels. [37]

While no interventional trials like MDRD exist in the dialysis population, Kaysen et al. explored the relationship between protein consumption, inflammation and serum albumin levels in an observational cohort. [41] They report that serum albumin levels are primarily associated not with nutritional intake but inflammation. A recent prospective study of 700 Dutch dialysis patients concurred. [42]

Do Nutritional Interventions Raise Serum Albumin Levels?

In keeping with our definition of malnutrition, a key test in assessing the utility of serum albumin as a measure of nutrition is whether nutritional supplementations can raise levels. Of the nine studies in which dialysis patients were randomized to oral nutritional interventions, all were modestly sized and only two were investigator blinded (see Table 3). Of the seven unblinded studies, four found no improvement in albumin levels after the intervention. Eustace et al. conducted the first blinded study in forty-seven (29-hemodialysis, 18-peritoneal dialysis) US dialysis patients who had a baseline serum albumin of 3.8 g/dL or less. [43] Subjects were randomized to essential amino acid tablets or placebo three times a day with meals. After three months, there was a statistically significant increase in serum albumin levels in the hemodialysis subgroup (mean increase with amino acids versus placebo: 0.26 vs. 0.04, p=0.02) with none in the peritoneal dialysis cohort. Of note, the mean baseline body mass index in the hemodialysis cohort was between 25 and 31 and in the peritoneal cohort between 23 and 24, suggesting that the cohort as a whole did not suffer from malnutrition. In the second blinded study, Hiroshige and colleagues [44] randomized 28 Japanese hemodialysis patients with serum albumin levels equal or less than 3.5 g/dl to either daily oral branched-chain amino acid oral supplements or placebo over a 12-month period. Using a crossover design, the mean baseline serum albumin of 3.3 g/dl rose to around 3.8 to 3.9 g/dl on the supplement. Interestingly, levels fell only marginally when supplements were stopped, and anthropometric measurements did not change at all, raising the distinct possibility that the rise in serum albumin was related to other factors.

The only interventional clinical trial in dialysis patients to have examined serum albumin in the context of hard clinical outcomes was the French Intradialytic Nutrition Evaluation Study (FineS). [45] Study investigators randomly assigned hemodialysis patients to intradialytic parenteral nutrition for 1 year versus no treatment, though both arms were also prescribed oral supplements. Two year mortality was the primary endpoint, and serum albumin a secondary one. While mortality was not influenced by the intervention, serum albumin level in both arms rose immediately, though not dramatically, and remained stable thereafter. Levels were generally equivalent between groups throughout the study period. There are a number of reasons to suspect that factors other than nutritional status influenced the rapid but relatively mild rise in serum albumin. First, baseline body mass indices in the cohort were within the normal range, making it unlikely that malnutrition was a problem in many study subjects. Second, the rise was relatively small (0.1 to 0.2 g/dl at most) despite significant nutritional supplementation. Third, the lack of study blinding raises the possibility that bias was introduced, perhaps by the introduction of extranutritional interventions that reduced underlying illnesses. In fact, the increase in serum albumin was much more impressive in the subgroup of subjects with high baseline C-reactive protein levels (reflective of inflammation). In addition, changes in serum albumin during the first 3 months, when the rise was most dramatic, were negatively correlated with c-reactive protein levels during the same period (r= -0.474, p<0.001).

In summary, the body of literature studying the effects of nutritional supplementation on serum albumin is limited by the inclusion of subjects without established malnutrition, the introduction of bias, and small sample sizes. The results are unpersuasive overall that nutritional supplementation significantly raises serum albumin levels.

The Use of Albumin as a Clinical, Research, and Quality Care Tool

Despite the sizeable amount of evidence indicating that serum albumin is not a reliable nutritional marker, it has nonetheless been mistakenly adopted for this very purpose. From a clinical standpoint, the National Kidney Foundation's Kidney Disease Outcomes Quality Initiative (K/DOQI) Clinical Practice Guidelines for Nutrition and The International Society of Renal Nutrition and Metabolism [46] recommended that serum albumin be routinely used as a measure of nutritional status. [47] Data from the Minnesota Experiment was used as supportive evidence. The Council on Renal Nutrition also recommended serum albumin as an important datum to identify malnutrition. Interestingly, a recent survey of dieticians found that serum albumin is the most commonly used measure of nutrition on dietary evaluation (>99%), while the history and physical is used much less often. [48] From a research standpoint, hundreds of scientific publications on nutrition in dialysis involve serum albumin, which is used prominently as a scientific nutritional biomarker.

Not surprisingly, serum albumin is being considered as a quality care index by a variety of payors. The Medicare ESRD Network Organizations Glossary suggests that albumin "may reflect the amount of protein intake in food". [49] CMS' Conditions for Coverage for Dialysis Units highlights serum albumin as the premier measure of nutrition along with body weight trends. [50] At least one large private dialysis organization uses albumin as a quality indicator, and it could very well be adopted in the future by CMS and other payors to determine performance and other value-based purchasing. Of course, this raises a number of concerns, not the least of which is that physicians' payments will be tied to a measure in most instances unrelated to what it was intended to measure. In addition, the focus on serum albumin could lead to additional cost and risk from nutrition interventions designed to raise the serum albumin. From the patient's standpoint, it could lead to "cherry picking" whereby caring for sicker patients (invariably those with lower serum albumin levels) would be avoided in order to meet performance expectations.

Does Serum Albumin Have any Clinical Utility?

Serum albumin has for some time offered a very strong—perhaps the strongest—predictor of mortality in dialysis patients. The association was initially reported in 1990 in a population of hemodialysis patients [51] and confirmed soon thereafter. [52] Since individuals born without any circulating albumin live generally healthy lives, [53] the relationship is not a causal one but rather likely related to the existence of underlying inflammatory conditions that lower albumin levels.

Unfortunately, the powerful inverse association between serum albumin and mortality has been mistakenly interpreted to suggest that malnutrition (as represented by low albumin) is very strongly linked with mortality in kidney disease patients (a presumption that may or may not be true). A common response therefore is to initiate nutritional supplements in patients with low albumin levels, despite their cost and lack of proven benefit. In fact, serum albumin does offer valuable information on which patients suffer from underlying illnesses. The difficulty is to use this information effectively. Aside from obvious conditions, a workup for low serum albumin should include such possible causes as dialysis access infections (even in old accesses that are not being used), dental and periodontal disease, *Helicobacter Pylori* infection, diverticulitis, peripheral vascular disease, occult malignancies, and possibly insulin resistance and metabolic acidosis. [22,54] Frequently an underlying cause may not be identified.

Summary

A host of experimental, clinical and observational evidence strongly support the premise that with rare exception (i.e. diets exceptionally low or absent in protein content), serum albumin is a poor marker of nutritional status. Therefore, reliance by clinicians, investigators, and payors on serum albumin as a measure of nutrition should be discouraged. Moreover, providing nutritional supplements to patients as a reflexive first step should be avoided altogether. Serum albumin can, however, provide clinicians with useful information than can lead to improved patient care and well-being if the underlying disorders are identified and treated.

References

[1]   Water Sanitation and Health – World Health Organization. [cited 23 Nov 2011]. Available from: http://www.who.int/water_sanitation_health/diseases/malnutrition/en/.

[2]   Rothschild MA, Oratz M, Schreiber SS. Albumin synthesis. 1. N Engl J Med. 1972;286:748-57.

[3]   Berson SA, Yalow RS, Schreiber SS, Post J. Tracer experiments with I131 labeled human serum albumin: distribution and degradation studies. J Clin Invest. 1953;32:746-68.

[4] Kelman L, Saunders SJ, Frith L, Wicht S, Corrigal A. Effects of dietary protein restriction on albumin synthesis, albumin catabolism, and the plasma aminogram. Am J Clin Nutr. 1972;25:1174-8.

[5] Rothschild MA, Oratz M, Schreiber SS. Serum albumin. Hepatology. 1988;8:385-401.

[6] Rothschild MA, Oratz M, Schreiber SS. Regulation of albumin metabolism. Annu Rev Med. 1975;26:91-104.

[7] Kirsch R, Frith L, Black E, Hoffenberg R. Regulation of albumin synthesis and catabolism by alteration of dietary protein. Nature. 1968;217:578-9.

[8] Sakuma K, Ohyama T, Sogawa K, Fujii-Kuriyama Y, Matsumura Y. Low protein--high energy diet induces repressed transcription of albumin mRNA in rat liver. J Nutr. 1987;117:1141-8.

[9] Coward WA, Whitehead RG, Lunn PG. Reasons why hypoalbuminaemia may or may not appear in protein-energy malnutrition. Br J Nutr. 1977;38:115-26.

[10] Morgan EH, Peters T, Jr. The biosynthesis of rat serum albumin. V. Effect of protein depletion and refeeding on albumin and transferrin synthesis. J Biol Chem. 1971;246:3500-7.

[11] Hoffenberg R, Black E, Brock JF. Albumin and gamma-globulin tracer studies in protein depletion states. J Clin Invest. 1966;45:143-52.

[12] Broom J, Fraser MH, McKenzie K, Miller JD, Fleck A. The protein metabolic response to short-term starvation in man. Clin Nutr. 1986;5:63-5.

[13] Fleck A, Raines G, Hawker F, et al. Increased vascular permeability: a major cause of hypoalbuminaemia in disease and injury. Lancet. 1985;1:781-4.

[14] Davies JW, Ricketts CR, Bull JP. Studies of plasma protein metabolism. I. Albumin in burned and injured patients. Clin Sci. 1962;23:411-23.

[15] Moshage HJ, Janssen JA, Franssen JH, Hafkenscheid JC, Yap SH. Study of the molecular mechanism of decreased liver synthesis of albumin in inflammation. J Clin Invest. 1987;79:1635-41.

[16] Coles GA, Peters DK, Jones JH. Albumin metabolism in chronic renal failure. Clin Sci. 1970;39:423-35.

[17] Bianchi R, Giuliano M, Toni M, Carmassi F. The metabolism of human serum albumin in renal failiure on conservative and dialysis therapy. Am J Clin Nutr. 1978:1615-26.

[18] Prinsen BH, Rabelink TJ, Beutler JJ, et al. Increased albumin and fibrinogen synthesis rate in patients with chronic renal failure. Kidney Int. 2003;64:1495-504.

[19] Kaysen GA, Schoenfeld PY. Albumin homeostasis in patients undergoing continuous ambulatory peritoneal dialysis. Kidney Int. 1984;25:107-14.

[20] Fish JC, Remmers AR, Jr., Lindley JD, Sarles HE. Albumin kinetics and nutritional rehabilitation in the unattended home-dialysis patient. N Engl J Med. 1972;287:478-81.

[21] Lecker S, Goldberg A, Mitch W. Protein degradation by the ubiquitin-proteasome pathway in normal and disease states. J Am Soc Nephrol. 2006;95:1807-19.

[22] Ballmer PE, McNurlan MA, Hulter HN, Anderson SE, Garlick PJ, Krapf R. Chronic metabolic acidosis decreases albumin synthesis and induces negative nitrogen balance in humans. J Clin Invest. 1995;95:39-45.

[23] Editorial: Classification of infantile malnutrition. Lancet. 1970;2:302-3.

[24] Weech A, EGoettsch, Reeves E. Nutritional Edema in the Dog. I. Development of hypoproteinemia on a diet deficient in protein. J Exper Med. 1935;61:299-317.

[25] Williams C. Kwashiorkor. Lancet. 1935;226:1151-2.

[26] Whitehead RG, Alleyne GA. Pathophysiological factors of importance in protein-calorie malnutrition. Br Med Bull. 1972;28:72-9.

[27] Krawinkel M. Kwashiorkor is still not fully understood. Bull World Health Organ. 2003;81:910-1.

[28] Rao KS. Evolution of kwashiorkor and marasmus. Lancet. 1974;1:709-11.

[29] Golden MH. Protein deficiency, energy deficiency, and the oedema of malnutrition. Lancet. 1982;1:1261-5.

[30] Whitehead RG, Coward WA, Lunn PG. Serum-albumin concentration and the onset of kwashiorkor. Lancet. 1973;1:63-6.

[31] Trowell HC, Davies JN, Dean RF. Kwashiorkor. II. Clinical picture, pathology, and differential diagnosis. Br Med J. 1952;2:798-801.

[32] Smith G, Robinson PH, Fleck A. Serum albumin distribution in early treated anorexia nervosa. Nutrition. 1996;12:677-84.

[33] Rigaud D, Hassid J, Meulemans A, Poupard AT, Boulier A. A paradoxical increase in resting energy expenditure in malnourished patients near death: the king penguin syndrome. Am J Clin Nutr. 2000;72:355-60.

[34] Okabe K. Assessment of emaciation in relation to threat to life in anorexia nervosa. Intern Med. 1993;32:837-42.

[35] Krantz MJ, Lee D, Donahoo WT, Mehler PS. The paradox of normal serum albumin in anorexia nervosa: a case report. Int J Eat Disord. 2005;37:278-80.

[36] Keys A, Brozek J, Henschel A, Mickelsen O, Taylor H. The Biology of Human Starvation. Minneapolis, MN: The University of Minnesota Press; 1950.

[37] Kopple JD, Levey AS, Greene T, et al. Effect of dietary protein restriction on nutritional status in the Modification of Diet in Renal Disease Study. Kidney Int. 1997;52:778-91.

[38] Aparicio M, Chauveau P, De Precigout V, Bouchet JL, Lasseur C, Combe C. Nutrition and outcome on renal replacement therapy of patients with chronic renal failure treated by a supplemented very low protein diet. J Am Soc Nephrol. 2000;11:708-16.

[39] Tom K, Young VR, Chapman T, Masud T, Akpele L, Maroni BJ. Long-term adaptive responses to dietary protein restriction in chronic renal failure. Am J Physiol. 1995;268:E668-77.

[40] Ihle BU, Becker GJ, Whitworth JA, Charlwood RA, Kincaid-Smith PS. The effect of protein restriction on the progression of renal insufficiency. N Engl J Med. 1989;321:1773-7.

[41] Kaysen GA, Dubin JA, Muller HG, Rosales L, Levin NW, Mitch WE. Inflammation and reduced albumin synthesis associated with stable decline in serum albumin in hemodialysis patients. Kidney Int. 2004;65:1408-15.

[42] Mutsert R, Grootendorst D, Indemans F, Boeschoten E, Krediet R, Dekker R. Assocation between serum albumin and mortality in dialysis patients is partly explained by inflammation, and not by malnutrition. J Renal Nutr. 2009;19:127-35.

[43] Eustace JA, Coresh J, Kutchey C, et al. Randomized double-blind trial of oral essential amino acids for dialysis-associated hypoalbuminemia. Kidney Int. 2000;57:2527-38.

[44] Hiroshige K, Sonta T, Suda T, Kanegae K, Ohtani A. Oral supplementation of branched-chain amino acid improves nutritional status in elderly patients on chronic haemodialysis. Nephrol Dial Transplant. 2001;16:1856-62.

[45] Cano NJ, Fouque D, Roth H, et al. Intradialytic parenteral nutrition does not improve survival in malnourished hemodialysis patients: a 2-year multicenter, prospective, randomized study. J Am Soc Nephrol. 2007;18:2583-91.

[46] Fouque D, Kalantar-Zadeh K, Kopple J, et al. A proposed nomenclature and diagnostic criteria for protein-energy wasting in acute and chronic kidney disease. Kidney Int. 2008;73:391-8.

[47] K/DOQI NKF. Clinical practice guidelines for nutrition in chronic renal failure. Am J Kidney Dis. 2000;35:S17-S104.

[48] Thompson, TG. Report to Congress on Medical Nutrition Therapy. [cited 23 NOV 2011] Available from: https://www.cms.gov/infoexchange/downloads/+ report%20to %20congress-medical%20nutrition%20therapy.pdf

[49] Medicare ESRD Network Organizations – Glossary. [cited 23 Nov 2011] Available from: http://www.cms.hhs.gov/manuals/downloads/eno114glossary.pdf.

[50] ESRD Basic Technical Surveyor Training – Interpretive Guidelines. [cited 23 23 NOV 2011] Available from: https://www.cms.gov/GuidanceforLawsAndRegulations+ /Downloads/esrdpgmguidance.pdf.

[51] Lowrie E, Lew N. Death risk in hemodialysis patients: The predictive value of commonly measured vairables and an evaluation of death rate differences between facilities. Am J Kidney Dis. 1990;15:458-82.

[52] Owen WF, Jr., Lew NL, Liu Y, Lowrie EG, Lazarus JM. The urea reduction ratio and serum albumin concentration as predictors of mortality in patients undergoing hemodialysis. N Engl J Med. 1993;329:1001-6.

[53] Koot BG, Houwen R, Pot DJ, Nauta J. Congenital analbuminaemia: biochemical and clinical implications. A case report and literature review. Eur J Pediatr. 2004;163:664-70.

[54] Grossman SB, Yap SH, Shafritz DA. Influence of chronic renal failure on protein synthesis and albumin metabolism in rat liver. J Clin Invest. 1977;59:869-78.

[55] Friedman A, Fadem S. Reassessment of albumin as a nutritional marker in kidney disease. J Am Soc Nephrol. 2010;21:223-30.

[56] Kuhlmann MK, Schmidt F, Kohler H. High protein/energy vs. standard protein/energy nutritional regimen in the treatment of malnourished hemodialysis patients. Miner Electrolyte Metab. 1999;25:306-10.

[57] Sharma M, Rao M, Jacob S, Jacob CK. A controlled trial of intermittent enteral nutrient supplementation in maintenance hemodialysis patients. J Ren Nutr. 2002;12:229-37.

[58] Kloppenburg WD, Stegeman CA, Hovinga TK, et al. Effect of prescribing a high protein diet and increasing the dose of dialysis on nutrition in stable chronic haemodialysis patients: a randomized, controlled trial. Nephrol Dial Transplant. 2004;19:1212-23.

[59] Akpele L, Bailey JL. Nutrition counseling impacts serum albumin levels. J Ren Nutr. 2004;14:143-8.

[60] Gonzalez-Espinoza L, Gutierrez-Chavez J, del Campo FM, et al. Randomized, open label, controlled clinical trial of oral administration of an egg albumin-based protein supplement to patients on continuous ambulatory peritoneal dialysis. Perit Dial Int. 2005;25:173-80.

[61] Leon JB, Albert JM, Gilchrist G, et al. Improving albumin levels among hemodialysis patients: a community-based randomized controlled trial. Am J Kidney Dis. 2006;48:28-36.

[62] Moretti H, Johnson A, Keeling-Hathaway T. Effects of protein supplementation in chronic hemodialysis and peritoneal dialysis patients. J Renal Nutr. 2009;19:298-303.

In: Issues in Dialysis
Editor: Stephen Z. Fadem

ISBN: 978-1-62417-576-3
© 2013 Nova Science Publishers, Inc.

Chapter XIII

The Chronic Kidney Disease-Mineral Bone Disorder (CKD-MBD) and Vascular Calcification

Keith A. Hruska[1,2,] Yifu Fang[1] and Toshifumi Sugatani[1]*

Departments of Pediatrics[1] and Internal Medicine[2] Division of Nephrology,
Washington University School of Medicine, St. Louis, Missouri, US

Abstract

The scientific progress in the pathogenesis of the CKD-MBD and vascular calcification that has accrued in recent years will be reviewed in this monograph. The factors regulating mesenchymal cell differentiation and their role in the neointimal calcification of atherosclerosis and the vascular media calcification observed in CKD and diabetes will be discussed. Bone regulatory proteins will be discussed regarding their role in bone mineralization and their participation in vascular calcification. This will include recent studies related to fetuin-A and the discovery of new skeletal hormones involved in regulating phosphate homeostasis and sensing skeletal hydroxyapatite precipitation. Finally, the relationship between skeletal mineralization and vascular mineralization will be discussed in terms of their links, especially through serum phosphate concentrations.

Introduction

The chronic kidney disease-mineral bone disorder (CKD-MBD) is a term coined in 2006 by the Kidney Disease Improving Global Outcomes Foundation (KDIGO) in recognition of the role mineral and skeletal disorders in the cardiovascular morbidity and mortality

---

[*] Corresponding Author: Keith A. Hruska, M.D. Department of Pediatrics, Washington University School of Medicine, 5th Fl MPRB/Room 5109, 660 S. Euclid Avenue, Hruska_k@kids.wustl.edu; (314) 286-2772-phone; (314) 286-2894- fax.

associated with CKD. [1] Embodied in the CKD-MBD concept is recent data demonstrating the phosphorus may be a cardiovascular risk factor through causation of vascular calcification, and that the skeleton is an endocrine organ whose hormonal functions are disturbed by CKD. The term replaces the broad use of secondary hyperparathyroidism and renal osteodystrophy which are now limited to their specific role as components of the syndrome.

Vascular calcification is a process that has been demonstrated during the progression of atherosclerosis with neointimal calcification, or with calcification of the tunica media. Intimal and medial calcification share similarities, but they may not share a common pathway and both are stimulated by chronic kidney disease (CKD). Primary medial calcification, or Mönckeberg's sclerosis (MS), has been associated with CKD, [2] aging, [3] and diabetes. [4] In CKD, MS was previously thought to be a passive process, [2] occurring as a direct consequence of an elevated calcium x phosphorous product. However, recent evidence discussed herein suggests that this is not the case. Rather, vascular calcification appears to be an active process involving a phenotypic drift towards an osteoblast-like cell secreting and mineralizing an extracellular matrix.

Understanding the pathogenesis of vascular calcification is essential as it is a frequent cause of morbidity and mortality for patients with CKD. [5] Indeed, the presence of vascular calcification occurs in all ages and stages of CKD. [6,7] However, the extent of coronary calcification appears to be more pronounced with a longer time on dialysis, older age, male gender, white race, diabetes, and higher serum calcium and phosphorous. [6] Coronary calcification is especially prone to be atherosclerotic and this form of VC has been shown to be due to differentiation of neointimal cells to an osteoblastic phenotype mineralizing their extracellular matrix akin to bone formation.

Differentiation of Mesenchymal Stem Cells

Osteoblasts, smooth muscle myocytes, adipocytes, fibroblasts and chondrocytes all share a common mesenchymal progenitor stem cell. Differentiation along the smooth muscle lineage requires crucial factors such as myocardin and myocardin related transcription factors (MRTFs), but the differentiated contractile state is plastic and in CKD dedifferentiation to a synthetic state is observed which allows for expression of features of other mesenchymal cell lineages, notably osteoblastic and chondrocytic. Differentiation along the osteogenic lineage requires crucial factors including the bone morphogenetic proteins (BMPs) [8] and Wnts. [9] The BMPs are part of the TGF-β superfamily that initiate signal transduction by binding to specific type II receptors, activating type I receptors, and affecting gene transcription through phosphorylation of regulatory Smad transcription factors. BMP induced osteogenesis requires lineage specific transcription factors such as *Runx2, Osx,* and *Msx1/2.*The transcriptome of these factors are key and include all of the proteins involved in osteoblast mediated bone formation. Mice genetically engineered to be deficient in *Runx2* or *Osx* show a complete lack of ossification, [10,11] while those deficient in *Msx 1/2* have significant skeletal abnormalities. [12,13]

The finding of *Runx2, Osx,* and *Msx1/2* expressed in calcified vessel walls has led to the theory that vascular calcification is also a tightly regulated, coordinated, and active osteoblastic process. An example of this in animals has been demonstrated in LDL receptor negative (LDLR -/-) mice fed a high fat diet. These animals developed vascular calcification associated with the expression of *Msx1* and *Msx2*. [14] In humans, expression of *Msx2* and *Runx2* along with the chondrogenic transcription factor *Sox9* has been described in calcified atherosclerotic samples. [15] In addition, increased expression of the target genes of these factors such as alkaline phosphatase, osteocalcin, bone sialoprotein, and type II collagen also occur. Furthermore, other bone regulatory proteins such as matrix Gla protein (MGP) and osteoprotegerin (OPG) (both discussed below) are downregulated in calcified vessels as compared to non-calcified vessels. [15] Deposition of bone matrix proteins has also been described in medial calcification associated with CKD. [16] These findings suggest that vascular calcification may in fact be an active process that simulates osteogenesis and bone formation.

The Vascular Smooth Muscle Cell

VSMCs normally reside in the vessel wall media in a differentiated state wherein their contractile properties regulate vascular tone. However, VSMC phenotype is characterized by the ability to reversibly enter a synthetic state of proliferation and production of large amounts of extracellular matrix. [17] The stimulus to change phenotype includes injury, various cytokines, growth factors, and certain components of the extracellular matrix. In the heightened synthetic state, VSMCs show decreased expression of contractile and adhesion proteins and a concomitant increase in cytoskeletal proteins. [18] In addition to various growth factors, culture of VSMC in medium supplemented with serum has been shown to stimulate the transition to the synthetic phenotype experimentally. [19] Transition into the synthetic state is thought to be involved in the pathogenesis of atherosclerosis and MS.

After serum stimulation, proliferating VSMC grow to form a confluent monolayer. [20] Subsequently, areas of the monolayer develop multicellular foci that form nodular aggregates consisting of non-proliferating, quiescent VSMC. Cells from these nodules appear to re-express markers of smooth muscle cell differentiation. Proliferating osteoblasts also form condensing nodules in culture as well. [21] Subpopulations of human and bovine aortic VSMCs have been shown to form these nodules and then spontaneously calcify. [22]

The addition of β-glycerophosphate, a phosphate donor, or high concentrations of inorganic phosphate have been shown to induce calcification in VSMCs *in vitro,* [23] and VSMCs from atherosclerotic donors showed increased expression of *Runx2*, OPN, and alkaline phosphatase. [24] Inorganic phosphate induced the expression of osterix and bone matrix proteins. [24] This action is stimulated through a sodium-phosphorous cotransporter in cultured VSMCs. [25,26] Thus, it appears that inorganic phosphate induces VSMCs toward an osteogenic phenotype *in vitro*. However, uremic serum also induces VSMCs to calcify, a process that is partly related to a factor that is independent of serum phosphate.

Thus, it has been demonstrated that vascular smooth muscle cells can be induced to calcify, and on occasion calcify spontaneously, in vitro. While this is important in the understanding of the pathogenesis of vascular calcification, the forces driving osteogenic differentiation in vivo are less clear. However, in addition to a higher incidence of vascular calcification, decreased bone formation is also a common finding in CKD, diabetes mellitus, and aging. Furthermore, recent findings in animal models suggest that decreased orthotopic bone mineralization, either by decreased bone formation or increased bone resorption, leads to increased pressure towards heterotopic mineralization. We will discuss what factors are involved in this "increased pressure", giving particular attention to phosphate.

Bone Metabolism and Vascular Calcification: A Possible Link

Matrix Gla Protein

MGP belongs to the family of mineral binding proteins that includes coagulation factors, anticlotting factors, and osteocalcin. MGP is a vitamin-K dependent protein, requiring the vitamin for γ-carboxylation of its glutamic acid residues resulting in production of carboxyglutamic acid (Gla) residues. The gla residues bind calcium and have been shown to inhibit hydroxyapatite precipitation. [27] The affinity of MGP binding to hydroxyapatite is enhanced by calcium and decreased by phosphate and magnesium. [27] MGP also appears to modulate endochondral bone formation. Overexpression of MGP blocks cartilage mineralization and inhibits endochondral ossification [28] while mice genetically engineered to be deficient in MGP have inappropriate mineralization of cartilage, disorganized chondrocyte columns, and osteopenia. [29] Mice genetically engineered to be deficient in MGP also develop extensive arterial calcification and die of arterial rupture. [29] Calcified arteries from these mice show decreased expression of smooth muscle cell markers and increased expression of bone specific markers such as *Runx2* and OPN. [30] This finding suggests that the vascular calcification associated with this mutation is not solely related to an inability to inhibit hydroxyapatite precipitation, but rather involves a more active process resulting in a dramatic phenotypic change in VSMCs. The function of MGP to bind BMPs in the matrix may relate to BMP activity and differentiation of neointimal cells to the osteochrondrogenic pathway, [31] although recent evidence does not support this possibility. [32]

Osteoprotegerin

Osteoprotegerin (OPG), a soluble circulating ligand of RANK, is an inhibitor of osteoclast differentiation and function and is part of the RANK/RANKL/OPG axis. Mice that are genetically engineered to be deficient in OPG (*opg-/opg-*) develop severe osteoporosis. [33] This likely occurred by uninhibited osteoclast function leading to excess bone resorption. Histomorphometric analysis of the bones of these mice reveals increased parameters of both bone resorption and bone formation, suggesting that the two processes may be coupled. [34] However, intravenous injection of recombinant OPG or transgenic overexpression of OPG is able to effectively reverse the osteoporotic phenotype. [35] In addition to the osteoporotic phenotype, OPG deficient mice also develop extensive vascular calcification. Furthermore, in contrast to the osteoporotic phenotype, only transgenic overexpression of OPG prevents vascular calcification. In other words, preventing bone resorption prevents the vascular calcification while reversing it does not. Of note, the increased bone resorption seen in these mice was not associated with an increased serum phosphate. [34] This may in part be due to the increased bone formation and mineral apposition rates seen in these mice. Furthermore, OPG deficient mice have markedly elevated RANKL as compared to wildtype. Elevated RANKL may be the link between bone and vascular calcification in this model as it has recently been shown to induce aortic myofibroblasts to form calcifying nodules with an osteogenic phenotype. [36] In addition, although normally not expressed in the vasculature, RANKL expression was increased in both the vessels of OPG deficient mice [35] and the aortic valves in human calcific aortic stenosis. [36]

The role of OPG in renal osteodystrophy and vascular calcification is less clear. Studies correlating serum OPG levels and histomorphometric parameters of bone turnover have been inconsistent.

Vitamin D

High dose vitamin D causes extensive arterial calcification in the rat. [37-39] Vertebrae from rats treated with 1,25 – hydroxyvitamin D3 have increased osteoblast number, increased mineral appositional rate, increased bone formation and decreased osteoclast number. [40] However, when vitamin D induces calcification in the rat, it is associated with a marked increase in the cross-linked N-teleopeptides, a marker of bone resorption. [39] Furthermore, treatment with OPG, an inhibitor of bone resorption, prevented vascular calcification and restored serum cross-linked N-teleopeptides back to control values. In addition, other agents known to inhibit bone resorption through different mechanisms than OPG also inhibited vitamin D induced vascular calcification. [38,41] Furthermore, 1,25 OH-vitamin D3 appears to promote the differentiation of osteoclasts through stimulation of RANKL in osteoblastic cells. [42] Thus, at least in these animal models, vascular calcification by vitamin D appears to be related to bone resorption. Why there is such a dichotomy in regards to the effects of vitamin D on bone metabolism is not clear, but may possibly be related to the dosage of the analog given. In addition, it is important to note that vitamin D also has effects on the vasculature as well. Indeed, low doses of paricalcitol and calcitriol stimulated smooth muscle cell differentiation and thereby inhibited aortic osteoblast gene expression in the atherosclerotic high fat fed *ldlr-/-*mouse and actually protected against vascular calcification. [43]

α2-HS glycoprotein/Fetuin-A

α2-HS glycoprotein (AHSG) or fetuin-A is a bone regulatory protein that shares homologies to the fetuin superfamily, proteins present abundantly in the fetal serum. [44] Fetuins have been shown to inhibit hydroxyapatite precipitation in vitro [45] as well as modulate the effects of the TGF-β superfamily on osteogenesis. [46] Fetuins can inhibit or stimulate osteogenesis, depending on their relative concentrations. [47] Mice that are genetically engineered to be deficient in fetuin-A are phenotypically normal but develop more extensive ectopic calcification than control when fed a mineral and vitamin D rich diet. [48]

In hemodialysis patients, serum fetuin-A levels are decreased and this decrease is associated with an increased risk of cardiovascular mortality and an impaired *ex vivo*ability to inhibit hydroxyapatite precipitation. [49] This decrease in fetuin-A levels is in part due to inflammation, as fetuin-A has been shown to be a negative acute phase reactant. [50] However, one must also not discount the effects of bone metabolism in this situation. Furthermore, it is also possible that the calcium based phosphate binders and vitamin D analogues given these patients to control secondary hyperparathyroidism may also serve to deplete fetuin-A levels via increased calcium and phosphorous incorporation into the fetuin-mineral complex.

BMP-7: Bone Formation, Phosphate, and Vascular Calcification

BMP-7, a member of the BMP family, is critical for renal, skeletal, and retinal development that is expressed in the adult primarily in the collecting tubule. Acute renal ischemia [51,52] and diabetic nephropathy [52,53] reduceBMP-7 expression. In CKD and renal osteodystrophy, treatment with BMP-7 restored normal bone turnover and osteoblast function [54,55] with either high or low turnover rates. Furthermore, BMP-7 has been shown to significantly reduce intimal calcification in the low density lipoprotein receptor deficient high fat fed atherosclerotic mouse (LDLR-/- high-fat)when CKD was induced. [56] Furthermore, LDLR -/- high-fat fed mice with CKD have low turnover osteodystrophy, [54] and restoration of bone metabolism was associated with a significant reduction in serum phosphate. [54] That renal osteodystrophy contributes to the serum phosphorus through excess bone resorption provides a link between bone turnover and vascular calcification.

When dietary phosphorous is ingested, it enters a rapidly exchangeable pool. A significant portion of this pool exists along the skeletal mineralizing surfaces where phosphorous is leaving the pool to be incorporated into bone crystals. When bone formation is reduced, the skeletal mineralizing surface is reduced, effectively reducing the volume of distribution of phosphorous, resulting in an increase in the serum phosphate associated with intake. By restoring normal bone turnover, BMP-7 increased the volume of distribution of phosphorous, resulting in a decrease in serum phosphate. Furthermore, since phosphorous has been shown to induce an osteogenic phenotype in VSMC cells *in vitro*, we propose that the reduction in serum phosphate is a mechanism by which BMP-7 prevents vascular calcification.BMP-7 has also been shown to maintain the VSMC phenotype *in vitro* after stimulation into the synthetic phenotype, [57] and BMP-7 stimulates the contractile phenotype in human VSMC derived from atherosclerotic donors. [58]

FGF-23: Regulator of Phosphorous Metabolism

Since phosphate homeostasis appears to be a central component of vascular calcification, understanding its regulation is essential. In addition to PTH and vitamin D, another hormone, FGF-23, plays a critical role in homeostasis. FGF-23 is a phosphaturic hormone produced by osteocytes. An FGF23 mutation blocking catabolism is causative of autosomal dominant hypophosphatemic rickets (ADHR). [59] Mesenchymal tumors causing tumor induced osteomalacia (TIO) produce high levels of FGF23. [60] FGF-23 inhibits the NaPi transport of the proximal tubule and inhibits expression of renal 1α-hydroxylase, resulting in inappropriately low levels of 1, 25-OH vitamin D3 when hypophosphatemia occurs. [61] FGF-23 levels are elevated in early in CKD. [62,63] This is a clarion demonstration that kidney disease affects the skeleton. Elevations in the levels of FGF-23 due to osteocytic secretion are enhanced by decreased clearance, which is a proximal tubular function. [62] Targeted deletion of the FGF-23 gene results in hyperphosphatemia, hypercalcemia, suppressed PTH, marked vascular calcification and low turnover osteopenia with accumulation of osteoid. [61] Mice homozygous died within 13 weeks of birth and autopsies revealed marked vascular calcification of the kidneys associated with an elevated BUN. While the suppressed PTH (secondary to elevated 1,25-OH vitamin D3 and calcium) could explain some of these abnormalities, it also suggests that FGF-23 may have additional effects on bone. Furthermore, the vascular calcification associated with FGF-23 deficiency was prevented by low dietary phosphorous.

Osteocalcin

A second skeletal hormone recently discovered, [64-66] is also affected by CKD induced inhibition of bone formation. Osteocalcin in its undercarboxylated form is a systemic regulator of energy metabolism through actions regulating insulin secretion, insulin action in adipose tissue, and leptin secretion. CKD is associated with a marked disturbance in energy metabolism, and the role of osteocalcin in this is unknown. However, the CKD phenotype of disordered energy metabolism is suggestive of a role for osteocalcin

Bone Metabolism and Vascular Calcification

Evidence suggests that changes in bone metabolism, either by increased bone resorption or decreased bone formation, leads to vascular calcification. Vascular calcification occurs both in the media and the intima, possibly by different processes. Treatment with BMP-7 in the LDLR -/- high fat mouse with CKD model resulted in reductions in intimal calcification through lowering phosphate by stimulating bone formation. It is also possible that if VSMC migration did not occur as part of the pathogenesis of atherosclerosis, then perhaps intimal calcification would also not occur. Indeed, intimal calcification does not occur in other animal models of vascular calcification.

Primary medial calcification occurs primarily in patients with CKD, diabetes mellitus, and as a part of aging. These three conditions also share a common characteristic of decreased bone formation. Indeed, animal models and human studies of aging [67,68] and diabetes [69,70] have demonstrated decreased bone volume and bone formation rates. Furthermore, treatment of LDLR -/- high fat fed mice (who have the metabolic syndrome or diabetes) with another bone anabolic, PTH (1-34)fragment also results in reduced vascular calcification. [71] While it is unknown what effect PTH (1-34) had on serum phosphate (presumably it would decrease it), it did result in an elevation of skeletal and serum OPN, a known inhibitor of vascular calcification. While other mechanisms may be involved in this protective effect of PTH (1-34), these findings further support the link between bone metabolism and vascular calcification.

With excess bone resorption, vascular calcification also occurs. We hypothesize that the pathogenesis involves reduced levels of serum fetuin-A, a known inhibitor of ectopic mineralization. However, since mice genetically engineered to be deficient in fetuin-A do not have significant ectopic calcification, reduced levels are likely not the sole factor involved in the pathogenesis. For example, high levels of serum RANKL may also be involved in the vascular calcification of the OPG deficient mouse. Furthermore, serum phosphate does not appear to be elevated in these animal models of vascular calcification. This may be related to a concomitant increase in bone formation rates seen in these models.

Conclusion: Implications for Chronic Kidney Disease

We have shown that prevention of secondary hyperparathyroidism results in low turnover renal osteodystrophy in CKD. [72] We propose that renal injury/disease produces a deficiency in Wnt and BMP activity in the skeleton and that secondary hyperparathyroidism develops as an adaptive process. [73,74] Furthermore, we propose that with a low turnover state in the skeleton, there is a decreased volume of distribution for phosphorous, resulting in an increase in the serum phosphate and greater stimulation of FGF23. Inorganic phosphate has been shown to induce an osteogenic phenotype in VSMC, resulting in a more active process of mineralization. The extent of vascular calcification indeed has been shown to be associated with higher serum phosphorous in humans with CKD. [6] Thus, treatment of positive phosphate balance in CKD may be required to decrease the high rates of associated cardiovascular mortality. Clearly vascular calcification is a significant problem for patients with CKD. In this manuscript we have provided evidence that bone metabolism affects the vasculature. While vascular calcification occurs without CKD, we propose that the central mechanism in most cases is abnormal bone metabolism. Complications likely specific to CKD include chronic inflammation leading to atherosclerosis and low serum fetuin-A levels and hyperphosphatemia from decreased excretion. Finally, one must not ignore the risk factors for atherosclerosis such as hypertension, hyperlipidemia, diabetes, and smoking towards vascular calcification.

Given that there is such significant morbidity and mortality associated with vascular calcification, it is essential to develop treatments to prevent or slow down the progression of this process. While attempts to adjust oral calcium, calcitriol analogues, and calcium in the dialysate are keys to management of renal osteodystrophy, institution of novel therapy early in CKD is probably required. We propose that bone anabolics such as BMP-7, Act-011, and anti-sclerostin antibodies may be novel therapeutic options for the treatment of low turnover osteopenia and the prevention of vascular calcification. Human studies must be performed to further assess this concept.

Acknowledgments

This work was supported by NIH grants (DK070790, AR41677, T32-DK062705) to KAH and research support from Shire, Genzyme, Abbott and Fresenius. We wish to thank Mat Davies, Richard Lund and Song Wang, past fellows in the Hruska lab for their hard work and research contributions to this effort.

Address for reprint requests: Keith A. Hruska, M.D., Department of Pediatrics, Campus Box 8208, 5th Fl MPRB, 660 S. Euclid Avenue, St. Louis, MO 63110.

References

[1] Moe S, Drueke T, Cunningham J, Goodman W, Martin K, Olgaard K, et al. Definition, evaluation, and classification of renal osteodystrophy: a position statement from kidney disease: Improving Global Outcomes (KDIGO). Kidney Int. 2006;69:1945-1953.

[2] Ejerblad S, Ericsson JLE, Eriksson I. Arterial lesions of the radial artery in uraemic patients. Acta Chir Scand. 1979;145:415-428.

[3] Elliott RJ, McGrath LT. Calcification of the human aorta during aging. Calcif Tissue Int. 1994;54:268-273.

[4] Edmonds ME. Medial arterial calcification and diabetes mellitus. Z Kardiol. 2000;89(Suppl 2):II/101-II/104.

[5] Blacher J, Safar ME, Guerin AP, Pannier B, Marchais SJ, London GM. Aortic pulse wave velocity index and mortality in end-stage renal disease. Kidney Int. 2003;63:1852-1860.

[6] Raggi P, Boulay A, Chasan-Taber S, Amin N, Dillon M, Burke SK, et al. Cardiac calcification in adult hemodialysis patients. A link between end-stage renal disease and cardiovascular disease? J Am Coll Cardiol. 2002;39:695-701.

[7] Goodman WG, Goldin J, Kuizon BD, Yoon C, Gales B, Sider D, et al. Coronary-artery calcification in young adults with end-stage renal disease who are undergoing dialysis. N Eng J Med. 2000;342:1478-1483.

[8] Cheng H, Jiang W, Phillips FM, Haydon RC, Peng Y, Zhou L, et al. Osteogenic Activity of the Fourteen Types of Human Bone Morphogenetic Proteins (BMPs). J Bone and Joint Surg. 2003;85:1544-1552.

[9] Kato M, Patel MS, Levasseur R, Lobov I, Chang BHJ, Glass DA, II, et al. Cbfa1-independent decrease in osteoblast proliferation, osteopenia, and persistent embryonic eye vascularization in mice deficient in Lrp5, a Wnt coreceptor. J Cell Biology. 2002;157:303-314.

[10] Komori T, Yagi H, Nomura S, Yamaguchi A, Sasaki K, Deguchi K, et al. Targeted disruption of Cbfa1 results in a complete lack of bone formation owing to maturational arrest of osteoblasts. Cell. 1997;89:755-764.

[11] Nakashima K, Zhou X, Kunkel G, Zhang Z, Deng JM, Behringer RR, et al. The novel zinc finger-containing transcription factor osterix is required for osteoblast differentiation and bone formation. Cell. 2002;108:17-29.

[12] Satokata I, Mass R. Msx1 deficient mice exhibit cleft palate and abnormalities of craniofacial and tooth development. Nat Genet. 1994;6:348-356.

[13] Satokata I, Ma L, Ohshima H, Bei M, Woo I, Nishizawa K, et al. Msx2 deficiency in mice causes pleiotropic defects in bone growth and ectodermal organ formation. Nat Genet. 2004;24(4):391-395.

[14] Towler DA, Bidder M, Latifi T, Coleman T, Semenkovich CF. Diet-induced diabetes activates an osteogenic gene regulatory program in the aortas of low density lipoprotein receptor-deficient mice. J Biol Chem. 1998;273:30427-30434.

[15] Tyson KL, Reynolds JL, McNair R, Zhang Q, Weissberg PL, Shanahan CM. Osteo/chondrocytic transcription factors and their target genes exhibit distinct patterns of expression in human arterial calcification. Arterioscler Thromb Vasc Biol. 2003;23:489-494.

[16] Moe SM, O'Neill KD, Duan D, Ahmed S, Chen NX, Leapman SB, et al. Medial artery calcification in ESRD patients is associated with deposition of bone matrix proteins. Kidney Int. 2002;61:638-647.

[17] Hedin U, Roy J, Tran PK, Lundmark K, Rahman A. Control of smooth muscle cell proliferation - the role of the basement membrane. Thromb Haemost. 1999;82(Suppl.):23-26.

[18] Worth NF, Rolfe BE, Song J, Campbell R. Vascular smooth muscle cell phenotypic modulation in culture is associated with reorganization of contractile and cytoskeletal proteins. Cell Motil Cytosk. 2001;49:130-145.

[19] Thyberg J. Differentiated properties and proliferation of arterial smooth muscle cells in culture. Int Rev Cytol. 1996;169:183-265.

[20] Brennan MJ, Millis AJ, Fritz KE. Fibronectin inhibits morphological changes in vascular smooth muscle cells. J Cell Physiol. 1982;112:284-290.

[21] Barone LM, Owen TA, Tassinari MS. Developmental expression and hormonal regulation of the rat matrix gla protein (MGP) gene in chondrogenesis and osteogenesis. J Cell Biochem. 1991;46:351-365.

[22] Boström K, Watson KE, Horn S, Worthman C, Herman IM, Demer LL. Bone morphogenetic protein expression in human atherosclerotic lesions. J Clin Invest. 1993;91:1800-1809.

[23] Shioi A, Nishizawa Y, Jono S, Koyama H, Hosoi M, Morii H. β-Glycerophosphate accelerates calcification in cultured bovine vascular smooth muscle cells. Arterioscler Thromb Vasc Biol. 1995;15:2003-2009.

[24] Mathew S, Tustison KS, Sugatani T, Chaudhary LR, Rifas L, Hruska KA. The mechanism of phosphorus as a cardiovascular risk factor in chronic kidney disease. J Am Soc Nephrol. 2008;19:1092-1105.

[25] Jono S, McKee MD, Murry CE, Shioi A, Nishizawa Y, Mori K, et al. Phosphate regulation of vascular smooth muscle cell calcification. Circ Res. 2000;87:e10-e17.

[26] Chen NX, O'Neill KD, Duan D, Moe SM. Phosphorus and uremic serum up-regulate osteopontin expression in vascular smooth muscle cells. Kidney Int. 2002;62:1724-1731.

[27] Roy ME, Nishimoto SK. Matrix Gla protein binding to hydroxyapatite is dependent on the ionic environment: calcium enhances binding affinity but phosphate and magnesium decrease affinity. Bone. 2002;31:296-302.

[28] Yagami K, Suh JY, Enomoto-Iwamoto M, Koyama E, Abrams WR, Shapiro IM, et al. Matrix GLA Protein Is a Developmental Regulator of Chondrocyte Mineralization and, When Constitutively Expressed, Blocks Endochondral and Intramembranous Ossification in the Limb. J Cell Biol. 1999;147:1097-1108.

[29] Luo G, Ducy P, McKee MD, Pinero GJ, Loyer E, Behringer RR, et al. Spontaneous calcification of arteries and cartilage in mice lacking matrix GLA protein. Nature. 1997;386:78-81.

[30] Steitz SA, Speer MY, Curinga G, Yang H-Y, Haynes P, Aebersold R., et al. Smooth muscle cell phenotypic transition associated with calcification. Circ Res. 2001;89:1147-1154.

[31] Bostrom K, Tsao D, Shen S, Wang Y, Demer LL. Matrix GLA Protein Modulates Differentiation Induced by Bone Morphogenetic Protein-2 in C3H10T1/2 Cells. J Biol Chem. 2001;276:14044-14052.

[32] O'Neill WC, Sigrist MK, McIntyre CW. Plasma pyrophosphate and vascular calcification in chronic kidney disease. Nephrol Dial Transplant. 2010;25:187-191.

[33] Bucay N, Sarosi I, Dunstan CR, Morony S, Tarpleyl J, Capparelli C, et al. Osteoprotegerin-deficient mice develop early onset osteoporosis and arterial calcification. Genes Dev. 1998;12:1260-1268.

[34] Nakamura M, Udagawa N, Matsuura S, Mogi M, Nakamura H, Horiuchi H, et al. Osteoprotegerin Regulates Bone Formation through a Coupling Mechanism with Bone Resorption. Endocrinology. 2003;144:5441-5449.

[35] Min H, Morony S, Sarosi I, Dunstan CR, Capparelli C, Scully S, et al. Osteoprotegerin reverses osteoporosis by inhibiting endosteal osteoclasts and prevents vascular calcification by blocking a process resembling osteoclastogenesis. J Exp Med. 2000;192:463-474.

[36] Kaden JJ, Bickelhaupt S, Grobholz R, Haase KK, Sarıkoc A, Kilic R, et al. Receptor activator of nuclear factor κB ligand and osteoprotegerin regulate aortic valve calcification. J Mol Cell Cardiol. 2004;36:57-66.

[37] Price PA, Faus SA, Williamson MK. Warfarin-induced artery calcification is accelerated by growth and vitamin D. Arterioscler Thromb Vasc Biol. 2000;20:317-327.

[38] Price PA, Faus SA, Williamson MK. Bisphosphonates Alendronate and Ibandronate Inhibit Artery Calcification at Doses Comparable to Those That Inhibit Bone Resorption. Arterioscler Thromb Vasc Biol. 2001;21:817-824.

[39] Price PA, June HH, Buckley JR, Williamson MK. Osteoprotegerin inhibits artery calcification induced by Warfarin and by Vitamin D. Arterioscler Thromb Vasc Biol. 2001;21:1610-1616.

[40] Erben RG, Scutt AM, Miao D, Kollenkirchen U, Haberey M. Short-Term Treatment of Rats with High Dose 1,25-Dihydroxyvitamin D3 Stimulates Bone Formation and Increases the Number of Osteoblast Precursor Cells in Bone Marrow. Endocrinology. 1997;138:4629-4635.

[41] Price PA, June HH, Buckley JR, Williamson MK. SB 242784, a Selective Inhibitor of the Osteoclastic V-H+-ATPase, Inhibits Arterial Calcification in the Rat. Circ Res. 2002;91:547-552.

[42] Kitazawa S, Kajimoto K, Kondo T, Kitazawa R. Vitamin D3 supports osteoclastogenesis via functional vitamin d response element of human RANKL gene promoter. J Cell Biochem. 2003;89:771-777.

[43] Mathew S, Lund RJ, Chaudhary LR, Geurs T, Hruska KA. Vitamin D receptor activators can protect against vascular calcification. J Am Soc Nephrol. 2008;19:1509-1519. PMCID:PMC2488263.

[44] Elzanowski A, Barker WC, Hunt LT, Seibel-Ross E. Cystatin domains in alpha-2-HS glycoprotein and fetuin. FEBS Lett. 1988;227(2):167-170.

[45] Schinke T, Amendt C, Trindl A, Poschke O, Muller-Esterl W, Jahnen-Dechent W. The serum protein α2-HS glycoprotein/fetuin inhibits apatite formation in vitro and in mineralizing calvaria cells. J Biol Chem. 1996;271(34):20789-20796.

[46] Demetriou M, Binkert C, Sukhu B, Tenenbaum HD, Dennis JW. Fetuin/alpha2-HS glycoprotein is transforming growth factor-beta type II receptor mimic and cytokine antagonist. J Biol Chem. 1996;271(22):12755-12761.

[47] Binkert C, Demetriou M, Sukhu B, Szweras M, Tennenbaum HC, Dennis JW. Regulation of osteogenesis by Fetuin. J Biol Chem. 1999;274:28514-28520.

[48] Schafer C, Heiss A, Schwarz A, Westenfeld R, Ketteler M, Floege J, et al. The serum protein α2-Heremans-Schmid glycoprotein/fetuin-A is a systemically acting inhibitor of ectopic calcification. J Clin Invest. 2003;112:357-366.

[49] Ketteler M, Bongartz P, Westenfeld R, Wildberger JE, Mahnken AH, Bohm R, et al. Association of low fetuin-A (AHSG) concentrations in serum with cardiovascular mortality in patients on dialysis: a cross-sectional study. Lancet. 2003;361:827-833.

[50] Lebreton JP, Joisel F, Raoult JP, Lannuzel B, Rogez JP, Humbert G. Serum concentration of human alpha 2-HS glycoprotein during the inflammatory process: evidence that alpha 2-HS glycoprotein is a negative acute-phase reactant. J Clin Invest. 1979;64(4):1118-1129.

[51] Simon M, Maresh JG, Harris SE, Hernandez JD, Arar M, Olson MS, et al. Expression of bone morphogenetic protein-7 mRNA in normal and ischemic adult rat kidney. Amer J Physiol. 1999;276:F382-F389.

[52] Wang S, Chen Q, Simon TC, Strebeck F, Chaudhary L, Morrissey J, et al. Bone morphogenetic protein-7 (BMP-7), a novel therapy for diabetic nephropathy. Kidney Int. 2003;63:2037-2049.

[53] Wang S, Hirschberg R. Loss of renal tubular BMP7 during the evolution of experimental diabetic nephropathy. J Am Soc Nephrol. 2000;11:655A.

[54] Davies MR, Lund RJ, Mathew S, Hruska KA. Low turnover osteodystrophy and vascular calcification are amenable to skeletal anabolism in an animal model of chronic kidney disease and the metabolic syndrome. J Am Soc Nephrol. 2005;16:917-928.

[55] Gonzalez EA, Lund RJ, Martin KJ, McCartney JE, Tondravi MM, Sampath TK, et al. Treatment of a murine model of high-turnover renal osteodystrophy by exogenous BMP-7. Kidney Int. 2002;61:1322-1331.

[56] Davies MR, Lund RJ, Hruska KA. BMP-7 is an efficacious treatment of vascular calcification in a murine model of atherosclerosis and chronic renal failure. J Am Soc Nephrol. 2003;14:1559-1567.

[57] Dorai H, Vukicevic S, Sampath TK. Bone morphogenetic protein-7 (osteogenic protein-1) inhibits smooth muscle cell proliferation and stimulates the expression of markers that are characteristic of SMC phenotype in vitro. J Cellular Physiol. 2000;184:37-45.

[58] Kokubo T, Ishikawa N, Uchida H, Chasnoff SE, Xie X, Mathew S, et al. CKD accelerates development of neointimal hyperplasia in arteriovenous fistulas. J Am Soc Nephrol. 2009;20:1236-1245. PMCID:PMC2689906.

[59] White KE, Evans WE, O'Riordan JLH, Speer MC, Econs MJ, Lorenz-Depiereux B, et al. Autosomal dominant hypophosphataemic rickets is associated with mutations in FGF23. Nat Genet. 2000;26:345-348.

[60] Shimada T, Mizutani S, Muto T, Yoneya T, Hino R, Takeda S, et al. Cloning and characterization of FGF23 as a causative factor of tumor-induced osteomalacia. Proc Natl Acad Sci. 2001;98:6500-6505.

[61] Shimada T, Kakitani M, Yamazaki Y, Hasegawa H, Takeuchi Y, Fujita T, et al. Targeted ablation of FGF23 demonstrates an essential physiological role of FGF23 in phosphate and vitamin D metabolism. J Clin Invest. 2004;113:561-568.

[62] Larsson T, Nisbeth U, Ljunggren O, Juppner H, Jonsson KB. Circulating concentration of FGF-23 increases as renal function declines in patients with chronic kidney disease, but does not change in response to variation in phosphate intake in healthy volunteers. Kidney Int. 2003;64:2272-2279.

[63] Weber TJ, Liu S, Indridason OS, Quarles LD. Serum FGF23 levels in normal and disordered phosphorus homeostasis. J Bone Miner Res. 2003;18:1227-1234.

[64] Lee NK, Sowa H, Hinoi E, Ferron M, Ahn JD, Confavreux C, et al. Endocrine Regulation of Energy Metabolism by the Skeleton. Cell. 2007;130:456-469.

[65] Fulzele K, Riddle RC, DiGirolamo DJ, Cao X, Wan C, Chen D, et al. Insulin Receptor Signaling in Osteoblasts Regulates Postnatal Bone Acquisition and Body Composition. Cell. 2010;142:309-319.

[66] Clemens TL, Karsenty G. The osteoblast: An insulin target cell controlling glucose homeostasis. J Bone Miner Res. 2011;26:677-680.

[67] Wang L, Banu J, Mcmahan CA, Kalu DN. Male rodent model of age-related bone loss in men. Bone. 2001;29:141-148.

[68] Clarke BL, Ebeling PR, Jones JD, Wahner HW, O'Fallon WM, Riggs BL, et al. Changes in quantitative bone histomorphometry in aging healthy men. J Clin Endo Metab. 1996;81:2264-2270.

[69] Suzuki K, Miyakoshi N, Tsuchida T, Kasukawa Y, Sato K, Itoi E. Effects of combined treatment of insulin and human parathyroid hormone(1-34) on cancellous bone mass and structure in streptozotocin-induced diabetic rats. Bone. 2003;33:108-114.

[70] Krakauer JC, McKenna MJ, Buderer NF, Rao DS, Whitehouse FW, Parfitt AM. Bone loss and bone turnover in diabetes. Diabetes. 1995;44:775-782.

[71] Shao JS, Cheng SL, Charlton-Kachigian N, Loewy AP, Towler DA. Teriparatide (Human Parathyroid Hormone (1-34)) Inhibits Osteogenic Vascular Calcification in Diabetic Low Density Lipoprotein Receptor-deficient Mice. J Biol Chem. 2003;278:50195-50202.

[72] Lund RJ, Davies MR, Brown AJ, Hruska KA. Successful treatment of an adynamic bone disorder with bone morphogenetic protein-7 in a renal ablation model. J Am Soc Nephrol. 2004;15:359-369.

[73] Hruska KA, Saab G, Chaudhary LR, Quinn CO, Lund RJ, Surendran K. Kidney-bone, bone-kidney, and cell-cell communications in renal osteodystrophy. Semin Nephrol. 2004;24:25-38.

[74] Hruska KA, Choi ET, Memon I, Davis TK, Mathew S. Cardiovascular risk in pediatric chronic kidney disease (CKD), the CKD-mineral bone disorder (CKD-MBD). Pediatr Nephrol. 2010;25:769-778.

In: Issues in Dialysis
Editor: Stephen Z. Fadem

ISBN: 978-1-62417-576-3
© 2013 Nova Science Publishers, Inc.

Chapter XIV

Update on Anemia and Kidney Disease

K. M. Goli[1], A. Pinkhasov[1], D. L. Landry[1], Y. Chait[2],
J. Horowitz[3], C. V. Hollot[4], R. P. Shrestha[2] and M. J. Germain[1,]*
[1]Baystate Medical Center, Division of Nephrology
[2]Department of Mechanical & Industrial Engineering,
University of Massachusetts at Amherst, US
[3]Department of Mathematics and Statistics, University of Massachusetts at Amherst, US
[4]Department of Electrical& Computer Engineering,
University of Massachusetts at Amherst, US

Abstract

In this chapter we will discuss the emerging issues and controversies in anemia management in Chronic Kidney Disease (CKD). The normal physiologic control of erythropoiesis and the pathophysiology in CKD will be discussed specifically with regards to current problems with dosing protocols and novel approaches to improve these issues. The causes and treatments of resistance to erythropoiesis stimulating agents (ESAs), hemoglobin "cycling" and variability will be addressed. The emerging safety concerns with ESAs and novel ESAs that may be safer will be discussed.

Historical Perspective

Anemia is highly prevalent in CKD and End Stage Renal Disease (ESRD) populations. Prior to the advent of ESAs, dialysis patients were heavily transfusion-dependent due to the symptoms of severe anemia. This changed in 1989 when the FDA approved the first ESA, thus ushering a new era of anemia management for patients with advanced CKD and ESRD. Administration of ESAs significantly decreased transfusion related complications and

---

* Corresponding Author. 100 Wason Avenue, Springfield, MA 01107; Michael.Germain@BHS.Org.

improved the quality of life. The first ESA available was epoetin alfa (Epogen/Procrit) and it was the only therapeutic option for over 10 years. Darbepoetin alfa became available in 2001. Over the last 22 years, the few studies that have been done have not demonstrated the hoped for cardiovascular benefits and have in fact shown potential risks of ESA treatment. There are new ESA products currently in development, with novel mechanisms of action that hold promise for greater safety and efficacy.

Physiological Aspects

Erythropoiesis is the process of generating new red blood cells (RBCs), which carry hemoglobin (Hgb). In healthy people, approximately 2.4 million new RBCs are produced each second, to maintain Hgb levels within fairly narrow limits [1] and thereby meet the body's oxygen demand. A feedback mechanism stimulates the production of the glycoprotein hormone erythropoietin (EPO). EPO, secreted primarily by the kidneys in response to hypoxia, stimulates the proliferation of RBC progenitors, and is the major regulating agent of erythropoiesis. In CKD, EPO production is compromised, and resistance to EPO action occurs, leading to inadaquate erythropoiesis, with anemia as the result. (Anemia is defined by the World Health Organization as Hgb concentrations lower than 13 g/dL in men and lower than 12 g/dL in women). While anemia in ESRD patients is primarily due to inadaquate production of EPO, there are other contributing factors, including resistance to EPO, blood loss, reduced RBC lifespan, bone marrow diseases, and iron deficiency. [2] Factors that stimulate the expression of EPO include hypoxia-inducible transcription factor 1 (HIF-1) and hepatocyte nuclear factor 4α; inhibitory factors include GATA-2 and nuclear factor κB (NFκB). [3] Novel investigational agents that target the above factors are the potential ESAs of the future.

What Is the Target Hemoglobin for Patients with CKD and End-Stage Renal Disease?

Since the inception of their use in 1989 [4] the safest and the most cost-effective dose of ESAs has remained an unanswered question. There is very little data studying the effects of ESAs on renal anemia in dialysis patients. Most of the data currently available come from observational cohort studies and several more recent randomized controlled trials (RCTs) in non-dialysis CKD patients. Some authors support the notion that such studies in CKD patients can be freely extrapolated to the ESRD population while others argue that anemia of CKD is generally a milder degree of illness on the same disease spectrum and therefore may not be as likely to show benefit in terms of mortality or cardiovascular events.

Review of RCTs in Hemodialysis Patients

The Normal Hematocrit Study was published in 1998 by Besarab *et al.*, and remains the only RCT evaluating ESA use in ESRD patients using "hard endpoints" such as death and cardiovascular morbidity. [5] This double-blinded study comprised 1233 prevalent ESRD patients with known ischemic heart disease or cardiomyopathy who were randomly assigned epoetin alfa to achieve either a goal hematocrit of 42% or 30%. After 29 months the study was terminated prematurely due to a trend towards increased mortality and nonfatal myocardial infarctions in the normal-hematocrit group (risk ratio of 1.3). The fact that the normal-hematocrit arm received higher doses of ESA, more intravenous iron and had lower Kt/V values during the study period may have also played a role in adverse outcomes. One important cautionary point regarding the above-mentioned results in this study is that – within each treatment arm – higher levels of hematocrit were associated with lower mortality rates.

The Era of Observational Study Data and Elevated Hemoglobin Targets

Despite the warnings raised by the Normal Hematocrit Study, a flurry of observational cohort studies published between 1999 and 2005 led to more aggressive anemia management in ESRD patients with a subsequent increase in achieved Hgb goals. The group from the University of Minnesota collaborated to publish several such studies from the Medicare database showing stable – if not improved – mortality rates for hemodialysis patients with HCT levels > 36% when compared to goal Hgb levels of 33-36% (risk ratio 0.92 in study by Li et al.). [6-8] Ofsthun et al. also reported from their Fresenius database that death and hospitalization were inversely associated with Hgb values and that there appeared to be "no apparent additional risk" when raising Hgb levels to > 12 g/dL. [9]

ESA Studies in CKD Patients

The CREATE study was a European multicenter, open-label RCT of epoetin beta in 603 advanced CKD patients (estimated GFR 24 mL/min) with baseline Hgb levels of 11-12.5 g/dL. [10] Group 1 patients received epoetin beta to achieve Hgb level of 13.0-15.0 g/dL while group 2 only received epoetin beta if the Hgb level fell below 10.5 g/dL (with goal of 10.5-11.5 g/dL). At the end of 3 year study, the primary end point – a composite of 8 cardiovascular events – was similar in both.

The CHOIR study was an open-label, multicenter RCT performed in the United States comprising 1432 patients with advanced CKD (estimated GFR 27 mL/min) and baseline Hgb < 11 g/dL. [11] Patients were randomized to receive epoetin alfa in order to achieve a goal Hgb of 13.5 g/dL (group 1) or 11.3 g/dL (group 2). The study was terminated early after the data and safety monitoring board determined that there was a < 5% chance that group 1 would achieve superiority in terms of the primary or secondary endpoints. In addition, 38.3% of all study participants withdrew from the study (16.9% patients went on to require renal replacement therapy and 21.4% for other reasons). Ultimately, there was no difference in the primary endpoint (time to death, myocardial infarction, hospitalization for congestive heart failure, or stroke) between groups. A secondary analysis of CHOIR published in 2010 found the dose of epoetin alfa and the inability to achieve target Hgb in either group was associated with increased hazard of a primary endpoint and that simply being in the higher Hgb arm was not a risk factor for adverse outcome (see ESA Resistance section).

The TREAT study remains the only double-blind, placebo-controlled RCT of anemia treatment in CKD patients to date. [12] This international, multicenter trial of 4038 diabetic CKD patients with baseline estimated GFR of 34 mL/min and Hgb of 10.4 g/dL had subjects randomized to a darbepoetin alfa arm for goal Hgb 13.0 g/dL versus a placebo arm that would only receive darbepoetin alfa if Hgb was less than 9.0 g/dL. Treatment was discontinued in this latter arm once the Hgb level was > 9.0 g/dL. The primary endpoint of death or cardiovascular event occurred in 632 treatment group patients and 602 patients assigned to placebo (HR 1.05; P=0.41). The outcome of death or development of ESRD had similar findings.

Interpretation of the Present Day Data, and Future Directions

The relationship between Hgb level and mortality is clearly not a straightforward one. While several high-quality RCTs have been published over the last 13 years in an effort to answer the question of what is the optimal hemoglobin level in a dialysis patient, there remains no consensus opinion. Initial reactions to the TREAT, CHOIR and CREATE studies led to a general assumption that all dialysis patients on ESAs with a Hgb level > 12 g/dL were at risk for increased cardiovascular morbidity and overall mortality until secondary analyses brought forward the concept of ESA hyporesponsiveness – and the high-risk medical conditions that often predispose to this – as well as the resultant elevated doses of ESA received that may be more likely contributing to mortality than a specific level of Hgb. Whether or not Hgb is even the right surrogate marker for patient outcomes in ESRD remains in question. Ultimately, it appears that no single study will answer the question of optimal target Hgb level in a dialysis patient but that patients will need to be evaluated and treated individually with the recognition that many factors play a role in the mortality of dialysis patients. Nevertheless, clinical practice guideline from NKF-KDOQI were updated in 2007 to recommend maintaining a Hgb range of 11-12 g/dL and strict avoidance of Hgb levels > 13 g/dL. [13]

In their recently updated guidelines for management of anemia in CKD patients, NICE (National Institute for Health and Clinical Excellence, UK) recommended Hgb range between 10 and 12 g/dL for adults, young people and children aged 2 years and older, and between 9.5 and 11.5 g/dL for children younger than 2 years of age, reflecting the lower normal range in that age group. [14] It will be interesting to see the new KDIGO guidelines on anemia management which are due for the later part of this year.

The lack of clear benefits of aiming for a higher Hgb goal than has been used in clinical practice has led the FDA (Food and Drug Administration) and CMS (Centers for Medicare and Medicaid Services) to readdress both the prescribing information and payment policy. CMS convened an advisory panel recently that was asked to determine whether blood transfusion posed a greater risk than ESA therapy to CKD patients. The panel did not find evidence to support the safety of ESAs over transfusions. The final ruling by CMS in May

2011 did not implement a National Coverage Decision (NCD) and therefore each Medicare Carrier or MAC (Medicare Administrative Contractor) can continue to have Local Coverage Decisions (LCDs) for payment of ESAs. [15] In June 2011 the FDA announced a change in the prescribing information (PI) in CKD for the ESAs that changed the dosing recommendations. It now states that ESAs should not be started until the Hgb is <10 g/dL in both ESRD and non-dialysis CKD patients. Once started, the dose should be held or decreased as the Hgb approaches 11 g/dL. For non-dialysis CKD patients ESAs should be prescribed only to avoid RBC transfusions when there is increased risk for transfusions in that patient. For dialysis patients the goal is to avoid RBC transfusions in all situations. [16] There was a boxed warning on the recent update of prescription information for epoetin alfa stating: In controlled trials, patients experienced greater risks for death, serious adverse cardiovascular reactions, and stroke when administered erythropoiesis-stimulating agents (ESAs) to target a hemoglobin level of greater than 11 g/dL. No trial has identified a hemoglobin target level, ESA dose, or dosing strategy that does not increase these risks. Use the lowest Epogen dose sufficient to reduce the need for red blood cell (RBC) transfusions. [17]

Originally, the Quality Incentive Payment (QIP) system under the bundled payment for dialysis financially penalized Hgb <10 g/dL twice as much as Hgb >12 g/dL., but CMS in November 2011 [18] adopted changes to the QIP for 2012. The proposal eliminates the <10 g/dL measure in an attempt to harmonize with the new PI. Undoubtedly these decisions will result in major changes to the management of anemia in CKD patients (dialysis and non-dialysis). If the clinician's ability to individualize treatment based on the patient's symptoms and medical conditions is severely restricted, the patient likely will suffer from more symptomatic anemia. To prevent transfusion and maintain patient's quality of life (QoL), more frequent monitoring of the Hgb, more careful attention to causes and treatment of ESA resistance, increased use of intravenous iron, and attempts to decrease intra-patient Hgb variability will be required.

Benefits and Risks of ESA Use

In addition to discussions concerning when to initiate ESAs and target Hgb levels, there also remains an ongoing debate concerning the risks and benefits of ESA use. Much of the data remains conflicting as researchers struggle to determine whether the results of numerous ESA studies are a reflection of the overall health and inflammatory status of patients requiring ESA use or of properties of the ESA itself.

What Are the Potential Benefits of ESA Use?

Anemia is present in the majority of ESRD patients and is associated with a decreased QoL. [19] Common impairments include fatigue, depression, shortness of breath and decreased physical activity. The CREATE study [20] reported improvements in QoL measures in the high Hgb (13-15 g/dL) group when compared to the low Hgb (11.0-12.5 g/dL) group in terms of general health and physical function, a result that is supported by 2 recent systematic reviews. [21,22] The TREAT study, however, showed only modest benefit in the FACT fatigue score in its high Hgb arm, with no other significant benefit in other QoL measures. [12]

The Canadian Erythropoietin Study Group's 1990 multicenter, double-blind, placebo-controlled RCT was recently reanalyzed (to comply with the FDA's newer statistical methods requirements). This analysis confirmed the original findings that the correction of severe anemia (Hgb < 9.0 g/dL) with Epoetin alfa in ESRD patients not only had clinically important improvements in fatigue, physical function and 6 minute walking tests, but also a significant decrease in need for transfusion at 8 weeks (58% in placebo v. 3% in Hgb target group of 9.5-11.0 g/dL). [23] Given the association of blood transfusion with risk for iron overload, transfusion reactions, transmission of viral infection, and possible induction of donor-specific HLA antibodies in potential future transplant recipients, the use of ESAs in anemic ESRD patients does appear to have benefit.

Left ventricular hypertrophy (LVH) is another common finding in ESRD patients and is associated with increased mortality. A 2009 meta-analysis of ESA treatment in over 1700 CKD and ESRD patients with severe anemia (Hgb < 10 g/dL) found a significant reduction in left ventricular mass index by 32.7 g/m^2 when Hgb levels were increased to $\leq$12 g/dL. [24] Patients presenting with moderate anemia (Hgb > 10 g/dL) did not show a significant benefit from this intervention or from more aggressive Hgb goals of > 12 g/dL. The correction of similar levels of moderate anemia in the CHOIR and CREATE trials also failed to show benefit in secondary endpoints of LVH and left ventricular mass index. [10,11]

What Are the Potential Risks Associated with ESA Use?

Two RCTs [12,25] have reported an increased risk of stroke in those patients assigned to a high Hgb goal (> 13.0 and > 13.5 g/dL, respectively) while an increased risk for vascular access thrombosis was reported in the Normal Hematocrit Study. [5] Others have reported the potential for inducing hypertension with ESAs; however, both the Normal Hematocrit Study and CREATE trial found no significant increase in blood pressure to support this claim.

Lastly, the issue of ESA use in patients with either an active or prior history of malignancy must be mentioned. In addition to an increased incidence of thrombotic events in patients with active cancer being treated with ESA, concerns regarding tumor progression and overall mortality in patients with breast, non-small cell lung, head and neck, lymphoid, and cervical cancers, when dosed to target a hemoglobin of $\geq$ 12 g/dL, [26] have been reported. The TREAT study also found an increased mortality rate in those patients with a prior (inactive) history of malignancy when treated with ESA. [12] This has led to extremely restricted use in patients with malignancies. There are now Black Box warnings in the ESA's prescribing information regarding these increased risks. [17]

Risk of Red Blood Cell Transfusions (RBCT) Versus ESA Therapy in CKD Patients

Since the achieved Hgb is a bell-shaped curve when treating CKD patients with an ESA, it is inevitable that when a lower Hgb is targeted there will be more patients who will require a RBCT. Threshold Hgb to perform a RBCT in a given patient a is controversial. If the person is asymptomatic and without significant cardiopulmonary disease [27] then a Hgb as low as 6-7 g/dL may be tolerated for chronic anemia. The Hgb threshold for transfusion in the pre-operative situation and in acute blood loss may be quite different.

In the transplant candidate population, it is important to examine the impact of anemia management and RBCT exposure on outcomes, time to transplant, death while awaiting a transplant, patient and graft survival post-transplant. By focusing only on the population that ultimately received a transplant, the true impact of RBCT in the transplant candidate population cannot be accurately evaluated. Consideration should be given to the potential differences in the impact of RBCT status/exposure on subpopulations such as women, older adults, and African Americans.

Relevant outcomes in these subpopulations include:

1) The impact of RBCT on panel reactive antibodies (PRA)
2) The impact of sensitization on transplant wait times, given the longer wait times in these subpopulations.
3) The potential differential impact of a longer wait time due to sensitization in older populations or populations with a higher burden of co-morbid conditions, e.g., mortality either awaiting a transplant or post-transplant.

Although in the pre-cyclosporine era there was evidence of a favorable impact of RBCT on those patients ultimately transplanted, the impact of RBCT on sensitization and prevention or delay of transplant in patients waiting for a transplant was less clear. It is possible that those transplant candidates who received RBCT and were ultimately transplanted may be less immunoresponsive/sensitized (manifested by lower PRA) than those that did not get transplanted. It may appear that RBCT has a positive impact on outcomes; however the more immunoresponsive (sensitized) transplant candidates would have been excluded, as they were not transplanted. Sensitized transplant candidates, manifested by higher PRA, who were ultimately transplanted may have been treated by different immunosuppressive regimens than less sensitized transplant candidates. In the current era of transplantation there is no evidence of a beneficial effect of RBCT on transplant outcomes, and transfused patients have a longer waiting time, higher mortality waiting for a transplant, and shorter graft survival. [28] Conclusions from 2010 USRDS (United States Renal Data System) report include: For transfused versus non-transfused patients, the Hazard Ratio was 4.04 for death and 0.72 for getting a transplant. Sensitized candidates wait longer for transplant, as 28% of wait-listed patients received a RBCT within 3 years of listing. Non-sensitized patients (PRA of 0% at listing) were as likely as mildly sensitized patients (PRA < 20%) to receive a transfusion. Highly sensitized patients (PRA 80 % +) were more likely to receive a transfusion within 3 years of listing, 41% within 3 years of listing. RBCT was associated with decreased likelihood of transplantation. PRA at transplant remains associated with adverse outcomes.

Another potential consideration is transfusion-associated infections or complications (e.g., hepatitis C, transfusion reactions, transfusion associated lung injury) which may preclude a patient from transplantation candidacy or be associated with considerable morbidity or mortality.

Current Dosing Algorithms with ESAs for Anemia Management in CKD

When Epoetin alpha (EPO) was first approved in 1989 for use in CKD, the dosing recommendations in the prescribing information (PI) [17] were based on the doses used in the registrational trials. The trials were done in dialysis patients with EPO given intravenously (IV) three times a week at the end of dialysis. The PI gives a starting dose based on body weight (50-100 U/kg 3 times a week). Although ESAs are approved for non-dialysis patients, the dosing recommendations in the PI are still based on three times a week dosing. Non dialysis CKD, peritoneal dialysis, and some HD patients are dosed subcutaneously (SQ) rather than IV. With subcutaneous dosing the frequency of dosing has been effective at weekly, bi-weekly, monthly or less frequently. [29] Among short-acting ESAs, efficacy of SQ administration in dialysis patients may be superior to that of IV administration. [30] However, in recent DOPPS (Dialysis Outcomes and Practice Patterns Study) data, when dosing was changed from SQ to IV, some of the dialysis units had no change in the effective dose while other dialysis units saw decreased efficacy with IV dosing. [31] Over a period of 6 months or more, the increased efficacy of SQ dosing vs IV may diminish.

In the PI, the recommendations are to decrease the dose by 25% when the Hgb exceeds or is anticipated to exceed the upper limit of the recommended range (10-12 g/dL). If the Hgb is falling or is below the target range then the dose is increased by 25%. The dose is held if the Hgb continues to rise above 12 g/dL. Dose adjustments are made monthly unless the Hgb rises more than 1 g/dL in a 2 week period. Dialysis units and non-dialysis ESA clinics have developed both written and computer based algorithms to improve anemia management. Most are based on the approach recommended in the PI. Some may make larger or smaller adjusted changes in the dose, and the dose may be held at different levels of Hgb. Dose adjustments may be made as frequently as weekly. The frequency of Hgb measurement in the algorithms also varies.

Even though EPO has a short half-life (6 hrs) the pharmacodynamics demonstrate an eight day lag in the response in the erythron. This allows the extended dosing intervals noted above and dictates a different method to anticipate the Hgb response in a dosing algorithm. More frequent Hgb measurements may allow more accurate estimation of response to the ESA, and a more timely response to a change in Hgb [32] but the frequency of dose changes and the incremental change in dose have to be taken into account along with the pharmacodynamics. Newer ESAs (darbepoetin, CERA) have longer half lives, but how this longer half-life affects the pharmacodynamics, dosing interval, and dosing algorithms is not well understood. For example CERA is dosed bimonthly or monthly, but EPO has also been effectively dosed at these extended intervals. [29]

The goals of an algorithm are to provide dosing that keeps the treated population in the target range for the greatest period of time. A secondary goal is to do that at the lowest feasible cumulative ESA dose. Optimally the intra-patient Hgb variability will be minimized. Observational studies have shown that an algorithm (written or computerized) that is applied in a systematic fashion (automatically by a computerized system or by a dedicated "anemia manager") will result in "better" anemia outcomes, lower EPO dose, more patients in target range, better intra-patient Hgb variability, and better dialysis unit performance on a population basis. [33-38]

Recent DOPPS data show a great deal of variability in anemia results in dialysis units that are not accounted for by patient factors. [34] This suggests that facility-specific algorithms (or the lack of, or inconsistent application of algorithms) may explain these results. To date few RCTs have been done to demonstrate superiority of one dosing algorithm over the PI or alternative algorithms. The AMIE algorithm has been one of the most studied and widely used and is based on simple dose adjustments based on ceiling and threshold Hgb levels. [35] Some of the Large Dialysis Organisations (LDOs) have developed and offered algorithms to their facilities, and in most cases they have been developed by trial and error at the local level. Recently more sophisticated computerized programs have been developed to individualize the dosing for the patient's individual response. Systems such as "artificial intelligence" have demonstrated some success in small pilot studies. [36,37] Recently we have demonstrated that with three times a week noninvasive real-time Hgb monitoring via the "Crit-Line" device (Hemometrics Inc. Ogden, UT), utilizing the AMIE algorithm, intra-patient Hgb variability could be decreased. [38] The device is now available with an FDA approved computerized algorithm that automatically uploads the real-time Hgb into the program and gives suggested EPO dosing (CLAM Hemometrics Inc. Ogden UT).

Since EPO sensitivity/resistance, iron stores, EPO utilization and administration, and RBC half-life have a significant impact on ESA response; optimally these factors would be accounted for in algorithm development. The development of individualized algorithms is further complicated by the individual's changing response over time. A patient can be responsive to an ESA at one time period and then resistant later (perhaps due to intercurrent medical events; e.g., infection, inflammation, poor PTH control, medication changes). Acute or chronic blood loss can further complicate management. The effect of dose holding versus a decrease in dose when the Hgb is above or approaching 12 gm/dL is controversial. Recent DOPPS survey data show that only a minority of dialysis facilities hold doses and that it varies by country (USA 24% of facilities to a low of 0% in Spain). [39] In animal studies, holding EPO doses resulted in neocytolysis and a rapid drop in Hgb. [40] This could result in iatrogenic cycling when a larger dose is restarted and then held again when the Hgb is above 12 gm/dl. Observational studies in dialysis patients have supported this hypothesis, except for one study. [41]

Erythropoiesis Modeling for ESA and Iron Dosing Protocols

Improvements in the performance of anemia management protocols (AMPs) require modeling of erythropoiesis and protocol design based feedback control principles. Erythropoiesis depends not only on iron and EPO, but also on a long list of other players including hepcidin, growth factors, vitamins, and cytokines. The current focus in erythropoiesis modeling and design of AMPs is on the causal relationship between ESAs and Hgb concentration. While iron administration is another common feature of AMPs, the lack of iron kinetics modeling is a likely reason that iron supplementation guidelines are not as well-studied.

AMP Design

Currently, institution-specific anemia management protocols follow the latest NKF-KDOQI guidelines and recommendations [42] to determine ESA and iron supplement dosing regimens. These protocols are rule-based and derived from expertise in managing ESRD patients and incorporating results from retrospective studies. The protocol plays the role of the kidneys by measuring Hgb levels and, in response, dispensing ESAs to affect erythropoiesis and ultimately to regulate Hgb. Thus, in designing an AMP, it is important to take into account the closed-loop nature of the AMP-Hgb relationship, and employ feedback control techniques. Indeed, AMPs can contribute to the oscillations in Hgb levels, as recognized by the clinical community, [43] and this is a consequence of the feedback interaction between AMPs and erythropoiesis. Recently, there has been effort to incorporate feedback control principles into the design of AMPs. Such efforts typically require a mathematical model of erythropoiesis. The challenge is to derive control-relevant models that are not overly complex, such as those found in detailed, physiologically-driven models, while capturing enough detail to be physiologically plausible. In what follows, we discuss such control-relevant models.

Pharmacokinetics

Typical pharmacokinetics (PK) models describing the absorption and disposition of ESAs consist of one or two compartments for intravenous administration, and three compartments for subcutaneous administration. [44] Intravenous administration results in faster absorption rate than subcutaneous administration. For single intravenous doses, the half-life of Epogen in CKD patients has been reported to be between 4 and 14 hours. [45 and references therein] For multiple-doses, some have reported short-term half-life reduction. [45] The pharmacokinetics of different Epoetin preparations produced in the US and Europe are similar. [46]

EPO levels can be modeled as the sum of endogenously-produced EPO (residual from compromised kidney function) and that due to ESA dosing. A PK model describing EPO level in response to dosing is described by

$$\frac{d}{dt}x(t) = -k_1 x(t) - \frac{V_{max}\frac{x(t)}{V_1}}{K_m + \frac{x(t)}{V_1}} + d(t)$$

$$E_p(t) = x(t) + E_{en}(t)$$

where E_p and E_{en} are total level and endogenously-produced EPO, respectively, x is the single-compartment state of ESA, and d is the intravenous dose level of ESA. The clearance of EPO is nonlinear, [45,47] and has been modeled above by a combination of a saturable relation (e.g., Michalis-Menten) and linear pathways. [44]

In the above model, k_1 is the linear clearance rate, $V_{\max}$ is the maximum nonlinear clearance, K_m is the value at which nonlinear clearance is 50% of its maximum value, and V_1 is the volume of distribution. In our experience with ESRD patients, the parameters $[k_1, V_{\max}, K_m, V_1]$ change with time due to intercurrent events, e.g., inflammation and bleeding.

Pharmacodynamics

Red blood cells are produced from pluripotent stem cells via processes of differentiation and maturation. EPO affects erythropoiesis by promoting cell survival at both the burst and colony forming unit-erythroid stages. [48] The overall stimulatory effects of E_p on this process is typically represented by a single Hill function or Michaelis-Menten kinetics [49,50]; we adopt the latter

$$k_{in}(t) = \frac{S_{\max} \frac{E_p(t)}{V_1}}{SC_{50} + \frac{E_p(t)}{V_1}}$$

where k_{in} is the cell production rate and $S_{\max}$ and SC_{50} are Michaelis-Menten parameters.

Using a compartmental model, the cell pool kinetics can be described by

$$\frac{d}{dt} R(t) = r_{in}(t) - \int_0^\infty r_{in}(t - \lambda) \ell(t - \lambda, \lambda) d\lambda$$

where R is the number of cells in the pool and $\ell(t, \tau)$ is the probability density function of cell lifespan τ of the cells entering the pool at time t. There exists little agreement about the type of cell lifespan models that are consistent with the physiology of erythropoiesis. The simplest of such models depicts the turnover of cells from one pool to the subsequent pool or death via senescence using a fixed lifespan of cells in that pool. More general cell lifespan models include the Gamma distribution [50] or Weibull distribution, [50] both also commonly used in survival analysis. [51] To model random destruction of RBCs in addition to lifespan, a survivor function $S(t)$ of the Verhulst-Pearl distribution form multiplied by an exponential factor is used in. [52]

Iron Kinetics

The precise mechanisms relating both EPO and iron to erythropoiesis are still not completely understood. [53] However, it is clear that an increase in ESA affects iron stores and the availability of iron for Hgb synthesis and other essential metabolic processes. [43] In CKD patients, iron metabolism is affected by inflammation, nutrition, blood loss, and the non-physiological pattern of ESA administration which has been particularly linked to functional iron deficiency. [54]

Earlier attempts to model iron kinetics involved multiple compartments, [55,56] however, such models require a large number of measurements in order to estimate the parameters. In the context of CKD, recent models use a single iron compartment [57] that depends on EPO levels and IV iron administration, or a nonlinear relation involving TSAT. [58] However, it is not clear if bone marrow iron stores and peripheral iron indices correlate well with the erythropoietic response [59] in the face of varying levels of inflammation and functional iron deficiency. The use of reticulocyte hemoglobin level, a readily available measurement, is now being promoted as an accurate predictor of the erythropoietic response to iron supplementation. [60]

The simplest approach to defining the total amount of hemoglobin H is to assume a constant amount of hemoglobin per red blood cell so that

$$H(t) = K_H RBC(t)$$

where K_H is the mean corpuscular hemoglobin (or MCH). While treating K_H as constant is reasonable for non-anemics, iron deficiencies in CKD patients make a time-varying K_H more appropriate. Modeling K_H as a function of reticulocyte hemoglobin and iron supplementation is certainly a worthwhile research topic.

Blood Volume Dynamics

Anemia management protocols seek to control hemoglobin concentration

$$[H(t)] = \frac{H(t)}{V_b}$$

where V_b is the blood volume. This is equivalent to controlling the hematocrit, which, as previously noted, is maintained at approximately 45% in healthy individuals. Thus, in addition to the total number of RBCs and MCH, anemia management calls for controlling blood volume, too.

In ESRD patients, the sodium balance is positive, leading to increased extracellular fluid volume. Both sodium and fluid are removed in hemodialysis, resulting in continuous fluctuations in blood volume V_b. These fluctuations underlie a fundamental limitation of current AMPs. By and large, AMPs can control RBC production and MCH, whereas hemodialysis controls blood volume, thus the management of the two, hemoglobin and blood volume, is conducted by two independent processes. For AMPs to become more effective, for example, to eliminate hemoglobin cycling, [61] it is imperative that the hemoglobin concentration should be regulated by relying on both erythropoiesis and fluid volume management. Total blood volume is not routinely measured in dialysis, and the only FDA-approved blood-volume measurement method requires RBC labeling [62] and has not been adopted in hemodialysis.

Preliminary Results

Our research group works on the design of AMPs using feedback control principles applied to the pharmacokinetics and pharmacodynamics described above. We take the RBC lifespan distribution as a 2nd-order Gamma distribution, and to avoid model over-parameterization, we use a time delay to capture the bioprocess involving the stimulatory effect of ESAs on proliferation and differentiation of progenitor cells into RBCs. As our focus has been only on the administration of ESAs, iron kinetics and blood volume dynamics were modeled as the constants K_H and V_b. A block diagram of this AMP-erythropoiesis feedback loop is shown in Figure 1.

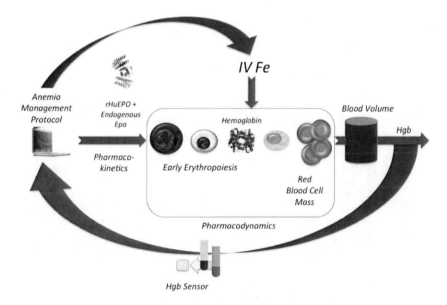

Figure 1. A block diagram representation of the AMP-erythropoiesis feedback control loop illustrating the coupled EPO/iron (IV Fe)/RBC dynamics. Control-relevant models allow for parameter estimation with only Hgb measurements.

An application of AMP design, based on feedback control theory and parameter estimation of our PK/PD model for a specific patient (#10 in our study) is shown in Figure 2. [63] A first observation is that, characteristically, this and virtually all other patient experience changes in the underlying erythropoiesis dynamics. This occurs due to inflammation or bleeding. An initial set of model parameters (model 1) accurately predicts hemoglobin response from days 550 to 675; but fails thereafter. At this point, it appears that the patient's PD has changed, either the iron content per cell constant (K_H) or RBC lifespan appears to have been increased. Our new protocol was designed based on model 1 to be robust to such model parameter uncertainty; indeed, the protocol guides the patient smoothly towards the target Hgb level of 11.25 g/dL. It is observed that the EPO doses needed to achieve target Hgb decreased substantially after the new AMP was implemented. An important feature of this AMP lies in its flexibility: its input data are current and past EPO and Hgb values, as well as desired Hgb target (11.25 g/dL in this example), which can be changed in response to the patient's condition. The protocol itself does not change. The protocol can be re-tuned periodically to the most recently estimated set of model parameters (Model 2). (See Figure 2.)

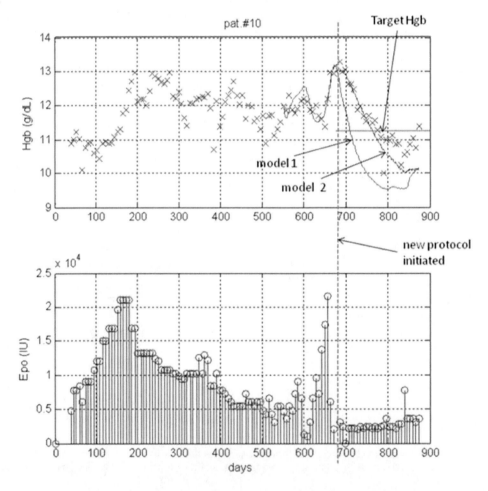

Figure 2. Hemoglobin (top) and IV EPO doses (bottom) traces of pat. #10 (day 1 is 1.1.2009). Prior to day 675, different AMPs have been used; our new protocol was initiated on day 675 with a target of 11.25 g/dL; model 1 and model 2 correspond to predicted responses using two different sets of estimated parameters.

However, such techniques may not be sufficient. Fluid volume balance and iron kinetics, two critical properties directly affecting hemoglobin levels, may be the underlying sources of variability observed in some patients.

To summarize, continuous advances in hemodialysis technology can offer improvements in the effectiveness of dialysis treatments in the face of limited resources. Similarly, new erythropoiesis stimulating protein preparations, HIF stabilizing agents, and therapeutic iron compounds may offer nephrologists with improved means for the treatment of anemia of CKD. Protocols for the administration of ESAs and iron continue to evolve; however, they are largely based on clinical studies and experience. The applications of mathematical modeling of erythropoiesis and feedback control techniques are currently under investigation by several groups, and when combined with carefully designed clinical studies have the potential to define a new paradigm for the design of clinical anemia management protocols.

ESA Resistance

Some patients are relatively resistant to ESAs and require large doses. This is clinically important, since a poor response to ESA therapy may be associated with increased mortality. [64] Evaluation for ESA resistance is recommended *if Hgb level is persistently less than 11 g/dL and if ESA doses are equivalent to epoetin greater than 500 IU/kg/wk.* [65] Although there is no universally accepted definition, the KDOQI definition of hyporesponsiveness [65] is widely used. Response to ESA is determined by dose, route of administration, frequency, iron stores, infection and inflammation etc. Figure 3 summarizes the causes of EPO resistance

Causes of EPO Resistance

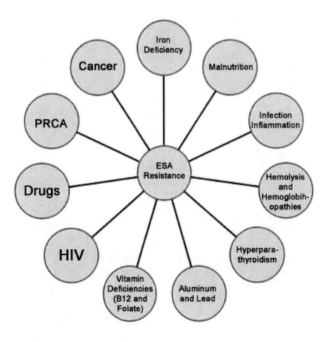

Figure 3. Causes of EPO Resistance.

Table 1. Causes, Clinical findings and Treatment of EPO resistance

Cause	Clinical findings	Treatment
Iron deficiency	High Dose EPO Ferritin < 1200 ng/mL TSAT < 20%	IV Iron. Check for occult bleeding and treat underlying cause.
Malnutrition	Low BMI hypoalbuminemia	Protein and micronutrient supplementation. Correct underlying cause of malnutrition.
Infection and inflammation	Check old AV grafts, periodontal disease, and old transplant kidney.	Treat underlying cause like removal of access referral to a dentist and transplant nephrectomy.
Hyperparathyroidism [77]	Elevated PTH	Treat hyperparathyroidism. If resistant to medical treatment consider parathyroidectomy.
Hemolysis and hemoglobinopathies [78,79]	Elevated LDH, low haptoglobin, increase in indirect bilirubin. Elevated reticulocyte index, positive coombs test.	Testing for hemoglobinopahties. Check for mechanical heart valves [80] and treat underlying disorder. Rule out autoimmune causes.
Drugs (antibiotics, antivirals, immunosuppressants, ACE/ARB etc.) [81,82,83]	Temporal relation of anemia and medications.	Discontinue offending drugs.
Folate and vitamin B12 deficiency	High MCV, elevated homocysteine and MMA.	Supplement folate and B12. [84]
Inadequate Dialysis	URR < 65%	Increase dialysis dose. Treat underlying cause of inadequate dialysis.
Pure Red Cell Aplasia (PRCA)	*ESA therapy > 4 weeks and with sudden rapid decline in Hb level at the rate of 0.5 to 1.0 g/dL/wk, or requirement of RBC transfusions > 1 to 2 per week; normal platelet and white blood cell counts; and absolute reticulocyte count < 10,000/µL*	Discontinue ESA's, RBC transfusions and immunosuppressive therapy. [85]
Malignancies: e.g., multiple myeloma, myelofibrosis and myelodysplastic syndromes.	*Refractory anemia.*	Treat underlying malignancy

Iron deficiency is the most common cause of ESA resistance. Three important mechanisms have been proposed to explain the iron deficiency in dialysis patients in addition to the increased demand of iron when erythropoiesis is stimulated by EPO. These include abnormal iron absorption, external blood loss and functional iron deficiency. [66] Functional iron deficiency is present when the usual tests for iron deficiency in dialysis patients do not indicate absolute iron deficiency (ferritin > 100 ng/ml; Tsat > 20%), but patients respond to additional iron administration with a rise in hematocrit at a stable EPO dose or maintain a stable hematocrit with a lower EPO dose. Patients with functional iron deficiency therefore have insufficient available iron to keep up with the demands of the stimulated erythropoiesis that occur when exogenous EPO is administered. [67]

Infection and Inflammation is the second most common cause of ESA resistance. Treatment of underlying infection usually restores the responsiveness. The existence of elements of malnutrition-inflammation complex syndrome (MICS) as indicated by a high malnutrition-inflammation score (MIS) and increased levels of proinflammatory cytokines such as IL-6 as well as decreased nutritional values such as low serum concentrations of total cholesterol, prealbumin, and TIBC correlates with EPO hyporesponsiveness in dialysis patients. [68] Occult infection of old nonfunctioning AVG is another common cause of erythropoietin resistance and chronic inflammatory state among dialysis patients. Resection of old nonfunctioning AVGs with occult infection is associated with resolution of markers of chronic inflammatory state. [69] Increased number of vascular access related infections and dialysis catheter insertions is also associated with higher EPO requirements. [70] Periodontitis is another occult source of inflammation in hemodialysis patients. [71] Patients who return to dialysis with failed transplants is another cause of ESA resistance [72] and transplant nephrectomy should be considered in these patients. [73] HIV and CMV seropositivity may also determine the EPO dose and Hgb levels in CKD patients. [74,75]

Insulin resistance: In recent study, insulin resistance is found to be associated with ESA resistance. Patients on hemodialysis who has diabetes and insulin resistance required larger doses of EPO. [76]

Non-iron Pharmacologic Agents

A number of non-iron pharmacologic agents have been evaluated as adjuvants to erythropoiesis stimulating agents (ESA). These include L-carnitine, androgens, pentoxifylline, and statins. While some centers are using these agents in EPO resistance patients, there are no good randomized controlled trials to support their use.

Role of Vitamin C in Anemia of CKD

Ascorbic acid may enhance iron availability by mobilizing iron from its storage sites [86] and through its role of incorporation of iron into the heme moiety. [87] Small randomized trials also suggest a potential benefit of ascorbic acid, although the effectiveness of this agent is unclear because of variability in results, particularly with different routes of administration. Safety concerns related to potential secondary oxalosis also exist in hemodialysis patients.

[88] A meta-analysis conducted to evaluate the efficacy and safety of ascorbic acid revealed that ascorbic acid use may result in an increase in hemoglobin concentration and transferrin saturation and decrease in EPO requirements. However, the available studies are limited by small numbers of subjects, short durations of follow-up and variable quality. [89]

Safety and Efficacy of IV Iron

ESRD individuals exhibit major differences in iron metabolism which include decreased duodenal iron absorption, decreased iron transport capacity because of a reduced transferrin concentration, increased iron loss due to frequent blood sampling, occult gastrointestinal bleeding and other means (such as losses of blood into dialysis tubing and dialyzers), and an increased rate of iron turnover to maintain the decreased red blood cell mass. [90] Alternatively, impaired capacity to mobilize iron from its stores can result in functional iron deficiency.

Role of Hepcidin

Oral iron is inferior to intravenous iron in patients on hemodialysis, in part because elevated serum levels of hepcidin prevent intestinal absorption of iron. Increased levels of hepcidin also impair the normal recycling of iron through the reticuloendothelial system. It is also proposed that increased hepcidin levels due to decreased renal clearance as well as due to inflammation may be a significant factor contributing to the development of anemia in CKD and should be considered in the development of new therapies for this disease. [91]

Efficacy of IV Iron

As described previously, RBC transfusions should be avoided in renal transplant candidates to prevent sensitization owing to the formation of preformed reactive antibodies. The Dialysis Patients' Response to IV Iron with Elevated Ferritin (DRIVE) study is a controlled, multicenter trial that randomly assigned hemodialysis patients to 1 g of ferric gluconate or no iron therapy if they were anemic, had serum ferritin of 500 to 1200 ng/ml, had TSAT $\leq$ 25%, and was receiving adequate EPO dosages. At randomization, EPO was increased 25% in both groups and further dosage changes were prohibited. At 6 weeks, hemoglobin increased significantly more in the intravenous iron group than in the control group. Hemoglobin response occurred faster and more patients responded after intravenous iron than in the control group. Ferritin <800 or >800 ng/ml had no relationship to the magnitude or likelihood of responsiveness to intravenous iron relative to the control group. The DRIVE study concluded that administration of ferric gluconate (125 mg for eight treatments) is superior to no iron therapy in anemic dialysis patients receiving adequate EPO dosages and have a ferritin 500 to 1200 ng/ml and TSAT <25% . [92] Later, DRIVE-II study which is a follow up observational extension of DRIVE study showed that ferric gluconate maintains hemoglobin and allows lower epoetin doses in anemic hemodialysis patients with low TSAT and ferritin levels up to 1200 ng/ml. [93] However critics pointed out that twelve weeks of safety data are clearly inadequate to justify the administration of IV iron to patients with underlying inflammatory processes, as seen in the DRIVE trials in high-sensitivity C-reactive protein elevated. Results from other studies also demonstrate that use of intravenous iron can lower ESA dose requirements in dialysis patients. [94] Although we have focused on the potential harm of excessive dose of ESAs, readers are reminded that the long-term safety of IV iron administration has never been established. [95] Ferumoxytol is a new intravenous iron preparation that is being used widely in United States. Among patients who were on HD, rapid intravenous injection of 510 mg of ferumoxytol led to greater Hgb increases compared with oral iron and with comparable tolerability. [96]

Hazards of Iron Therapy

Literature indicates that excessive iron load may cause several toxic side effects. Rare acute adverse events like anaphylactic reactions may occur. Low-molecular-weight iron dextrans (e.g. ferrous gluconate and iron sucrose) have a markedly lower incidence of associated severe anaphylactoid reactions than high-molecular-weight iron dextrans. Furthermore, iron overload may lead to ventricular arrhythmia and heart failure [97] and causes low density lipoprotein (LDL) oxidation, endothelial dysfunction and an increased infection rate thereby stimulating atherosclerosis. [97,98] These findings suggest that iron administration may contribute to cardiovascular complications in CKD and dialysis patients. In a recent article, therapeutically administrated iron induced an increase in intramonocytic ferritin levels. It also showed that cumulative iron loading negatively impacts the innate immune effector function and likewise increases the risk for infectious complications. [99] High doses of ESA's need to be avoided because of safety issues as shown in recent trials. However, there is no evidence to support the assumption that achieving a target hemoglobin concentration in patients on dialysis with evidence of ongoing inflammation by using less ESA and more IV iron will prove safer than trying to achieve that target with more ESA or any other potential strategy. Well designed, randomized clinical trials with clinically relevant endpoints and the adequate collection of safety information are needed to address this concern. [95]

Iron Supplementation and Monitoring Parameters

According to the KDOQI guidelines, sufficient iron should be given to maintain ferritin > 200 ng/ml and TSAT >20% or CHr >29 pg/cell during ESA treatment and that these indices should be used in monitoring. [42] According to the Japanese Society for Dialysis Therapy (JSDT) guidelines, to prevent iron overload and its complications, iron therapy should be instituted only when both TSAT <20% and ferritin <100 ng/ml, thus using lower dose of iron and giving it less frequently than in western countries. [100-101] However, in patients with CKD and ESRD, TSAT and Ferritin are poor indicators of body iron load. [102] The Drive Study as described above clearly demonstrated improvement of anemia in dialysis patients with high ferritin 500-1200 ng/ml and TSAT < 25%. [92] Other indices have been studied like hypochromic red blood cells, cellular hemoglobin in reticulocytes or reticulocyte hemoglobin content (CHr) and reticulocyte hemoglobin equivalent (Ret He) and are gaining popularity but are not yet widely used [103-104] due to limitations in instrumentation as in the case with CHr. [42] According to the NICE (National Institute for Health and Clinical Excellence) guidelines, patients with CKD whose ferritin level is greater than 100 ng/ml, iron deficiency should be defined as TSAT <20% or percentage of hypochromic red cells >6% where the test is available. [105] Currently there is no consensus regarding the timing of IV iron therapy initiation and on monitoring iron indices. Based on the lack of consensus, an individualized approach should be utilized while keeping in mind the hazards of iron therapy which are described above. The new KDIGO guidelines on anemia management are due to be out this year which will hopefully clarify some of the above issues.

Hemoglobin Variability, Cycling and Mortality

Interpatient hemoglobin variability is defined as the width of the hemoglobin (Hgb) level distribution curve for a population at a single point in time and that could be quantified as the standard deviation (SD) of that range. The 3 major factors contributing to this variability were perceived as the variability in Hgb level target/action threshold, variability in anemia management penetration, effectiveness, and variability in individual patient responses to ESAs and intravenous iron. [106] Intrapatient Hb level variability is the variation in Hgb levels over time in a single patient. [107] Hgb cycling is defined as periodic fluctuation in Hgb levels in an individual patient. [61] A hemoglobin cycle was defined as a series of measured hemoglobin levels in an individual patient that oscillated over time, in which the levels decreased or increased over time, and then reversed direction and approximately retraced the initial trajectory. [61]

Measuring Hemoglobin Variability

In clinical practice, it is generally the intrapatient Hgb variability is important, whereas for quality assurance purposes, both interpatient and intrapatient Hgb variability are relevant. Various non temporal and temporal methods are described to measure hemoglobin variability. [108]

The Impact of Hemoglobin Cycling on Patients' Health and Mortality

The impact of hemoglobin cycling on patients' health outcomes is not known. The frequent cycling of hemoglobin concentrations in hemodialysis patients treated with ESA's is an artificial phenomenon as it is not seen in normal healthy homeostasis. Hemoglobin fluctuations may potentially cause pathologic tissue changes for a variety of reasons. Reduced hemoglobin concentration leads to left ventricular dilatation and hypertrophy. This results at least in part from changes in intracardiac cellular growth signaling. It was hypothesized that as hemoglobin levels rise and fall in hemodialysis patients, the disordered activation and resetting of cardiac growth signals could result in pathologic alterations in cardiac structure and function. Similarly, other tissues and organs throughout the body may also be sensitive to injury related to variability in hemoglobin level and oxygen delivery. [61]

Several reports linked the hemoglobin variability as an independent marker of mortality. [109] Some suggested that it is actually the number of months with the hemoglobin values below the target range, rather than the hemoglobin variability itself is the cause of increased mortality. [110] This created confusion among the physicians about their own ESA dosing algorithms, by contributing to Hgb level variability, could be placing patients at risk, and also whether efforts to minimize time spent with a low Hgb level through the use of escalating ESA doses could favorably affect outcomes. [111] NHCT, CHOIR, CREATE and TREAT trials further increased this confusion.

A recent retrospective observational study concluded that after adjustment for confounding disease severity, evidence supporting an association between interpatient Hgb level variability and mortality is weak and inconsistent. [112] Around the same time another prospective cohort study demonstrated that facility-level hemoglobin SD was associated strongly and positively with patient mortality, not tightly linked to numerous patient characteristics, but related strongly to facility anemia management practices. It concluded that facility-level hemoglobin variability may be modifiable and its optimization may improve hemodialysis patient survival. [34] While this controversy persists, it is reasonable to adopt the strategies to decrease intra- and interpatient Hgb variability until we have further studies to clarify.

Strategies to Decrease Intra- and Interpatient Hb Variability [13,108,111]

- Weekly Hgb level monitoring rather than biweekly or monthly
- More frequent review of ESA dose (biweekly rather than monthly)
- ESA administered by intravenous (rather than subcutaneous) route
- Narrower target Hgb level range (10.5-11.5 rather than 10-12g/dL)
- Lower upper target Hgb level
- Smaller (25% increase or decrease rather than doubling or withholding) titrations in ESA dose
- Preemptive adjustments in ESA dose based on trends within the target range
- Preemptive increase in ESA dose for infections, bleeding, surgeries, and after hospitalization
- Optimal iron management (avoid iron deficiency with maintenance protocols)
- Consider long acting ESAs for patients with frequent missed dialysis treatments
- Develop and refine facility-specific anemia treatment algorithms
- Dedicated anemia management nurse
- Identifying and treating the underlying causes of ESA hypo-responsiveness.

Innovative Investigational Agents to Treat Anemia of CKD

- Hematide
- Hypoxia-Inducible transcription Factor (HIF) Stabilizers
- GATA inhibitors.
- Hemopoetic cell phosphatase inhibitors
- Sotatercept

Hematide: It is a synthetic erythropoietin-mimetic agent which is a dimeric peptide conjugated to a PEG moiety. Its amino acid sequence is unrelated to native EPO and it is immunologically distinct but with the same functional and biological properties. It is partially cleared by the kidney and has a prolonged half-life allowing for monthly injections. [113] One of its advantages is lower immunogenicity compared with conventional ESAs as a study by Macdougall et al. concluded that Hematide can correct anemia in patients with pure red-cell aplasia caused by antierythropoietin antibodies. [114]

Hypoxia-Inducible transcription Factor (HIF) Stabilizers: are the orally-active inhibitors of HIF prolyl hydroxylase. In a study by Bernhardt et al., 12 hemodialysis patients were given an orally active prolyl-hydroxylase inhibitor, FG-2216, with an increase in plasma EPO levels, indicating that FG-2216 can stimulate endogenous EPO production via manipulation of the HIF system. [115] There are controversies on safety of their use.

GATA inhibitors: GATA-4 participates in the switch of the primary EPO production site from the fetal liver to the adult kidney. [116] GATA-1, 2 and 3 transcription factors specifically bind to the GATA element in the human EPO gene promoter and negatively regulate EPO gene expression. [117] Therefore, disrupting this negative signal is a potential future strategy for anemia management. Molecule K-11706, which is orally administered, restored the hemoglobin concentration, reticulocyte counts, EPO levels, and erythropoiesis suppressed by IL-1 beta or TNF-alfa in a mouse model of anemia. [118]

Hemopoietic cell phosphatase inhibition: SHP-1, also known as hemopoietic cell phosphatase (HCP), binds to the negative regulatory domain of the EPO receptor leading to dephosphorylation of JAK-2 and subsequent down-regulation of EPO intracellular signal transduction. [119] Studies of CD 34 + cells from HD patients who responded poorly to EPO showed that when compared to EPO-responsive patients, EPO –hyporesponsive patients' CD34+ cells showed increased mRNA and protein expression of SHP-1. The treatment of CD34+ cells with SHP-1 inhibitor resulted in partial recovery of erythroid colony formation. Inhibition of SHP-1 may also be beneficial in improving responsiveness to rHuEPO. [120]

Sotatercept (ACE-011) is a novel therapeutic agent that has been shown to increase levels of red blood cells and hemoglobin as well as stimulate new bone formation. Sotatercept is a soluble activin receptor type 2A IgG-Fc fusion protein that inhibits certain members of the TGF-beta superfamily. It is not an EPO based product or EPO-mimetic and does not bind to the EPO-receptor. A phase IIa, multicenter, double-blinded, RCT ongoing to evaluate the effect of sotatercept on anemia in patients with ESRD. [121]

Conclusion

There are many unanswered questions concerning anemia management in CKD as evidenced by the discussion above. Many of these questions will need to be addressed by large RCTs. In the meanwhile clinicians must understand the current state of knowledge and use their best judgment weighing the risks and benefits of treatment. These are restricted however by policies by the payers for ESA dosing that are not aligned across the country. Added to this confusion are current guidelines by KDOQI and pending guidelines by KDIGO. CMS has imposed Quality Incentive Payments (QIP) on dialysis units that penalize for Hgb values below 10 g/dL and above 12 g/dL. Recent changes in the prescribing information (PI) for ESA mandated by the FDA give dosing guidelines that are in conflict with these goals (no ESA for Hgb $\geq$ 10 g/dL). These dosing guidelines will likely result in increased Hgb cycling and variability which is the opposite of the FDA goals. There are no indications for patient's symptoms of quality of life. The clinician must work within these constraints to provide the best care possible for their individual patients.

References

[1] Guyton AC, Hall JE. Guyton and Hall Textbook of Medical Physiology. 11th ed. Philadelphia: Elsevier Saunders; 2006.

[2] Nurko S. Anemia in chronic kidney disease: causes, diagnosis, treatment, Cleve Clin J Med. 2006;73(3):289-97.

[3] Jelkmann W. Control of erythropoietin gene expression and its use in medicine. Methods Enzymol. 2007;435:179-97.

[4] Eschbach JV, Egrie JC, Downing MR, et al. Correction of the anemia of end-stage renal disease with recombinant human erythropoietin. Results of a combined phase I and II clinical trial. N Engl J Med. 1987;316:73-78.

[5] Besarab A, Bolton WK, Browne JK, et al. The effects of normal as compared with low hematocrit values in patients with cardiac disease who are receiving hemodialysis and epoetin. N Engl J Med. 1998 Aug 27;339(9):584-590.

[6] Li S, Collins AJ. Association of hematocrit value with cardiovascular morbidity and mortality in incident hemodialysis patients. Kidney Int. 2004;65:626-633.

[7] Collins AJ, Li S, St Peter W, et al. Death, hospitalization, and economic associations among incident hemodialysis patients with hematocrit values of 36 to 39%. J Am Soc Nephrol. 2001;12:2465-2473.

[8] Ma JZ, Ebben J, Xia H, Collins AJ. Hematocrit level and associated mortality in hemodialysis patients. J Am Soc Nephrol. 1999;10:610-619.

[9] Ofsthun N, Labrecque J, Lacson E, et al. The effects of higher hemoglobin levels in mortality and hospitalization in hemodialysis patients. Kidney Int. 2003;63:1908-1914.

[10] Drueke TB, Locatelli F, Clyne N, et al. Normalization of hemoglobin level in patients with chronic kidney disease and anemia. N Engl J Med. 2006;355:2071-2084.

[11] Singh AK, Szczech L, Tang KL, et al. Correction of anemia with epoetin alfa in chronic kidney disease. N Engl J Med. 2006;355:2085-2098.

[12] Pfeffer MA, Burdmann EA, Chen CY, et al. The TREAT Investigators. A trial of darbepoetin alfa in type 2 diabetes and chronic kidney disease. N Engl J Med. 2009;361:2019-2032.

[13] National Kidney Foundation. KDOQI Clinical Practice Guideline and Clinical Practice Recommendations for Anemia in Chronic Kidney Disease: 2007 Update of Hemoglobin Target. Am J Kidney Dis. 2007;50:471-530.

[14] Anemia management in people with chronic kidney disease – NICE Clinical Guideline 114 2011; Feb. [cited 20 Jul 2011]. Available from: http://www.nice.org.uk/+ nicemedia/live/13329/52853/52853.pdf.

[15] Proposed Decision Memo for Proposed Decision Memo for Erythropoiesis Stimulating Agents (ESAs) for Treatment of Anemia in Adults with CKD Including Patients on Dialysis and Patients not on Dialysis (CAG-00413N). [cited 2 Jul 2011]. Available from: http://www.cmms.hhs.gov/medicare-coverage-database/details/nca-proposed-decision-memo.aspx?NCAId=245&ver=9&NcaName=Erythropoiesis+Stimulating+ Agents+(ESAs)+for+Treatment+of+Anemia+in+Adults+with+CKD+Including+Patient s+on+Dialysis+and+Patients+not+on+Dialysis&MEDCACId=56&bc=BEAAAAAAE AAA&.

[16] Response to citizen petition regarding epoetin alfa (Docket No. FDA-2009-P-0426). [cited 2 Jul 2011]. Available from: http://www.mtppi.org/new/FDA_Response.pdf.

[17] Highlights of Prescribing Information – Epogen® (epoetin alfa). [cited 22 Jul 2011]. Available from: http://pi.amgen.com/united_states/epogen/epogen_pi_hcp_english.pdf.

[18] Centers for Medicare & Medicaid Services. Medicare Program; End-Stage Renal Disease Prospective Payment System and Quality Incentive Program. Department of Health and Human Services. 42 CFR Parts 413 and 414 Federal Register 2011;76(218):70228-70316. [cited 23 Nov 2011]. Available from: http://www.gpo.gov/fdsys/pkg/FR-2011-11-10/pdf/2011-28606.pdf.

[19] Evans RW, Manninen DL, Garrison LP Jr, et al. The quality of life of patients with end-stage renal disease. N Engl J Med. 1985;312:553-559.

[20] Drueke TB, Locatelli F, Clyne N, et al. Normalization of hemoglobin level in patients with chronic kidney disease and anemia. N Engl J Med. 2006;355:2071-2084.

[21] Gandra SR, Finkelstein FO, Bennett AV, Lewis EF, Brazg T, Martin ML. Impact of erythropoiesis-stimulating agents on energy and physical function in nondialysis CKD patients with anemia: a systematic review. Am J Kidney Dis. 2010;55(3):519.

[22] Johansen KL, Finkelstein FO, Revicki DA, Gitlin M, Evans C, Mayne TJ. Systematic review and meta-analysis of exercise tolerance and physical functioning in dialysis patients treated with erythropoiesis-stimulating agents. Am J Kidney Dis. 2010;55:535.

[23] Keown PA, Churchill DN, Poulin-Costello M, et al. Dialysis patients treated with Epoetin alfa show improved anemia symptoms: A new analysis of the Canadian Erythropoietin Study Group trial. Hemodial Int. 2010;14:168-173.

[24] Parfrey PS, Lauve M, Latremouille-Viau D, Lefebvre P. Erythropoietin therapy and left ventricular mass index in CKD and ESRD patients: a meta-analysis. Clin J Am Soc Nephrol. 2009;4:755.

[25] Parfrey PS, Foley RN, Wittreich BH, et al. Double-blind comparison of full and partial anemia correction in incident hemodialysis patients without symptomatic heart disease. J Am Soc Nephrol. 2005;16:2180-2189.

[26] Bohlius J, Schmidlin K, Brillant C, et al. Recombinant human erythropoiesis-stimulating agents and mortality in patients with cancer: a meta-analysis of randomised trials. Lancet. 2009;373:1532-42.

[27] Guidelines for Transfusion of Red Blood Cells – Adults. New York State Council on Human Blood and Transfusion Services. [cited 23 Nov 2011]. Available from: http://www.wadsworth.org/labcert/blood_tissue/txrbcadultsfinal1104.pdf.

[28] Snyder JJ. Continued use of Transfusion in the Transplant Waitlist Population, Even Among Non-Sensitized Candidates. [cited 2011 Jun 16]. Available from: http://www.usrds.org/2010/pres/b_cs/F-FC303_Snyder_BloodTransufsions.pdf.

[29] Spinowitz B, Germain M, Benz R, Wolfson M, McGowan T, Tang KL, Kamin M. Epoetin Alfa Extended Dosing Study Group. A randomized study of extended dosing regimens for initiation of epoetin alfa treatment for anemia of chronic kidney disease. Clin J Am Soc Nephrol. 2008 Jul;3(4):1015-21.

[30] Kaufman JS, Reda DJ, Fye CL, et al. Subcutaneous compared with intravenous epoetin in patients receiving hemodialysis. Department of Veterans Affairs Cooperative Study Group on Erythropoietin in Hemodialysis Patients. N Engl J Med. 1998 Aug 27;339(9):578-83.

[31] Pisoni RL, et al. XLVII European Renal Association/European Dialysis and Transplant Association Congress (ERA-EDTA 2010). Free Communication Session 24; OSu054.

[32] Gawada AE, Nathanson BH, Jacobs AA, Aranoff GR, Germain MJ and Brier ME. Determining Optimum Hemoglobin Sampling for Anemia Management from Every-Treatment Data. Clin J Am Soc Nephrol. 2010;5:1939–1945.

[33] Miskulin DC, Weiner DE, Tighiouart H, et al. Computerized decision support for EPO dosing in hemodialysis. Am J Kidney Dis. 2009;54:1081-1088.

[34] Pisoni RL, Bragg-Gresham JL, Fuller DS, et al. Facility-level interpatient hemoglobin variability in hemodialysis centers participating in the Dialysis Outcomes and Practice Patterns Study (DOPPS): associations with mortality, patient characteristics, and facility practices. Am J Kidney Dis. 2011;57(2):266-275.

[35] Will EJ, Richardson D, Tolman C, Bartlett C. Development and exploitation of a clinical decision support system for the management of renal anaemia. Nephrol Dial Transplant. 2007;22 [Suppl 4]:iv31–iv36.

[36] Brier ME, Gaweda AE, Dailey A, Aronoff GR, Jacobs AA. Randomized trial of model predictive control for improved anemia management. Clin J Am Soc Nephrol. 2010;5(5):814-20.

[37] McCarthy JT, Rogers JL, Hocum CL, Gallaher EJ, Gudgell SF, Albright RC. [F-FC272] Use of the Mayo Clinic Anemia Management System (MCAMS) Decreases Darbepoetin Use by 30% in Chronic Hemodialysis (CHD) Patients. ASN Renal Week. J Am Soc Nephrol. 2010;21.

[38] Ho WR, Germain MJ, Garb J, Picard S, Mackie M-K, Bartlett C, Will EJ. Use of 12 month haemoglobin monitoring with a computer algorithm reduces haemoglobin. Nephrol Dial Transplant. 2010;25:2710-2714.

[39] Van Wyck D. The Changing Landscape of Anemia Management. Presented at: National Kidney Foundation 2011 Spring Clinical Meeting (NKF 2011). Session 291.

[40] Rice L, Alfrey CP, Driscoll T, et al. Neocytolysis contributes to the anemia of renal disease. Am J Kidney Dis. 1999;33:59-62.

[41] Singh AK. Should we keep hemoglobin levels as a viable outcome measure? Nephrol News Issues. 2010 Mar;24(3):15-6, 18.

[42] KDOQI Clinical Practice Guidelines and Clinical Practice Recommendations for Anemia in Chronic Kidney Disease. [cited 23 Nov 2011]. Available from: http://www.kidney.org//professionals//KDOQI//guidelines_anemia//index.htm.

[43] Unger EF, Thompson AM, Blank MJ, Temple R. Erythropoiesis stimulating agents–time for a reevaluation. N Engl J Med. 2010;362(3):189-92.

[44] Olsson-Gisleskog P, Jacqmin P, Perez-Ruixo JJ. Population pharmacokinetics meta-analysis of recombinant human erythropoietin in healthy subjects. Clin Pharmacokinet. 2007;46(2):159-73.

[45] Heatherington AC. Clinical pharmacokinetic properties of rHuEPO: a review. In Molineux G, Foote MA, Elliott SG, eds. Erythropoietins and Erythropoiesis, Milestones in Drug Therapy. birkhäuser Verlag/Switzerland; 2003:87-112.

[46] Lissy M, Ode M, Roth K. Comparison of the Pharmacokinetic and Pharmacodynamic Profiles of One US-Marketed and Two European-Marketed Epoetin Alfas: A Randomized Prospective Study. Drugs RD. 2011;11(1):61-75.

[47] Besarab A. Physiological and pharmacodynamic considerations for route of Epo administration. Semin Nephrol. 2000;20(4):364-74.

[48] Erslev AJ, Besarab A. Erythropoietin in the pathogenesis and treatment of the anemia of chronic renal failure. Kidney Int. 1997;51(3):622-30.

[49] Krzyzanski W, Woo S, Jusko WJ. Pharmacodynamic models for agents that alter production of natural cells with various distributions of lifespans. J Pharmacokinet Pharmacodyn. 2006;33(2):125-66.

[50] Freise KJ, Widness JA, Schmidt RL, Veng-Pedersen P. Modeling time variant distributions of cellular lifespans: increases in circulating reticulocyte lifespans following double phlebotomies in sheep. J Pharmacokinet Pharmacodyn. 2008;35(3):285–323.

[51] Collett D. Modelling Survival Data in Medical Research. Chapman & Hall; 1994.

[52] Uehlinger DE, Gotch FA, Sheiner LB. A pharmacodynamic model of erythropoietin therapy for uremic anemia. Clin Pharmacol Ther. 1992;51(1):76-89.

[53] Li H, Ginzburg YZ. Crosstalk between Iron Metabolism and Erythropoiesis. Adv Hematol. 2010;2010:605435.

[54] Handelman GJ and Levin NW. Iron and anemia in human biology: a review of mechanisms. Heart Fail Rev. 2008;13(4):393-404.

[55] Nooney G. Erythron-Dependent Model of Iron Kinetics. Biophys J. 1966 Sep;6(5):601-9.

[56] Franzone PC, Paganuzzi A, Stefanelli M. A mathematical model of iron metabolism. J Math Biol. 1982;15(2):173-201.

[57] Banks HT, Bliss KM, Kotanko P, Tran H. A computational model of red blood cell dynamics in patients with chronic kidney disease. in preparation.

[58] Bellazzi R, Siviero C, Bellazzi R. Mathematical modeling of erythropoietin therapy in uremic anemia. Does it improve cost-effectiveness? Haematologica. 1994;79(2):154-64.

[59] Stancu S, Bârsan L, Stanciu A, Mircescu G. Can the response to iron therapy be predicted in anemic nondialysis patients with chronic kidney disease? Clin J Am Soc Nephrol. 2010;5(3):409-16.

[60] Ng HY, Chen HC, Pan LL, et al. Clinical interpretation of reticulocyte hemoglobin content, RET-Y, in chronic hemodialysis patients. Nephron Clin Pract. 2009;111(4):c247-5.

[61] Fishbane S, Berns JS. Hemoglobin cycling in hemodialysis patients treated with recombinant human erythropoietin. Kidney Int. 2005;68(3):1337-43.

[62] Dworkin HJ, Premo M, Dees S. Comparison of red cell and whole blood volume as performed using both chromium-51-tagged red cells and iodine-125-tagged albumin and using I-131-tagged albumin and extrapolated red cell volume. Am J Med. Sci. 2007;334(1):37-40.

[63] Germain MG, Vogt WC, Shrestha RP, Nichols B, Hollot CV, Horowitz J, Chait Y. The engineering of anemia management protocols in chronic kidney disease. ASN Renal Week 2010, Denver, CO.

[64] Bradbury BD, Danese MD, Gleeson M, Critchlow CW. Effect of Epoetin alfa dose changes on hemoglobin and mortality in hemodialysis patients with hemoglobin levels persistently below 11 g/dL. Clin J Am Soc Nephrol. 2009;4(3):630.

[65] KDOQI guidelines. Am J Kidney Dis. Suppl 3 2006 May;47(5):S81-S85.

[66] Nissenson AR, Strobos J. Iron deficiency in patients with renal failure. Kidney Int. Suppl 1999 Mar;69:S18-21.

[67] Cavill I, Macdougall IC. Erythropoiesis and iron supply in patients treated with erythropoietin. Erythropoiesis. 1992;3:50−55.

[68] Kalantar-Zadeh K, McAllister C, Lehn R, Lee G, Nissenson A, Kopple J. Effect of malnutrition-inflammation complex syndrome on EPO hyporesponsiveness in maintenance hemodialysis patients. Am J Kidney Dis. 2003;42:761-773.

[69] Nassar GM, Fishbane S, Ayus JC. Occult infection of old nonfunctioning arteriovenous grafts: a novel cause of erythropoietin resistance and chronic inflammation in hemodialysis patients. Kidney Int. Suppl 2002 May;(80):49-54.

[70] Roberts TL, Obrador GT, St Peter WL, Pereira BJ, Collins AJ. Relationship among catheter insertions, vascular access infections, and anemia management in hemodialysis patients. Kidney Int. 2004;66(6):2429.

[71] Kadiroglu AK, Kadiroglu ET, Sit D, et al. Periodontitis is an important and occult source of inflammation in hemodialysis patients. Blood Purif. 2006;24:400-404.

[72] Solid CA, Foley RN, Gill JS, Gilbertson DT, Collins AJ. Epoetin use and Kidney Disease Outcomes Quality Initiative hemoglobin targets in patients returning to dialysis with failed renal transplants. Kidney Int. 2007;71(5):425.

[73] López-Gómez JM, Pérez-Flores I, Jofré R, Carretero D, Rodríguez-Benitez P, Villaverde M, Pérez-García R, Nassar GM, Niembro E, Ayus JC. Presence of a failed kidney transplant in patients who are on hemodialysis is associated with chronic inflammatory state and erythropoietin resistance. J Am Soc Nephrol. 2004;15(9):2494.

[74] Shrivastava D, Rao TK, Sinert R, Khurana E, Lundin AP, Friedman EA. The efficacy of erythropoietin in human immunodeficiency virus-infected end-stage renal disease patients treated by maintenance hemodialysis. Am J Kidney Dis. 1995 Jun;25(6):904-9.

[75] Betjes MG, Weimar W, Litjens NH. CMV seropositivity determines epoetin dose and hemoglobin levels in patients with CKD. J Am Soc Nephrol. 2009 Dec;20(12):2661-6.

[76] Abe M, Okada K, Soma M, Matsumoto K. Relationship between insulin resistance and erythropoietin responsiveness in hemodialysis patients. Clin Nephrol. 2011 Jan;75(1):49-58.

[77] Rao DS, Shih MS, Mohini R. Effect of serum parathyroid hormone and bone marrow fibrosis on the response to erythropoietin in uremia. N Engl J Med. 1993;328(3):171.

[78] Cheng IK, Lu HB, Wei DC, Cheng SW, Chan CY, Lee FC. Influence of thalassemia on the response to recombinant human erythropoietin in dialysis patients. Am J Nephrol. 1993;13:142-148.

[79] Tomson CR, Edmunds ME, Chambers K, Bricknell S, Feehally J, Walls J. Effect of recombinant human erythropoietin on erythropoiesis in homozygous sickle-cell anaemia and renal failure. Nephrol Dial Transplant. 1992;7:817-821.

[80] Evers J. Cardiac hemolysis and anemia refractory to erythropoietin: on anemia in dialysis patients. Nephron. 1995;71(1):108.

[81] Albitar S, Genin R, Fen-Chong M, Serveaux MO, Bourgeon B. High dose enalapril impairs the response to erythropoietin treatment in haemodialysis patients. Nephrol Dial Transplant. 1998;13(5):1206.

[82] Ertürk S, Nergizoğlu G, Ateş K, Duman N, Erbay B, Karatan O, Ertuğ AE. The impact of withdrawing ACE inhibitors on erythropoietin responsiveness and left ventricular hypertrophy in haemodialysis patients. Nephrol Dial Transplant. 1999;14(8):1912.

[83] Bamgbola O. Resistance to erythropoietin-stimulating agents: etiology, evaluation, and therapeutic considerations. Pediatr Nephrol. 2011 Mar 20. [Epub ahead of print]

[84] Bamgbola OF, Kaskel F. Role of folate deficiency on erythropoietin resistance in pediatric and adolescent patients on chronic dialysis. Pediatr Nephrol. 2005;20:1622–1629.

[85] Rossert J, Macdougall I, Casadevall N. Antibody-mediated pure red cell aplasia (PRCA) treatment and re-treatment: multiple options. Nephrol Dial Transplant. 2005 May;20 Suppl 4:iv23-26.

[86] Bridges KR, Hoffman KE. The effects of ascorbic acid on the intracellular metabolism of iron and ferritin. J Biol Chem. 1986;261(30):14273-14277.

[87] Goldberg A. The enzymic formation of haem by the incorporation of iron into protoporphyrin; importance of ascorbic acid, ergothioneine and glutathione. Br J Haematol. 1959;5:150-157.

[88] Canavese C, Petrarulo M, Massarenti P, et al. Longterm, low-dose, intravenous vitamin C leads to plasma calcium oxalate supersaturation in hemodialysis patients. Am J Kidney Dis. 2005;45(3):540-549.

[89] Deved V, Poyah P, James MT, Tonelli M, Manns BJ, Walsh M, Hemmelgarn BR, Alberta Kidney Disease Network. Ascorbic acid for anemia management in hemodialysis patients: a systematic review and meta-analysis. Am J Kidney Dis. 2009 Dec;54(6):1089-97.

[90] Besarab A, Coyne DW. Iron supplementation to treat anemia in patients with chronic kidney disease. Nat Rev Nephrol. 2010 Dec;6(12):699-710.

[91] Nemeth E. Targeting the hepcidin-ferroportin axis in the diagnosis and treatment of anemias. Adv Hemato. 2010:750643.

[92] Coyne DW, Kapoian T, Suki W, Singh AK, Moran JE, Dahl NV, Rizkala AR; DRIVE Study Group. Ferric gluconate is highly efficacious in anemic hemodialysis patients with high serum ferritin and low transferrin saturation: results of the Dialysis Patients' Response to IV Iron with Elevated Ferritin (DRIVE) Study. J Am Soc Nephrol. 2007 Mar;18(3):975-84.

[93] Kapoian T, O'Mara NB, Singh AK, Moran J, Rizkala AR, Geronemus R, Kopelman RC, Dahl NV, Coyne DW. Ferric gluconate reduces epoetin requirements in hemodialysis patients with elevated ferritin. J Am Soc Nephrol. 2008;19:372–379.

[94] Besarab A, et al. Optimization of epoetin therapy with intravenous iron therapy in hemodialysis patients. J. Am. Soc Nephrol. 2000;11:530–538.

[95] Spiegel DM, Chertow GM. Lost without directions: Lessons from the anemia debate and the drive study. Clin J Am Soc Nephrol. 2009;4:1009–1010.

[96] Provenzano R, Schiller B, Rao M, Coyne D, Brenner L, Pereira BJ. Ferumoxytol as an intravenous iron replacement therapy in hemodialysis patients. Clin J Am Soc Nephrol. 2009;4:386–393.

[97] Kletzmayr J, Hörl WH. Iron overload and cardiovascular complications in dialysis patients. Nephrol Dial Transplant. 2002;17(Suppl 2):25–29.

[98] Hayat A. Safety issues with intravenous iron products in the management of anemia in chronic kidney disease. Clin Med Res. 2008;6:93–102.

[99] Sonnweber T, Theurl I, Seifert M, Schroll A, Eder S, Mayer G, Weiss G. Impact of iron treatment on immune effector function and cellular iron status of circulating monocytes in dialysis patients. Nephrol Dial Transplant. 2011;26:977–987.

[100] Tsubakihara Y, Nishi S, Akiba T, Hirakata H, Iseki K, Kubota M, Kuriyama S, Komatsu Y, Suzuki M, Nakai S, Hattori M, Babazono T, Hiramatsu M, Yamamoto H, Bessho M, Akizawa T. 2008 Japanese Society for Dialysis Therapy: guidelines for renal anemia in chronic kidney disease. Ther Apher Dial. 2010 Jun;14(3):240-75.

[101] Yamamoto H, Tsubakihara Y. Limiting Iron Supplementation for Anemia in Dialysis Patients-The Basis for Japan's Conservative Guidelines. Semin Dial. 2011 May;24(3):269-71.

[102] Ferrari P, Kulkarni H, Dheda S, Betti S, Harrison C, St Pierre TG, Olynyk JK. Serum iron markers are inadequate for guiding iron repletion in chronic kidney disease. Clin J Am Soc Nephrol. 2011 Jan;6(1):77-83. Epub 2010 Sep 28.

[103] Rehu M, Ahonen S, Punnonen K. The diagnostic accuracy of the percentage of hypochromic red blood cells (%HYPOm) and cellular hemoglobin in reticulocytes (CHr) in differentiating iron deficiency anemia and anemia of chronic diseases. Clin Chim Acta. 2011 Sep 18;412(19-20):1809-13. Epub 2011 Jun 14.

[104] Brugnara C, Schiller B, Moran J. Reticulocyte hemoglobin equivalent (Ret He) and assessment of iron-deficient states. Clin Lab Haematol. 2006 Oct;28(5):303-8.

[105] Anemia management in people with chronic kidney disease – NICE Clinical Guideline. 2011;114:12. [cited 17 Jul 2011]. Available from: http://www.nice.org.uk/+nicemedia/live/13329/52853/52853.pdf.

[106] Lacson E Jr, Ofsthun N, Lazarus M. Effect of variability in anemia management on hemoglobin outcomes in ESRD. Am J Kidney Dis. 2003;41:111-124.

[107] Berns JS, Elzein H, Lunn RI, Fishbane S, Meisels IS, DeOreo PB. Hemoglobin variability in epoetin-treated hemodialysis patients. Kidney Int. 2003;64:1514-1521.

[108] Kalantar-Zadeh K, Aronoff GR. Hemoglobin variability in anemia of chronic kidney disease. J Am Soc Nephrol. 2009;20:478-487.

[109] Yang W, Israni RK, Brunelli SM, Joffe MM, Fishbane S, Feldman HI. Hemoglobin variability and mortality in ESRD. J Am Soc Nephrol. 2007;18:3164-3170.

[110] Gilbertson DT, Ebben JP, Foley RN, Weinhandl ED, Bradbury BD, Collins AJ. Hemoglobin level variability: associations with mortality. Clin J Am Soc Nephrol. 2008;3:133-138.

[111] Wish JB. Hemoglobin variability as a predictor of mortality: What's a practitioner to do? Am J Kidney Dis. 2011 Feb;57(2):190-3.

[112] Weinhandl ED, Peng Y, Gilbertson DT, Bradbury BD, Collins AJ. Hemoglobin variability and mortality: confounding by disease severity. Am J Kidney Dis. 2011;57(2):255-265.

[113] Stead RB, Lambert J, Wessels D, Iwashita JS, Leuther KK, Woodburn KW, Schatz PJ, Okamoto DM, Naso R, Duliege AM. Evaluation of the safety and pharmacodynamics of Hematide, a novel erythropoietic agent, in a phase 1, double-blind, placebo-controlled, dose-escalation study in healthy volunteers. Blood. 2006 Sep 15;108(6):1830-4. Epub 2006 May 23.

[114] Macdougall IC, Rossert J, Casadevall N, Stead RB, Duliege AM, Froissart M, Eckardt KU. A peptide-based erythropoietin-receptor agonist for pure red-cell aplasia. N Engl J Med. 2009 Nov 5;361(19):1848-55.

[115] Bernhardt WM, Wiesener MS, Scigalla P, Chou J, Schmieder RE, Günzler V, Eckardt KU. Inhibition of prolyl hydroxylases increases erythropoietin production in ESRD. J Am Soc Nephrol. 2010 Dec;21(12):2151-6. Epub 2010 Nov 29.

[116] Dame C, Sola MC, Lim KC, Leach KM, Fandrey J, Ma Y, Knöpfle G, Engel JD, Bungert J. Hepatic erythropoietin gene regulation by GATA-4. J Biol Chem. 2004 Jan 23;279(4):2955-61. Epub 2003 Oct 28.

[117] Imagawa S, Yamamoto M, Miura Y. Negative regulation of the erythropoietin gene expression by the GATA transcription factors. Blood. 1997 Feb 15;89(4):1430-9.

[118] Nakano Y, Imagawa S, Matsumoto K, Stockmann C, Obara N, Suzuki N, Doi T, Kodama T, Takahashi S, Nagasawa T, Yamamoto M. Oral administration of K-11706 inhibits GATA binding activity, enhances hypoxia-inducible factor 1 binding activity, and restores indicators in an in vivo mouse model of anemia of chronic disease. Blood. 2004 Dec 15;104(13):4300-7. Epub 2004 Aug 24.

[119] Klingmüller U, Lorenz U, Cantley LC, Neel BG, Lodish HF. Specific recruitment of SH-PTP1 to the erythropoietin receptor causes inactivation of JAK2 and termination of proliferative signals. Cell. 1995 Mar 10;80(5):729-38.

[120] Akagi S, Ichikawa H, Okada T, Sarai A, Sugimoto T, Morimoto H, Kihara T, Yano A, Nakao K, Nagake Y, Wada J, Makino H. The critical role of SRC homology domain 2-containing tyrosine phosphatase-1 in recombinant human erythropoietin hypo-responsive anemia in chronic hemodialysis patients. J Am Soc Nephrol. 2004 Dec;15(12):3215-24.

[121] Raje N, Vallet S. Sotatercept, a soluble activin receptor type 2A IgG-Fc fusion protein for the treatment of anemia and bone loss. Curr Opin Mol Ther. 2010 Oct;12(5):586-97.

In: Issues in Dialysis
Editor: Stephen Z. Fadem

ISBN: 978-1-62417-576-3
© 2013 Nova Science Publishers, Inc.

Chapter XV

Accumulation of Toxic Metals and Trace Elements in Chronic Dialysis Patients

Tzung-Hai Yen[1,2], Dan-Tzu Lin-Tan[1,2] and Ja-Liang Lin[1,2,]*

[1]Department of Nephrology and Division of Clinical Toxicology, Chang Gung Memorial Hospital, Taipei, Taiwan; [2]School of Medicine, Chang Gung University, Taoyuan, Taiwan, ROC

Abstract

This chapter highlights key issues related to accumulation of toxic metals and trace elements in chronic dialysis patients, with special emphasis on lead and cadmium, but excluding aluminum. In a meta-analysis study, it has been demonstrated that blood levels of lead, cadmium, chromium, copper, and vanadium were higher in maintenance hemodialysis patients than control counterparts. Clinical evidences have suggested that elevated blood lead levels were associated with hypertension-related morbidity and mortality, and accelerated age-related renal function impairment in the general population. In earlier studies, we have showed that environmental exposure to lead was related to progressive renal insufficiency in patients with and without diabetes, and that chelation therapy may retard the progression of renal insufficiency in these patients. In a large-scale, cross-sectional, prospective study, we have showed that blood lead levels were associated with inflammation, malnutrition, and 1-year mortality in 211 diabetic patients treated with maintenance hemodialysis. In another 18-month study, we have revealed that high blood lead level was associated with increased hazard ratios for all-cause, cardiovascular-cause, and infection-cause 18-month mortality in 927 maintenance hemodialysis patients. In a peritoneal dialysis population, we also revealed that blood lead levels were associated with residual renal function and hyperparathyroidism, and were related to increased hazard ratio for all-cause 18-month mortality. Cadmium can cause kidney damage even at very low levels of exposure. In patients with end-stage renal disease, cadmium may accumulate in bone tissue, increasing the bone cadmium

---

[*] Correspondence: Professor Ja-Liang Lin, MD. Department of Nephrology and Division of Clinical Toxicology, Chang Gung Memorial Hospital, 199 Tung Hwa North Road, Taipei 105, Taiwan. Tel: +886 3 3281200 ext 8892; Fax: +886 3 3287490; E-mail: jllin99@hotmail.com

content in these patients. In a study, we have demonstrated that environmental cadmium exposure was significantly associated with inflammation and malnutrition in maintenance hemodialysis patients. Following adjustment for potential confounders, blood cadmium levels were negatively correlated with serum albumin levels, but were positively correlated with high sensitivity-C reactive protein. Overall, a 10-fold increase in blood cadmium levels was associated with a 0.06 g/dL decrease in serum albumin levels. This is of particular importance in diabetics, because there may exist a positive association between cadmium exposure and the severity of diabetes, as well as diabetes-related organ damage. In another study, we have confirmed that elevated blood cadmium levels were associated with increased hazard ratio for 18-month all-cause mortality in diabetic patients undergoing maintenance hemodialysis.

Introduction

Patients with end-stage renal disease are characterized by functional and biochemical disturbances that result primarily from the diminished renal capacity to remove organic solutes from the body. Most research on uremic toxicity has focused on retention and removal of these organic compounds. However, subtle changes in the concentration of inorganic compounds, including toxic metals and trace elements, may also cause functional or biochemical disturbances.

In chronic dialysis patients, the most important factors for toxic metal and trace element concentration are the degree of renal failure and the modality of renal replacement therapy. Accumulation of toxic metals and trace elements in dialysis patients may result from environmental exposure or contaminated dialysate. Chronic dialysis patients are at great risk for excess of toxic metals and trace elements, because they are at exposed to very high titers of dialysate, and thus even otherwise trivial concentration gradients of toxic metals between blood and dialysate may lead to substantial systemic toxicities. [1] Furthermore, the lack of endogenous renal clearance in dialysis patients may also predispose to accumulation of the environmental toxic metals and trace elements from the general environment, even if not present in the dialysate. [1] In a recent meta-analysis, [2] it has been demonstrated that blood levels of lead, cadmium, chromium, copper, and vanadium were higher in maintenance hemodialysis patients than control counterparts.

Lead

Lead is known for its toxic effects on human beings. Clinical evidence [3,4] suggests that blood lead levels were associated with all-cause and cardiovascular-cause mortality in the general population. The phasing out of leaded gasoline for transportation vehicles between 1973 and 1995 and the removal of lead from paint by federal mandate by 1978 has resulted in substantial lowering of mean blood lead levels in all segments of the US population. However, because lead is a persistent metal, it is still present in the environment - in water, brass plumbing fixtures, soil, dust, and imported products manufactured with lead. Diagnosis of lead toxicity has traditionally been based on significantly elevated blood lead levels. However, data now implicates low-level exposures and blood lead levels previously considered normal as causative factors in cognitive dysfunction, neurobehavioral disorders, neurological damage, hypertension, and renal impairment. [5,6] For example, a recent epidemiological investigation [7] demonstrated that US adults with low blood lead levels (<10 µg/dL) still had high cardiovascular-cause mortality rate in those subjects with blood lead levels >3.61 µg/dL and <10 µg/dL. Furthermore, many epidemiology studies showed that blood lead levels accelerate age-related renal function impairment in the general population. [8-10]

In a series of prospective investigations, we have shown that environmental exposure to lead was related to progressive renal insufficiency in patients with [11] and without [12-14] diabetes, and chelation therapy may retard renal disease progression in these patients. In a study 87 patients with type 2 diabetes and diabetic nephropathy, as defined by serum creatinine level 1.5 - 3.9 mg/dL, with normal body lead burden and no lead exposure history were observed over a 12-month period. Thirty subjects with high-normal body lead burden (80 - 600 µg) were randomly assigned to a chelation and control group. For 3 months, the 15 chelation-group patients underwent lead-chelation therapy with calcium disodium ethylenediaminetetraacetic acid (EDTA) weekly until body lead burden fell < 60 µg, and the 15 control group subjects received a weekly placebo. During the following 12 months, renal function was regularly assessed at 3-month intervals. The primary outcome was an elevation of serum creatinine to 1.5 times baseline value during the observation period. It was found that 36 patients achieved primary outcomes. It was found that basal blood lead levels and body lead burden were the most important risk factors in predicting progressive diabetic nephropathy. Following chelation, the rates of decline in glomerular filtration rates in the chelation group and the control group, respectively, were 5.0 ± 5.7 and 11.8 ± 7.0 ml/min/1.73m^2 (P = 0.0084) during follow-up, although both groups had similar rates of progression of renal function during the 12-month observation period. It was concluded that low-level environmental lead exposure accelerates progressive diabetic nephropathy and lead-chelation therapy can decrease its rate of progression. [11]

In another study, 202 non-diabetic patients with similar stage of chronic kidney disease who had a normal body lead burden and no history of exposure to lead were observed for 24 months. After the observation period, 64 subjects with a high normal body lead burden were randomly assigned to the chelation or control groups. For three months, the patients in the chelation group received lead-chelation therapy with calcium disodium EDTA, and the control group received placebo. During the ensuing 24 months, repeated chelation therapy was administered weekly to 32 patients with high-normal body lead burden (80 - 600 µg) unless on repeated testing the body lead burden fell < 60 µg; the other 32 patients served as controls and received weekly placebo infusions for 5 weeks every 6 months. It was found that the primary end point occurred in 24 patients during the observation period; the serum creatinine levels and body lead burden at base line were the most important risk factors. The glomerular filtration rate improved significantly by the end of the 27-month intervention period in patients receiving chelation therapy: the mean change in the glomerular filtration rate in the patients in the chelation group was 2.1 ± 5.7 ml/min/1.73m^2, as compared with -6.0 $\pm$ 5.8 ml/min/1.73m^2 in the controls (P < 0.001). The rate of decline in the glomerular filtration rate in the chelation group was also lower than that in the controls during the 24-month period of repeated chelation therapy or placebo. It was concluded that low-level environmental lead exposure may accelerate progressive renal insufficiency in non-diabetic patients with chronic kidney disease. Repeated chelation therapy may improve renal function and slow the progression of renal insufficiency. [14]

In the following investigation, 108 chronic kidney disease patients with low-normal body lead burden (< 80 µg) and no lead exposure history were observed for 24 months. Following the observation, 32 patients with low-normal body lead burden (20 - 80 µg) were randomly assigned to chelation and control groups. The chelation group patients were given calcium disodium EDTA chelation therapy for 3 months and repeated chelation therapy during the following 24 months to maintain their body lead burden < 20 µg, while the control group patients underwent placebo therapy. It was found that the primary endpoint occurred in 14 patients during the observation period. Baseline body lead burden was the important risk factor in determining progressive renal insufficiency. The mean glomerular filtration rate change in chelation group patients was 6.6 ± 10.7 ml/min/1.73m^2, compared with -4.6 ± 4.3 ml/min1.73m^2 in the control group patients (P < 0.001) at the end of the intervention period. The mean decrease in glomerular filtration rate per year of chelation group patients was lower than that of control group patients during the repeated chelation period. It was concluded that environmental exposure to lead, even at low level, might accelerate progressive renal insufficiency of non-diabetic patients with chronic kidney disease. [12]

In a 4-year repeated chelation study, 116 non-diabetic patients with similar stage of chronic kidney disease, high-normal body lead burden (60 - 600 µg) and no lead exposure history were randomly assigned to a chelation or control group. For 3 months, the 58 chelation group patients received initial lead-chelation therapy with calcium disodium EDTA, and the 58 control group patients received placebos. During the ensuing 48 months, repeated chelation therapy was administered weekly to chelation group patients unless, on repeated testing, body lead burden was < 60 µg; the control group patients received weekly placebo infusions for 5 weeks at 6-month intervals. It was again found that mean change in the glomerular filtration rate in the chelation group was -1.8 ± 8.8 ml/min/1.73 m^2, as compared with -12.7 ± 8.4 ml/min/1.73 m^2 in the control group (P < 0.0001) at study end. The rate of decline in glomerular filtration rate was lower in the chelation than control group, although both groups had similar decline rates before chelation. At the end of the study, 18 patients (including 15 control group patients) had elevated serum creatinine levels to two times the baseline values. Both Cox and Kaplan-Meier analysis demonstrated that repeated chelation therapy was the important determining factor for slowing progression of renal insufficiency. It was concluded that repeated chelation therapy could slow progression of renal insufficiency in non-diabetic patients with high-normal body lead burden. [13]

In patients with end-stage renal disease, lead had been shown to accumulate in bone and increased blood lead levels were found in maintenance hemodialysis patients. [15,16] Some clinical studies [16,17] showed an association between blood lead levels and hemoglobin level, diastolic blood pressure, and intact parathyroid hormone level in maintenance hemodialysis patients. According to the United States Renal Data System report in 2010 [18], adjusted rates of all-cause mortality were 6.4 - 7.8 times higher for dialysis patients than for individuals in the general population, with most of the reported deaths attributed to cardiovascular-cause. Recent evidence from clinical studies [19-22] showed that chronic inflammation, a nontraditional risk factor for cardiovascular disease, is common in maintenance hemodialysis patients and may cause protein energy malnutrition and progressive atherosclerosis. Malnutrition and inflammation, two relatively common and concurrent conditions in maintenance hemodialysis patients, was identified as the main cause

Accumulation of Toxic Metals and Trace Elements in Chronic Dialysis Patients   255

of poor short-term survival in such populations. [23] Correcting inflammation has the potential to decrease the epidemic of cardiovascular disease in maintenance hemodialysis patients. Therefore, it is important to identify correctable factors associated with inflammation in maintenance hemodialysis patients. However, the correlation between blood lead levels and mortality, inflammation and/or malnutrition in chronic dialysis patients remains unknown.

In a large-scale, cross-sectional, 12-month, prospective study involving 211 diabetic patients undergoing maintenance hemodialysis, 34, 112, and 65 patients, respectively, were found to have abnormal (> 20 µg/dL), high-normal (10 - 20 µg/dL), and low-normal (< 10 µg/dL) blood lead levels measured at baseline. It was found initially that patients with abnormal blood lead levels had a greater proportion of malnutrition (14.7% versus 1.5% and 11.6%, P = 0.01) and inflammation (76.5% versus 52.3% and 50.9%, P = 0.01) than patients with low- and high-normal blood lead levels. Furthermore, backward stepwise regression analysis found that high-sensitivity C-reactive protein level correlated positively and albumin level correlated negatively with blood lead levels after adjustment for other confounders. Sixteen patients died at the end of the study. Kaplan-Meier analysis showed that patients with an abnormal blood lead levels had greater cumulative mortality than patients with low and low-normal blood lead levels (P = 0.004). In was concluded [24] that blood lead levels may correlate with systemic inflammation and malnutrition in diabetic maintenance hemodialysis patients, and may also contribute to the one-year, all-cause mortality in this population.

In another 18-month study, 927 maintenance hemodialysis patients were analyzed. Baseline variables and blood lead levels were measured before hemodialysis and categorized as three equal groups: high (> 13.08 µg/dL), middle (8.80 - 13.08 µg/dL), and low (< 8.80 µg/dL). Mortality and cause of death were recorded for longitudinal analyses. It was found that at baseline, after related variables were adjusted, logarithmic transformation of blood lead level was negatively related to log ferritin and positively related to the vintage of hemodialysis and the percentage of urban area patients. By the end of the follow-up, 59 patients had died. Kaplan-Meier survival analysis showed that the high blood lead level group had greater mortality than the low blood lead level group (log-rank test, P < 0.001). After adjustment for potential variables, Cox multivariate analysis demonstrated that by using the low blood lead level as the reference, high blood lead levels were associated with increased hazard ratios for all-cause (hazard ratio 4.70; 95% confidence interval 1.92 - 11.49; P = 0.003), cardiovascular-cause (hazard ratio 9.71; 95% confidence interval 2.11 - 23.26; P = 0.005), and infection-cause (hazard ratio 5.35; 95% confidence interval 1.38 - 20.83; P = 0.046) 18-month mortality in patients on maintenance hemodialysis. Moreover, there was a significant trend (P = 0.032) of hazard ratios for all-cause mortality trend tests among the three study groups. It was concluded that high blood lead level was associated with increased hazard ratios for all-cause, cardiovascular-cause, and infection-cause 18-month mortality in maintenance hemodialysis patients. [25]

The reason why blood lead levels or corrected blood lead levels increased the risk of mortality in patients on maintenance hemodialysis remains unknown. Some studies performed on animals [26,27] have shown that chronic exposure to low-dose lead results in the generation of reactive oxygen species and the expression of angiotensin II. It reduces nitric oxide availability, and increases blood pressure. [27] Low-level exposure to lead also promotes hydroxyl radical generation and lipid peroxidation, [28] enhances vascular reactivity to sympathetic stimulation, and diminishes DNA repair, which may be relevant for rapidly dividing cells in the inflamed arterial wall. [29,30] Moreover, rats chronically exposed to low levels of lead were successfully treated with antioxidants; [27,28] thus, oxidative stress plays a primary role in low levels of lead exposure. [30,31] Overproduction of reactive oxygen species in patients on maintenance hemodialysis has been implicated in increased long-term complications, including accelerated inflammation or malnutrition in patients on maintenance hemodialysis, [32-34] and infection-cause and cardiovascular-cause mortality in these patients. However, further study is needed to clarify the definite pathogenesis.

Finally, in another 18-month, cross-sectional, prospective study [35], blood lead levels were measured in 315 chronic peritoneal dialysis patients at baseline, and patients were categorized as high (> 8.66 µg/dL), middle (5.62 - 8.66 µg/dL) and low (< 5.62 µg/dL) blood lead levels. It was found initially that patients with high blood lead levels had a trend of higher parathyroid hormone and lower residual renal function than other groups. Stepwise multiple regression analysis found that parathyroid hormone positively correlated and residual renal function negatively correlated with logarithmic-transformed blood lead levels in chronic peritoneal dialysis patients after adjustment for other confounders. At the end of follow-up, 37 (11.7%) patients had died. Kaplan-Meier analysis showed that patients with high blood lead levels had greater cumulative mortality than patients with middle and low blood lead levels (P = 0.008). Cox multivariate regression analysis showed that, using the low blood lead levels group as the reference, basal high blood lead levels (hazard ratio = 3.745, 95% confidence interval = 1.218 - 11.494, P = 0.001) and middle blood lead levels (hazard ratio = 1.867, 95% confidence interval = 1.618 - 2.567, P = 0.001) were associated with increased hazard ratio for all-cause mortality for chronic peritoneal dialysis patients. There is a significant trend (P < 0.001) of hazard ratio for mortality trend tests among the three study groups. It was concluded [35] that blood lead levels may correlate with residual renal function and hyperparathyroidism, and may contribute to increased hazard ratio for the 18-month, all-cause mortality in chronic peritoneal dialysis patients.

Why high blood lead level is associated with a high mortality rate in chronic peritoneal dialysis patients remains unknown. However, exposure to low level lead may cause oxidative stress, inflammation [26,28,36] and overproduction of reactive oxygen species, which may in turn induce malnutrition, anemia and atherosclerosis in end-stage renal disease patients. [23,32] Therefore, it is possible that basal blood lead level degrees were related to the 18-month all-cause mortality of chronic peritoneal dialysis patients in the current study. However, after adjustment for age, residual renal creatinine clearance, important factors to determine mortality of chronic peritoneal dialysis patients, [37] and related variables, basal blood lead level degrees are still associated with mortality. Hence, other pathogeneses may exist between blood lead levels and mortality in chronic peritoneal dialysis patients. Several other mechanisms may also underlie the toxic effects of lead [28,29,36]; the definite pathogenesis of blood lead levels associated with mortality requires further investigation.

Cadmium

Battery factories, zinc smelters, pigment plants and soldering activities cause occupational exposure to cadmium. The most significant contemporary source results from the production of nickel-cadmium batteries. [38,39] Occupational exposure occurs mainly through the respiratory route, but may also involve the gastrointestinal route to a lesser degree. Environmentally, the main source of cadmium exposure is tobacco smoke for the smoker, followed by diet for the non-smoker. [40-42] Dietary cadmium is a growing concern. Cadmium gets into soil from the use of fertilizers and as a result of zinc-mining processes, in which cadmium is a discarded impurity. In Taiwan, since the 1970s, at least 200 hectares of farm-land have been polluted by the heavy metal cadmium. [43] Consequently, the cadmium pollution has led to contamination the rice production and caused acute social panic. According to the recent investigation performed by the Taiwan Environmental Protection Administration most of the cadmium pollution incidents in Taiwan resulted from the wastewater discharge of stearate cadmium factories. To prevent the cadmium pollution incidents from spreading, the Taiwan Environmental Protection Administration has either forced these factories to close down or assisted them in improving their production processes since the 1980s. Unfortunately, accidental incidents of cadmium pollution still emerge in an endless stream, despite the strict governmental controls placed on these questionable factories. [43] Therefore, many of the maintenance hemodialysis patients in Taiwan might also be in cadmium overload.

Previous studies [44-46] have suggested that cadmium was associated with renal dysfunction, bone disease, cardiovascular disease and cancer. The link between cadmium exposure and all-cause mortality in populations exposed to relatively high cadmium levels, including workers with occupational exposure [47] and individuals living in heavily polluted areas, [48] has been well demonstrated. In the general US population with exposure to low cadmium levels, a nationwide study [49] has demonstrated that the hazard ratios [95% confidence interval (CI)] for all-cause, cancer, cardiovascular disease, and coronary heart disease mortality associated with a 2-fold higher creatinine-corrected urinary cadmium were, respectively, 1.28 (95% CI, 1.15-1.43), 1.55 (95% CI, 1.21-1.98), 1.21 (95% CI, 1.07-1.36), and 1.36 (95% CI, 1.11-1.66) for men. Interestingly, in another US general population analysis [50], participants with higher levels of both blood lead and cadmium had increased risk for estimated glomerular filtration rate <60 mL/min/1.73 m^{2}compared to those with lower levels of both metals.

In one of our studies, 954 maintenance hemodialysis patients were divided into four equal-sized groups based on blood cadmium levels. It was found initially that abnormal blood cadmium levels$\geq$ 1 µg/L) were exhibited in 26.8% (256/954) of studied subjects. More subjects in the highest quartile group were malnourished (chi-square = 23.27, P < 0.0001) and had inflammatory changes (chi-square = 13.99, P = 0.0029) than in the lowest quartile group. Stepwise multiple regression analysis revealed a significant inverse correlation between serum albumin and blood cadmium levels. Notably, a 10-fold increase in blood cadmium levels was associated with a 0.06 g/dL decrease in serum albumin levels (P = 0.0060). Multivariate regression analysis also demonstrated a positive correlation between inflammatory risk (high-sensitivity C-reactive protein > 3 mg/L) and blood cadmium levels. The risk ratio of inflammation with a 10-fold increase in blood cadmium levels was 1.388 (95% confidence interval: 1.025 - 1.825, P = 0.0336). It was therefore concluded that environmental cadmium exposure was significantly associated with malnutrition, inflammation and even protein-energy wasting in maintenance hemodialysis patients. [51]

In terms of pathogenesis, a substantial body of evidence exists indicating a relationship between cadmium and inflammation and toxic effects. In animal studies, proinflammatory cytokines, including tumor necrosis factor-α, interleukin-1α and interleukin-6, were significantly enhanced following cadmium injection. [52,53] Cadmium exposure could induce lipid peroxidation in the heart, lung, liver and spleen [54,55] as well as increasing oxidative stress in tissue, which can be reduced by anti-oxidants such as tetramethylthiourea and N-acetyl-cysteine. [56,57] An in vitro experiment also indicated that Na-K-ATPase was inhibited by cadmium, which may play a role in the pathogenesis of renal and cardiovascular damage. [58] Blood lead and cadmium, at levels considerably below current safety standards, were associated with the increased prevalence of peripheral arterial disease [59] and heart-related diseases [46] in the general population. Moreover, cadmium exposure also increases high-sensitivity C-reactive protein levels in humans. [59]

The above findings indicate that environmental cadmium exposure is closely associated with malnutrition and inflammation in maintenance hemodialysis patients. Since protein-energy wasting is a strong predictor of the extent of sickness as well as morbidity and mortality in maintenance hemodialysis patients, [60] and since a higher percentage of patients with raised blood cadmium levels exhibited this condition, blood cadmium levels provide useful information for such patients. Regular measurements of blood cadmium levels have the potential to assess protein-energy wasting in long-term hemodialysis patients.

Recent epidemiological studies also suggest a positive association between exposure to the environmental low-level cadmium and the severity of diabetes and diabetes-related organ damages. [61] In patients with end-stage renal disease, cadmium has been shown to accumulate in the bone and increase blood cadmium levels in maintenance hemodialysis patients. [2,62,63]

In another of our studies, 212 diabetic maintenance hemodialysis patients were categorized into three equal groups according to basal blood cadmium levels, i.e. high (> 0.889 µg/L; n = 71), middle (0.373-0.889 µg/L; n = 70) and low (< 0.373 µg/L; n = 71) blood cadmium levels groups. The mortality and cause of death were recorded and analyzed longitudinally. It was found that patients with high blood cadmium levels had trends of higher white blood cell counts, glycosylated hemoglobin, phosphate and blood lead levels than other group patients. At the end of the follow-up, 31 patients had died. Kaplan-Meier analysis showed that patients with high blood cadmium levels suffered higher cumulative mortality than other groups (log-rank test, P = 0.036). Cox multivariate regression analysis demonstrated that logarithmic blood cadmium levels were associated with increased hazard ratio for the all-cause mortality (hazard ratio = 2.336, 95% confidence interval = 1.099 - 4.964, P = 0.027) in these patients. Similarly, if patients with low blood cadmium levels were set as reference, there was an increase in hazard ratio for mortality in patients with high blood cadmium levels (hazard ratio = 2.865, 95% confidence interval = 1.117 - 7.353, P = 0.043). It was concluded that blood cadmium levels were associated with increased hazard ratio for 18-month, all-cause mortality in diabetic patients undergoing maintenance hemodialysis. [64]

The possible pathogenesis of the association between blood cadmium level and mortality in diabetic patients with maintenance hemodialysis remains unknown. Exposure to low-level cadmium may cause oxidative stress, overproduction of reactive oxygen species and inflammation in patients with end-stage renal disease, which may cause malnutrition, infection and progressive atherosclerosis and increase hazard ratio for mortality in long-term dialysis patients. [32,33] Moreover, an in vitro experiment has indicated that Na-K-ATPase is inhibited by cadmium, which may play a role in the pathogenesis of renal and cardiovascular damage. [58] Cadmium has direct toxic effects on pancreatic function, and reduces the secretion of insulin. [61] In a mice study, [65] cadmium exposure causes abnormal adipocyte differentiation, expansion and function, which might lead to development of insulin resistance, hypertension and cardiovascular disease. Hence, the current investigation indicated that blood cadmium level is associated with increased HBA1c in diabetic maintenance hemodialysis patients. Subsequently, the increased HBA1c is related to the increased hazard ratio of mortality of diabetic maintenance hemodialysis patients. [66] However, further investigation is needed to evaluate the definite pathogenesis in these patients.

Chromium

Chromium can affect saccharide (potentiated insulin action via interaction with insulin receptor on the cell surface) and lipid metabolism (inhibition of hydroxymethylglutaryl-CoA reductase with a hypolipidemic effect). [67] It has been shown that the concentration of chromium was also increased in the bone of end-stage renal failure patients. [68] Additional research is needed in this area before a solid conclusion can be made.

Copper

Chronic copper poisoning may lead to liver disorders. It has been found that blood copper levels were elevated in uremic patients regardless of dialysis modality [69] and this elevation was not accounted for by an increase in plasma ceruloplasmin. Further study is needed in this area.

Vanadium

Vanadium has been reported to inhibit a number of enzyme activities such as those of those of the sodium pump. [70,71] The main excretory pathway of this element is via the kidney. It has been reported [72] that the tap water from Kanagawa prefecture, Japan, had the highest vanadium concentrations among the 21 cities in Japan and the US. As a result, the hemodialysis patients exhibited extremely high levels of serum vanadium as compared with healthy adults. Again, further research is also needed in this aspect.

Conclusion

Toxic metals and trace elements excess may cause or contribute to protean manifestations of systemic disease. Chronic dialysis patients may be at an increased risk of toxic metals and trace element excess, and this in turn may contribute to the increased morbidity and mortality observed in this population. Although more clinical data are needed, this hypothesis seems worthy of thorough investigation, given that excesses of most toxic metal and trace elements are potentially treatable.

References

[1] Rucker D, Thadhani R, Tonelli M. Trace element status in hemodialysis patients. Semin Dial. 2010;23(4):389-395.

[2] Tonelli M, Wiebe N, Hemmelgarn B, Klarenbach S, Field C, Manns B, Thadhani R, Gill J. Trace elements in hemodialysis patients: a systematic review and meta-analysis. BMC Med. 2009;7:25.

[3] Lustberg M, Silbergeld E. Blood lead levels and mortality. Arch Intern Med. 2002;162(21):2443-2449.

[4] Schober SE, Mirel LB, Graubard BI, Brody DJ, Flegal KM. Blood lead levels and death from all causes, cardiovascular disease, and cancer: results from the NHANES III mortality study. Environ Health Perspect. 2006;114(10):1538-1541.

[5] Yen TH, Lin JL, Weng CH, Tang CC. Colic induced by lead. CMAJ 2010;182(9):E381.

[6] Yen TH, Lin-Tan DT, Lin JL. Chronic renal failure induced by lead. Kidney Int. 2011;79(6):688.

[7] Menke A, Muntner P, Batuman V, Silbergeld EK, Guallar E. Blood lead below 0.48 micromol/L (10 microg/dL) and mortality among US adults. Circ. 2006;114(13):1388-1394.

[8] Staessen JA, Lauwerys RR, Buchet JP, Bulpitt CJ, Rondia D, Vanrenterghem Y, Amery A. Impairment of renal function with increasing blood lead concentrations in the general population. The Cadmibel Study Group. N Engl J Med. 1992;327(3):151-156.

[9] Payton M, Hu H, Sparrow D, Weiss ST. Low-level lead exposure and renal function in the Normative Aging Study. Am J Epidemiol. 1994;140(9):821-829.

[10] Kim R, Hu H, Rotnitzky A, Bellinger D, Needleman H. A longitudinal study of chronic lead exposure and physical growth in Boston children. Environ Health Perspect. 1995;103(10):952-957.

[11] Lin JL, Lin-Tan DT, Yu CC, Li YJ, Huang YY, Li KL. Environmental exposure to lead and progressive diabetic nephropathy in patients with type II diabetes. Kidney Int. 2006;69(11):2049-2056.

[12] Lin JL, Lin-Tan DT, Li YJ, Chen KH, Huang YL. Low-level environmental exposure to lead and progressive chronic kidney diseases. Am J Med. 2006;119(8):707 e701-709.

[13] Lin-Tan DT, Lin JL, Yen TH, Chen KH, Huang YL. Long-term outcome of repeated lead chelation therapy in progressive non-diabetic chronic kidney diseases. Nephrol Dial Transplant. 2007;22(10):2924-2931.

[14] Lin JL, Lin-Tan DT, Hsu KH, Yu CC. Environmental lead exposure and progression of chronic renal diseases in patients without diabetes. N Engl J Med. 2003;348(4):277-286.

[15] Krachler M, Wirnsberger GH. Long-term changes of plasma trace element concentrations in chronic hemodialysis patients. Blood Purif. 2000;18(2):138-143.

[16] Colleoni N, Arrigo G, Gandini E, Corigliano C, D'Amico G. Blood lead in hemodialysis patients. Am J Nephrol. 1993;13(3):198-202.

[17] Kessler M, Durand PY, Huu TC, Royer-Morot MJ, Chanliau J, Netter P, Duc M. Mobilization of lead from bone in end-stage renal failure patients with secondary hyperparathyroidism. Nephrol Dial Transplant. 1999;14(11):2731-2733.

Accumulation of Toxic Metals and Trace Elements in Chronic Dialysis Patients   261

[18] U.S. Renal Data System, USRDS 2010 Annual Data Report. Atlas of Chronic Kidney Disease and End-Stage Renal Disease in the United States, National Institutes of Health, National Institute of Diabetes and Digestive and Kidney Diseases, Bethesda, MD, 2010.

[19] Wanner C, Metzger T. C-reactive protein a marker for all-cause and cardiovascular mortality in haemodialysis patients. Nephrol Dial Transplant. 2002;17 Suppl 8:29-32; discussion 39-40.

[20] Pecoits-Filho R, Nordfors L, Lindholm B, Hoff CM, Schalling M, Stenvinkel P. Genetic approaches in the clinical investigation of complex disorders: malnutrition, inflammation, and atherosclerosis (MIA) as a prototype. Kidney Int. Suppl 2003;(84):S162-167.

[21] Pupim LB, Caglar K, Hakim RM, Shyr Y, Ikizler TA. Uremic malnutrition is a predictor of death independent of inflammatory status. Kidney Int. 2004;66(5):2054-2060.

[22] Kalantar-Zadeh K, Block G, Humphreys MH, Kopple JD. Reverse epidemiology of cardiovascular risk factors in maintenance dialysis patients. Kidney Int. 2003;63(3):793-808.

[23] Kalantar-Zadeh K. Recent advances in understanding the malnutrition-inflammation-cachexia syndrome in chronic kidney disease patients: What is next? Semin Dial. 2005;18(5):365-369.

[24] Lin JL, Lin-Tan DT, Yen TH, Hsu CW, Jenq CC, Chen KH, Hsu KH, Huang YL. Blood lead levels, malnutrition, inflammation, and mortality in patients with diabetes treated by long-term hemodialysis. Am J Kidney Dis. 2008;51(1):107-115.

[25] Lin JL, Lin-Tan DT, Hsu CW, Yen TH, Chen KH, Hsu HH, Ho TC, Hsu KH. Association of blood lead levels with mortality in patients on maintenance hemodialysis. Am J Med. 2011;124(4):350-358.

[26] Rodriguez-Iturbe B, Sindhu RK, Quiroz Y, Vaziri ND. Chronic exposure to low doses of lead results in renal infiltration of immune cells, NF-kappaB activation, and overexpression of tubulointerstitial angiotensin II. Antioxid Redox Signal. 2005;7(9-10):1269-1274.

[27] Vaziri ND. Mechanisms of lead-induced hypertension and cardiovascular disease. Am J Physiol Heart Circ Physiol. 2008;295(2):H454-465.

[28] Ding Y, Gonick HC, Vaziri ND. Lead promotes hydroxyl radical generation and lipid peroxidation in cultured aortic endothelial cells. Am J Hypertens. 2000;13(5 Pt 1):552-555.

[29] Nawrot TS, Staessen JA. Low-level environmental exposure to lead unmasked as silent killer. Circulation. 2006;114(13):1347-1349.

[30] Aykin-Burns N, Franklin EA, Ercal N. Effects of N-acetylcysteine on lead-exposed PC-12 cells. Arch Environ Contam Toxicol. 2005;49(1):119-123.

[31] Ding Y, Vaziri ND, Gonick HC. Lead-induced hypertension. II. Response to sequential infusions of L-arginine, superoxide dismutase, and nitroprusside. Environ Res. 1998;76(2):107-113.

[32] Morena M, Delbosc S, Dupuy AM, Canaud B, Cristol JP. Overproduction of reactive oxygen species in end-stage renal disease patients: a potential component of hemodialysis-associated inflammation. Hemodial Int. 2005;9(1):37-46.

[33] Yao Q, Pecoits-Filho R, Lindholm B, Stenvinkel P. Traditional and non-traditional risk factors as contributors to atherosclerotic cardiovascular disease in end-stage renal disease. Scand J Urol Nephrol. 2004;38(5):405-416.

[34] Lin TH, Chen JG, Liaw JM, Juang JG. Trace elements and lipid peroxidation in uremic patients on hemodialysis. Biol Trace Elem Res. 1996;51(3):277-283.

[35] Lin JL, Lin-Tan DT, Chen KH, Hsu CW, Yen TH, Huang WH, Huang YL. Blood lead levels association with 18-month all-cause mortality in patients with chronic peritoneal dialysis. Nephrol Dial Transplant. 2010;25(5):1627-1633.

[36] Vaziri ND, Sica DA. Lead-induced hypertension: role of oxidative stress. Curr Hypertens Rep. 2004;6(4):314-320.

[37] Marron B, Remon C, Perez-Fontan M, Quiros P, Ortiz A. Benefits of preserving residual renal function in peritoneal dialysis. Kidney Int. Suppl 2008;(108):S42-51.

[38] Jarup L, Hellstrom L, Alfven T, Carlsson MD, Grubb A, Persson B, Pettersson C, Spang G, Schutz A, Elinder CG. Low level exposure to cadmium and early kidney damage: the OSCAR study. Occup Environ Med. 2000;57(10):668-672.

[39] Borjesson J, Bellander T, Jarup L, Elinder CG, Mattsson S. In vivo analysis of cadmium in battery workers versus measurements of blood, urine, and workplace air. Occup Environ Med. 1997;54(6):424-431.

[40] Lin JL, Lu FH, Yeh KH. Increased body cadmium burden in Chinese women without smoking and occupational exposure. J Toxicol Clin Toxicol. 1995;33(6):639-644.

[41] Wu HM, Lin-Tan DT, Wang ML, Huang HY, Wang HS, Soong YK, Lin JL. Cadmium level in seminal plasma may affect the pregnancy rate for patients undergoing infertility evaluation and treatment. Reprod Toxicol. 2008;25(4):481-484.

[42] Lin JL, Lin-Tan DT, Chu PH, Chen YC, Huang YL, Ho TC, Lin CY. Cadmium excretion predicting hospital mortality and illness severity of critically ill medical patients. Crit Care Med. 2009;37(3):957-962.

[43] Lu LT, Chang IC, Hsiao TY, Yu YH, Ma HW. Identification of pollution source of cadmium in soil: application of material flow analysis and a case study in Taiwan. Environ Sci Pollut Res Int. 2007;14(1):49-59.

[44] Jarup L, Berglund M, Elinder CG, Nordberg G, Vahter M. Health effects of cadmium exposure--a review of the literature and a risk estimate. Scand J Work Environ Health. 1998;24 Suppl 1:1-51.

[45] Jarup L. Cadmium overload and toxicity. Nephrol Dial Transplant. 2002;17 Suppl 2:35-39.

[46] Voors AW, Shuman MS, Johnson WD. Additive statistical effects of cadmium and lead on heart-related disease in a North Carolina autopsy series. Arch Environ Health. 1982;37(2):98-102.

[47] Pesch B, Haerting J, Ranft U, Klimpel A, Oelschlagel B, Schill W. Occupational risk factors for renal cell carcinoma: agent-specific results from a case-control study in Germany. MURC Study Group. Multicenter urothelial and renal cancer study. Int J Epidemiol. 2000;29(6):1014-1024.

[48] Nishijo M, Morikawa Y, Nakagawa H, Tawara K, Miura K, Kido T, Ikawa A, Kobayashi E, Nogawa K. Causes of death and renal tubular dysfunction in residents exposed to cadmium in the environment. Occup Environ Med. 2006;63(8):545-550.

[49] Menke A, Muntner P, Silbergeld EK, Platz EA, Guallar E. Cadmium levels in urine and mortality among U.S. adults. Environ Health Perspect. 2009;117(2):190-196.

[50] Navas-Acien A, Tellez-Plaza M, Guallar E, Muntner P, Silbergeld E, Jaar B, Weaver V. Blood cadmium and lead and chronic kidney disease in US adults: a joint analysis. Am J Epidemiol. 2009;170(9):1156-1164.

[51] Hsu CW, Lin JL, Lin-Tan DT, Yen TH, Huang WH, Ho TC, Huang YL, Yeh LM, Huang LM. Association of environmental cadmium exposure with inflammation and malnutrition in maintenance haemodialysis patients. Nephrol Dial Transplant. 2009;24(4):1282-1288.

[52] Min KS, Kim H, Fujii M, Tetsuchikawahara N, Onosaka S. Glucocorticoids suppress the inflammation-mediated tolerance to acute toxicity of cadmium in mice. Toxicol Appl Pharmacol. 2002;178(1):1-7.

[53] Kayama F, Yoshida T, Elwell MR, Luster MI. Role of tumor necrosis factor-alpha in cadmium-induced hepatotoxicity. Toxicol Appl Pharmacol. 1995;131(2):224-234.

[54] Yiin SJ, Chern CL, Sheu JY, Lin TH. Cadmium-induced liver, heart, and spleen lipid peroxidation in rats and protection by selenium. Biol Trace Elem Res. 2000;78(1-3):219-230.

[55] Manca D, Ricard AC, Tra HV, Chevalier G. Relation between lipid peroxidation and inflammation in the pulmonary toxicity of cadmium. Arch Toxicol. 1994;68(6):364-369.

[56] Dong W, Simeonova PP, Gallucci R, Matheson J, Flood L, Wang S, Hubbs A, Luster MI. Toxic metals stimulate inflammatory cytokines in hepatocytes through oxidative stress mechanisms. Toxicol Appl Pharmacol. 1998;151(2):359-366.

[57] Kirschvink N, Martin N, Fievez L, Smith N, Marlin D, Gustin P. Airway inflammation in cadmium-exposed rats is associated with pulmonary oxidative stress and emphysema. Free Radic Res. 2006;40(3):241-250.

[58] Kramer HJ, Gonick HC, Lu E. In vitro inhibition of Na-K-ATPase by trace metals: relation to renal and cardiovascular damage. Nephron. 1986;44(4):329-336.

[59] Navas-Acien A, Selvin E, Sharrett AR, Calderon-Aranda E, Silbergeld E, Guallar E. Lead, cadmium, smoking, and increased risk of peripheral arterial disease. Circulation. 2004;109(25):3196-3201.

[60] Kalantar-Zadeh K, Kopple JD, Block G, Humphreys MH. A malnutrition-inflammation score is correlated with morbidity and mortality in maintenance hemodialysis patients. Am J Kidney Dis. 2001;38(6):1251-1263.

[61] Edwards JR, Prozialeck WC. Cadmium, diabetes and chronic kidney disease. Toxicol Appl Pharmacol 2009;238(3):289-293.

[62] Vanholder R, Cornelis R, Dhondt A, Lameire N. The role of trace elements in uraemic toxicity. Nephrol Dial Transplant. 2002;17 Suppl 2:2-8.

[63] Chen B, Lamberts LV, Behets GJ, Zhao T, Zhou M, Liu G, Hou X, Guan G, D'Haese PC. Selenium, lead, and cadmium levels in renal failure patients in China. Biol Trace Elem Res. 2009;131(1):1-12.

[64] Yen TH, Lin JL, Lin-Tan DT, Hsu CW, Chen KH, Hsu HH. Blood cadmium level's association with 18-month mortality in diabetic patients with maintenance haemodialysis. Nephrol Dial Transplant. 2011;26(3):998-1005.

[65] Kawakami T, Sugimoto H, Furuichi R, Kadota Y, Inoue M, Setsu K, Suzuki S, Sato M. Cadmium reduces adipocyte size and expression levels of adiponectin and Peg1/Mest in adipose tissue. Toxicology. 2010;267(1-3):20-26.

[66] Oomichi T, Emoto M, Tabata T, Morioka T, Tsujimoto Y, Tahara H, Shoji T, Nishizawa Y. Impact of glycemic control on survival of diabetic patients on chronic regular hemodialysis: a 7-year observational study. Diabetes Care. 2006;29(7):1496-1500.

[67] Zima T, Mestek O, Tesar V, Tesarova P, Nemecek K, Zak A, Zeman M. Chromium levels in patients with internal diseases. Biochem Mol Biol Int. 1998;46(2):365-374.

[68] D'Haese PC, Couttenye MM, Lamberts LV, Elseviers MM, Goodman WG, Schrooten I, Cabrera WE, De Broe ME. Aluminum, iron, lead, cadmium, copper, zinc, chromium, magnesium, strontium, and calcium content in bone of end-stage renal failure patients. Clin Chem. 1999;45(9):1548-1556.

[69] Sondheimer JH, Mahajan SK, Rye DL, Abu-Hamdan DK, Migdal SD, Prasad AS, McDonald FD. Elevated plasma copper in chronic renal failure. Am J Clin Nutr. 1988;47(5):896-899.

[70] Hosokawa S, Yoshida O. Serum vanadium levels in chronic hemodialysis patients. Nephron. 1993;64(3):388-394.

[71] Hosokawa S, Yoshida O. Vanadium in patients undergoing chronic haemodialysis. Nephrol Dial Transplant. 1989;4(4):282-284.

[72] Tsukamoto Y, Saka S, Kumano K, Iwanami S, Ishida O, Marumo F. Abnormal accumulation of vanadium in patients on chronic hemodialysis therapy. Nephron. 1990;56(4):368-373.

In: Issues in Dialysis
Editor: Stephen Z. Fadem

ISBN: 978-1-62417-576-3
© 2013 Nova Science Publishers, Inc.

Chapter XVI

Adequacy of Dialysis

James Tattersall
Leeds Teaching Hospitals, Leeds, UK

Abstract

For over thirty years urea clearance, quantified by Kt/V has been used as the rational basis to prescribe and quantify dialysis. The minimal level for adequacy has been defined at a Kt/V of around 1.2 for thrice weekly HD and 1.7 per week for peritoneal dialysis. While there have been significant improvements, dialysis still provides less than 10% of normal renal clearance and outcome remains poor compared to other chronic diseases. Over this time, dialysis research has concentrated on improving the efficacy of dialysis and its outcome.

Over the last ten years, it has become apparent that increasing Kt/V does not result in improving outcome using conventional treatment schedules. The focus has switched to more frequent and longer dialysis sessions, increasing the clearance of higher molecular weight solutes and addressing the bone mineral abnormalities, hypertension and fluid overload which is responsible for the cardiovascular complications of dialysis.

The concept of adequacy must change to cope with longer and more frequent dialysis schedules, the contribution of residual renal function and to quantify the clearance of phosphate and higher molecular weight solute. The inconvenience of the treatment and impact on quality of life should be taken into account. A measure of fluid overload should be included. New developments such as online clearance and bioimpedance provide practical tools to make the process easier and more accurate.

Introduction

What Is Adequate Dialysis?

Dialysis aims to restore health when kidney function is insufficient on its own. Ideally, dialysis should completely replace renal function at low cost and no adverse effects or inconvenience to the patient. With current dialysis techniques, this ideal is impossible. With hemodialysis, complete replacement of the clearance, salt and water homeostatic functions of the kidney can be achieved, but only if treatment duration is long and frequent (e.g. at least 8 hours daily). With peritoneal dialysis, clearance can be increased at the expense of larger exchange fluid volumes and frequency. Even with high fluid volumes, the peritoneal membrane permeability to solutes and water is an insurmountable barrier which limits urea clearance to less than 20% of normal renal function. For solutes other than urea clearance is limited to less than 10% of normal renal function. With current dialysis techniques, the risks of adverse effects on the patient are increased as efficacy increases (e.g. by increasing fluid volumes, flow rates, artificial membrane surface area, treatment time and frequency).

Until we have implantable, or at least wearable, artificial kidney systems, capable of replacing renal function continuously and safely without tethering the patient to a power or fluid source, dialysis remains a compromise between cost, inconvenience and risk of adverse effects on the one hand and efficacy on the other. Current dialysis techniques generally provide 5-10% of normal renal function, sufficient to control symptoms and observable adverse effects of uremia, at least in the short or medium term.

An adequate dialysis could be considered the best compromise between acceptable health, cost, inconvenience and adverse effects. This compromise may be found between the minimum treatment required to maintain health and the maximum tolerated by the patient. A fully informed patient is best placed to choose the dialysis strategy and dose which best fulfills these expectations.

Few studies have attempted to capture the patient's wishes, expectations and priorities in renal replacement therapy. Where this has been attempted, patients tend to give higher priority to home treatment, flexible scheduling and reduced treatment time than to survival and absence of symptoms. [1]

Optimal or Adequate?

An optimal dialysis could be considered as the dialysis treatment which is tuned to improve health to the maximum possible extent, regardless of cost. In the optimal dialysis there would be no further benefit to health by increasing treatment efficacy. The optimal dialysis may consider inconvenience of the treatment and any adverse effects.

With dialysis techniques in current common use, an optimal dialysis is not clearly different from an adequate dialysis. Two landmark randomized controlled trials (RCT) were unable to show any benefit to health on increasing dialysis dose above those commonly accepted as adequate for hemodialysis and peritoneal dialysis.

It is probable that more frequent and longer dialysis may prove to be optimal, but any negative impact on quality of life may be difficult to account. There are studies underway attempting to quantify these effects.

The concept of dialysis adequacy depends on measurable surrogate outcomes such as clearance, generation rates and concentrations of solutes representative of uremic toxins. Real outcomes such as quality of life, hospitalization rates, functional status and quality of life are clearly of overriding importance, but more difficult to analyze as it is difficult to separate the effects of dialysis from other influences such as age and co-morbidity.

Clearance

The concept of clearance is central to nephrology as a means of understanding and measuring kidney function. The clearance concept emerged in the early part of the 20th century. Clearance of any solute is defined as the minimum volume of plasma water containing the mass of the solute excreted in one minute. [2]

In steady state (e.g. for patients not on dialysis or receiving continuous dialysis and whose overall clearance is not changing), clearance (K, in units of volume/time, e.g. ml/minute) is the ratio of generation rate (G, in units of mass/time, e.g. mg/minute) and concentration in plasma water (C, in units of mass/volume, e.g. mg/ml) as in Equation 1.

In intermittent dialysis, concentration in plasma water varies with time, falling during dialysis (when clearance is high relative to generation rate) and increasing between dialysis sessions when clearance is low or absent (Equation 2).

Predicting concentration of a solute from generation rate (G), clearance rate (K).	
Steady state.	Equation 1. $C = \frac{G}{K}$
Changing concentration in intermittent treatments, V=volume of distribution, t=time, C0=initial concentration, Ct= concentration after time t.	Equation 2. $C_t = \frac{G}{K} + \left(\frac{G}{K} - C_0\right) e^{-\frac{Kt}{V}}$

Dialysis Dose

Dialysis adequacy is defined in terms of the dose of dialysis, a concept similar to treatment by a drug. Dialysis dose is quantified through the parameters of a kinetic model derived from the principles of pharmacokinetics, which includes clearance, familiar as a means of quantifying renal function. Other components of dose include duration, frequency and a normalizing factor such as body weight or, more commonly, distribution volume or surface area. The models are described later in the chapter.

Kt/V

The Kt/V is central to prescribing and quantifying dose of intermittent treatments. It is the exponential term in Equation 2. In hemodialysis, Kt/V quantifies a single dialysis treatment and combines K, the urea clearance, t the duration of the dialysis session and V, the urea distribution volume (equal to the body water volume). Urea clearance is used because it is relatively easy to measure and its generation rate, G is proportional to dietary protein intake. Also urea is the only solute which is able to pass easily between intracellular and extracellular water, so it behaves approximately according to a simple model, where it is assumed that urea it is distributed evenly throughout the entire body water volume. This assumption greatly simplifies the measurement and calculation of Kt/V.

Kt/V can be predicted using K from the dialyzer datasheet, t as the prescribed session length and V from the Watson equation (Equation 13, Equation 14). This is the 'prescribed'

Kt/V. The K from the dialyzer datasheet overestimates the 'in-vivo' clearance during dialysis by about 30% (as described later in this chapter). This error in prescribed Kt/V is offset by the Watson equation overestimating V, also by about 30%.

Kt/V can be calculated independently from pre- and post-dialysis urea concentrations using a kinetic model as described later in the chapter. The equilibrated Kt/V (eqKt/V) takes the peripheral retention of urea into account. The eqKt/V can be calculated by using a post-dialysis urea concentration sample taken about 30 minutes after dialysis. This allows time for the urea to become equilibrated or evenly distributed throughout the body water, satisfying the assumption of the single-pool model. Alternatively the 30 minute 'equilibrated' concentration can be estimated from pre- and immediate post-dialysis samples using Equation 20. In peritoneal dialysis, Kt/V is the weekly urea clearance divided by body water volume.

**Table 1. Various measures of urea clearance suitable
for different dialysis schedules and modalities**

Measure	Definition G in mg/minute, C in mg/ml, V in ml.	units	Serum concentration as C	Normal renal function	peritoneal dialysis	hemodialysis (anuric)*
StdKt/V	G x 10080/(V x C)	week^{-1}	Average pre-dialysis concentration	20	1.7	2.1
SRI	G x 10080/(V x C)	week^{-1}	Peak concentration	20	1.7	1.8
EKR	G / C	ml/min	Time Average concentration (TAC)	70	6	12
TAC:TAD	G / C	ml/min	Time average deviation (TAD) + TAC	70	6	9

*4 hours, three times per week, spKt/V=1.2, V=65.6liters, BSA=1.73m^2.

Frequency and Duration

As a quantifier of a single dialysis session, Kt/V is incomplete on its own. It can only be used to compare treatments which have the same number of sessions per week and the same duration of dialysis. The rate at which urea is removed by dialysis (flux) is proportional to the instantaneous plasma water concentration. As plasma urea concentration falls during dialysis, the flux falls in proportion. This fall is most significant in short infrequent treatments and smaller in longer or more frequent (i.e. more continuous) treatments. In comparing or interpreting Kt/V, it is generally assumed that the dialysis is provided as three sessions of around 4 hours duration per week (12 hours per week).

A further problem relates to the use of a single-pool model to calculate Kt/V. In reality, urea is not evenly distributed within body water during dialysis. It is retained to some extent in peripheral, poorly-perfused areas of the body (e.g. resting muscles). This reduces the mass of urea removed by dialysis and causes Kt/V to be an overestimate. This overestimation is greater in shorter, more intensive treatments.

To overcome these limitations, a standard weekly Kt/V (stdKt/V) [3], solute removal index (SRI) [4], equivalent renal clearance (EKR) [5] and TAC:TAD [6] have been proposed.

These measures all return to the conventional clearance concept, quantified as the ratio of mass generation rate (G) to concentration in plasma water (C), [7] accounted or averaged over a week. These measures are, in effect, equivalent to the measure of continuous renal function expressed in units of volume/time. SRI and stdKt/V take body size into account by dividing clearance by body volume (V), so their units are time^{-1}. These measures vary according to their definition of plasma water concentration. Concentration can be considered as the average of pre-dialysis concentration, time-average average concentration (TAC), maximum (peak) and the time average deviation (TAD). The time average deviation is calculated as the average absolute difference between each instantaneous concentration and the TAC.

These weekly dose measures can be calculated from V, C and G returned from the two-pool model (described later in the chapter), thereby avoiding overestimation due to retention of urea in peripheral compartments. Each of the dose measures can include renal function.

EKR and TAC:TAD are in the familiar clearance units of ml/min and can be normalized to 1.73 m^2 surface area (SA) by multiplying by 1.73/SA or to 40 liters volume by multiplying by 40/V.

When there is no residual renal function and all dialysis sessions have equal Kt/V, the stdKt/V can be calculated without using the two-pool model using Equation 3. The retention of urea in peripheral compartments is taken into account by using the equilibrated (eqKt/V).

Calculation of stdKt/V. t=dialysis session time, N=number of treatments per week. [8]	$$\text{Equation 3. } stdKt/V = \dfrac{10080\frac{1-e^{-eqKt/V}}{t}}{\frac{1-e^{-eqKt/V}}{Kt/V}+\frac{10080}{Nt}-1}$$

Equation 3 makes use of a peculiarity of stdKt/V in that stdKt/V is insensitive to timing of the individual sessions. A weekly schedule of three dialysis sessions performed consecutively on the same day will have the same stdKt/V as one where the three sessions are spaced evenly. This is because the very high pre-dialysis concentration after six days without dialysis is offset by much lower pre-dialysis concentrations for the sessions which follow immediately after. [9]

EKR, SRI and TAC:TAD are calculated using the two-pool model and are sensitive to the timing of the individual sessions.

SRI and TAC:TAD are the most sensitive to the dialysis 'un-physiology' (or intermittency and unequal spacing). By using averages, TAC:TAD is relatively immune from random measurement errors and is more reproducible when the spacing between dialysis sessions are variable. SRI and TAC:TAD have the intellectual tidiness of returning approximately the same value for recommended minimum dose in hemodialysis and peritoneal dialysis and also the level of renal function when we usually start dialysis (TAC:TAD = 6-9ml/min, SRI=1.7-1.8week^{-1}).

Flexible Schedules

In home hemodialysis, a patient may prefer a flexible schedule to fit in with their lifestyle. For example, dialysis sessions may be timed to fit in with irregularly scheduled work or family commitments. If the patient is travelling, they may need to fit in with the dialysis schedules of different facilities. The length, frequency, K and start time of the individual sessions may be varied independently.

If the patient has access to appropriate software, they can ensure that they have an adequate weekly dialysis despite these variations in treatment. The patient can have extra session or increase K or t for individual sessions to offset the effect of skipped or shortened session. Such software will need to use one of the weekly dose measures which are sensitive to schedule variations (e.g. TAC:TAD or SRI).

Continuous Treatments

The weekly dose measures stdKt/V, SRI, EKR and TAC:TAD are equally suitable for continuous treatments such as peritoneal dialysis. Because TAD is zero and the various measures of creatinine are the same for continuous treatments, each of the weekly dose measures will give the same result, depending on their units. In a typical peritoneal dialysis, both SRI and stdKt/V will be about 1.8 week^{-1}. Both EKR and TAC:TAD will be about 6 ml/min.

For historical reasons, the weekly doses, SRI and stdKt/V, are known as 'Kt/V' in continuous treatments. This continuous treatment weekly 'Kt/V' should not be confused with the hemodialysis per-session 'Kt/V' which has different units.

In continuous treatments, the disequilibrium that occurs in intermittent treatments is absent and a two-pool model is not required. Also, it is easier to quantify the clearance of solutes other than urea. For historical reasons, the dose of peritoneal dialysis is also quantified as weekly creatinine clearance (in liters/week/1.73m^2).

Renal Function

Recent research has shown that residual renal function is retained for some years after the start of dialysis, contributes significantly to total urea clearance in the majority of patients and is a significant predictor of outcome. [10,11,12] In peritoneal dialysis, variations in renal function seem to account for all or almost all of the association between total clearance and outcome. Increasing small solute clearance by dialysis has little or no impact on survival. [13]

Urea is re-absorbed by the renal tubules. This causes urea clearance to be about 40% lower than GFR. Creatinine is excreted into the tubules, causing creatinine clearance to overestimate GFR by the about the same amount. The mean of urea and creatinine clearance by 24 hour urine collections have been shown to be a reasonable approximation to GFR.

The clearance of certain toxins, including potassium and phosphate can be higher than GFR due to tubular excretion. The kidneys have the capability to excrete protein-bound uremic toxins, such as p-cresol, which are cleared poorly by peritoneal dialysis and hardly at all by hemodialysis.

The kidneys also have beneficial functions other than excreting solute. These include hormonal and homeostatic functions and the excretion of water. Therefore, any measure of renal function based on small solute clearance may significantly underestimate its beneficial impact.

As a continuous clearance, renal function is not easily comparable to a measure of intermittent dialysis such as the per-session Kt/V in hemodialysis. For example, with GFR above 12 ml/minute, any measure of concentration will be lower than could be achieved by three sessions per week of hemodialysis, even if Kt/V is infinite. On the other hand, renal clearance can be included in the two-pool model used to compute any of the continuous dose measures (SRI, stdKt/V, EKR or TAC:TAD).

In a study of 30 non-anuric patients treated by peritoneal dialysis, the renal clearance of solutes other than urea was greater than the peritoneal clearance. Of the solutes studied, only the concentration of p-cresol correlated with symptoms (0). [14]

It is obvious that assessment of dialysis adequacy should take account of renal function in non-anuric patients. Renal function could have a significant impact on the uremic state, even when urea clearance is less than 1 ml/min and 24 hour urine volume less than 200 ml/day.

Table 2. Clearance of various solutes in peritoneal dialysis

solute	Clearance ml/min	
	Renal	Peritoneal
Urea	3.1	6.7
Creatinine	5.4	4.5
Phosphate	2.8	3.6
Beta-2-microglobulin	1.8	0.5
p-cresol	1.2	0.5

Different Solutes

Until recently, dialysis adequacy focused on measures of small solutes such as urea and creatinine. This is because it is relatively easy to control and quantify small solute clearance. Early research in three times weekly dialysis suggested that improving Kt/V up to around 1.0 resulted in improved survival. However further increases in Kt/V have not resulted in improved survival, at least with conventional hemodialysis schedules. [15] In peritoneal dialysis, all, or most, of any advantage of higher Kt/V has been shown to be associated with more residual renal function, rather than increasing dialysis dose.

We now have the opportunity to increase the clearance of larger solutes such as beta-2-microglobulin using larger and more porous dialyzers and by adding filtration to dialysis as in online hemodiafiltration. These improvements have minimal cost and have been shown to effectively reduce beta-2-microglobulin concentration in plasma. Unlike urea, beta-2-microglobulin is toxic and lower levels are associated with improved outcome. [16] The use of high-flux membranes, which increases beta-2-microglobulin clearance, has been shown to improve survival, at least in high-risk patients. [17]

Much of the excess mortality rate in dialysis patients is due to cardiovascular problems and associated with high serum phosphate levels. Longer dialysis sessions have been shown to reduce phosphate levels. In peritoneal dialysis, longer dwell times have been shown to increase phosphate clearance.

Urea is a highly atypical solute and not at all representative of uremic toxins. Urea is not particularly toxic and is relatively easy to remove by dialysis due to its low molecular weight and high diffusivity. There are specific urea channels in cell membranes which allow urea to pass through cell membranes virtually unimpeded. Urea is reabsorbed in the renal tubules so its clearance rate by the kidneys is lower than for other solutes. In contrast, other solutes are harder to clear by dialysis and renal clearance is relatively more important.

The efficiency of hemodialysis is much reduced for non-urea solutes which are distributed in both intra- and extra- cellular fluid. This is because solute in cells is relatively inaccessible to the dialysis process. Solute is not cleared from erythrocyte water as blood passes through the dialyzer. There is a significant solute rebound as it slowly diffuses out of cells after dialysis. Single pool kinetic modeling and calculation of single-pool Kt/V is only meaningful for urea which diffuses rapidly through cell membranes. The mass of urea removed by hemodialysis is relatively easy to increase by increasing blood and dialysate flow. Clearance of other solutes is relatively less dependent on blood flow and more dependent on dialyzer membrane surface area and permeability and on treatment time.

Urea diffuses relatively easily across the peritoneum. Urea clearance by peritoneal dialysis is influenced mainly by the volume and frequency of the dialysate exchanges. Other solutes diffuse more slowly through the peritoneum; their clearance is limited by the peritoneal surface area and treatment time, which cannot so easily be manipulated.

Certain known uremic toxins are bound to plasma albumin and not cleared at all by conventional hemodialysis. Peritoneal dialysis remove 5-10g day of albumin which provide about 1 ml/min of bound solute clearance. It is currently possible to modify hemodialysis to clear bound toxin. [18] These bound-toxin dialysis methods are currently expensive and not in routine use. Further research is needed to investigate potential benefits of bound toxin clearance.

Table 3. Comparative physical properties of selected solutes

Solute	Molecular weight	Distribution	Renal clearance, relative to GFR	Diffusion rate relative to urea
Urea	60	Body water	0.7	1
Creatinine	113	Body water	1.3	0.8
Phosphate	94	Mostly intracellular	0.8	0.8
Beta-2-microglobulin	12,000	Extracellular	0.5	0.06

Table 3 lists some properties of four commonly measured dialyzable solutes. It is obvious that clearance by dialysis should be quantified for a range of typical solutes and certainly not just urea.

Salt and Water

The importance and assessment of fluid overload is described by Richard Glassock (Chapter 9). The control of fluid overload is one of the main and probably the most important function of dialysis. Assessment of dialysis adequacy must include a measure of fluid overload. Until recently, this was by clinical assessment and blood pressure. Now we have bioimpedance, which can be used to measure the absolute volume of fluid overload. [19]

Clearance in Hemodialysis

The theory and principles of clearance from water passing through a dialyzer is well understood. Clearance from water is measured routinely as part of the quality assurance of the manufacturing process. The dialyzer manufacturers are legally required to measure and quote the clearance of a range of solutes. Diffusion theory can be used to model and predict the clearance under conditions not directly measured.

For solute to be cleared by the dialyzer, it must be carried into the dialyzer by flow at the 'blood' inlet (Qb), diffuse into the dialysate across the membrane and be carried out of the dialyzer by flow at the dialysate outlet (Qd). Clearance has the same units as flow (e.g. ml/minute) and is limited by the lowest of the three determining flows, Qb, Qd and a solute-specific diffusion term, the overall clearance (KoA, also in ml/min). The KoA is related to the density and size of pores in the membrane, the membrane surface area and the distance through which solute must diffuse. The KoA is the theoretical limit for dialyzer clearance, when blood and dialysate flow are infinite.

The Koa will vary depending on solute, lower for solutes of greater molecular weight which diffuse more slowly. For solutes which are small enough to pass through the pores unimpeded, KoA is approximately inversely proportional to the square-root of the solute's molecular weight. The KoA can calculated form measurements of dialyzer clearance (Kid) using Equation 4. [20] Alternatively, Equation 4 can be used to calculate KoA from data quoted in the datasheet that must accompany every pack of dialyzers.

Using Equation 5, a predicted Kid can be calculated from KoA for any value of Qb and Qd. This predicted Kid is used to prescribe dialysis and, by comparing with actual clearance measured during dialysis, for quality control and trouble-shooting).

Michael's equations, relating dialyzer clearance (Kid) to flow into the 'blood' inlet (Qb), dialysate outlet and the KoA.	
Calculating KoA	Equation 4. $KoA = \dfrac{Qb}{1-\frac{Qb}{Qd}} \times \ln\left[\dfrac{1-\frac{Kd}{Qd}}{1-\frac{Kd}{Qb}}\right]$
Predicting K	Equation 5. $Kd = \dfrac{1-e^{KoA\times\frac{Qb-Qd}{Qb\times Qd}}}{\frac{1}{Qb}-\frac{1}{Qd}\times e^{KoA\times\frac{Qb-Qd}{Qb\times Qd}}}$

The Effect of Convection on Dialyzer Clearance

Ultrafiltration carries solute through the dialyzer membrane and will affect Kid. This effect is depends on the ultrafiltration rate (Qi), the sieving coefficient (SC), initial Kid (at zero Qi), blood and dialysate flow.

The mass of solute transferred across the membrane by filtration also depends on the concentration of solute in the blood compartment of the dialyzer. This concentration is reduced by diffusion, so the effect of convection is reduced when KoA is high relative to blood flow. Also, the mass transfer by convection has the effect of reducing the concentration difference across the membrane, which reduces the rate of diffusion. The overall effect of convection on Kid is greater for larger solutes which have lower KoA and is almost non-existent for small solutes such as urea, which diffuse more easily.

The effect of ultrafiltration on dialyzer clearance can be included using Equation 6 and Equation 7. [21]

Fichu's equations, for predicting the effect of filtration on dialyzer clearance. It is assumed that the dialysate is prepared on-line by filtration of dialysate, and take account of the fact that the dialysate flow will be reduced by the filtrate flow. SC is the solute-specific sieving coefficient for the dialyzer, K0 is the value of Kid at zero ultrafiltration rate, e.g. estimated using equation 5.	
post-dilution	Equation 6. $Kd = K0 + \dfrac{Qb - K0}{Qb} \times Qf \times Sc$
pre-dilution	Equation 7. $Kd = K0 + \dfrac{\frac{Qb \times Qd}{Qb + Qd} - K0}{Qd} \times Qf \times Sc$

More realistic models of dialyzer function exist, which take boundary layers and other factors into account. [22]

Difference between 'In-vitro' and 'In-vivo' Clearance

The clearance quoted in the dialyzer datasheet is measured 'in-vitro', i.e. using water instead of blood. For urea, the 'in-vivo' clearance from blood during hemodialysis of a patient is typically about 30% lower than the 'in-vitro' clearance using the same dialyzer, Qb, and Qd. This difference is masked in the calculation of Kt/V by an error of a similar magnitude in the estimation of V using the Watson equations (Equation 13 and Equation 14).

This difference is partly due to the presence of protein in the blood and that the fact that only the blood water (about 84% of the total volume of blood) is cleared. This accounts for about half of the difference between in-vitro and in-vivo clearance. The remainder of the difference appears to be due to a reduction in the diffusion component, KoA, by about 45%. This is thought to be due to membrane fouling as plasma protein may be drawn into the membrane pores due to filtration and block them. Another possibility is that diffusion of solute through plasma is slower than through water, due to the 'crowding' effect of the plasma proteins.

For solutes other than urea, the erythrocyte membrane effectively prevents any significant clearance from erythrocytes as they pass through the dialyzer. Therefore, only the plasma water flow (around 60% of the total blood flow) is cleared.

To predict 'in-vivo' clearance, first calculate effective blood using Equation 10 or Equation 11. Then calculate the 'in-vivo' KoA by multiplying the 'in-vitro' KoA by 0.55. Finally, use effective blood flow as Qb and 'in-vivo' KoA in Equation 5.

Equations to calculate effective blood water flow (Qb_{Eff}) for 'in-vivo' clearance. Hct is the hematocrit and tprot is the total protein concentration in g/l.

Plasma water fraction	Equation 8. $fPw = 0.984 - 0.000718 \times tprot$
Whole blood water fraction	Equation 9. $fBw = (1 - Hct) \times fPw + Hct \times 0.72$
Effective blood flow for urea clearance	Equation 10. $Qbeff = Qb \times fBw$
Effective blood flow for all other solutes	Equation 11. $Qbeff = Qb \times (1 - Hct) \times fPw$

Additional factors which may reduce 'in-vivo' clearance are:

- Dialyser fiber clotting, reducing the surface area available for diffusion.
- Blood flow may be lower than displayed on the dialysis machine front panel. This is because peristaltic pumps lose efficiency as the inflow ('arterial') pressure falls. This inflow pressure falls during 'in-vivo' dialysis due to the viscosity of blood (which is much higher than water) and to the resistance offered by the fistula needles.
- Access recirculation reduces effective clearance by reducing the solute concentration in the dialysate compartment and reducing the concentration gradients which drive diffusion. In access recirculation, the inflow 'arterial' blood is diluted by the presence of dialyzed blood which has passed directly from the outflow 'venous' needle via the access and without passing through the systemic circulation. Access recirculation may occur when the inflow needle is incorrectly placed downstream of the outflow needle or when the extracorporeal blood flow exceeds the access flow.
- Cardio-pulmonary recirculation is unavoidable when a fistula or graft is used as the access. A proportion of the dialyzed blood re-entering the access passed through the heart and lungs and back to the access via the artery supplying the access. This will predictably reduce the mass of solute cleared by reducing concentration at the dialyzer inlet by a factor of CO/Kid, where CO is cardiac output.

Clearance in Peritoneal Dialysis

For solute to be cleared by peritoneal dialysis, it must be carried to the peritoneal capillaries via the circulation, pass through the peritoneal capillary walls, diffuse through the peritoneal interstitial tissue and mesothelium into the peritoneal dialysate and drained via the catheter.

As with hemodialysis, the mechanism of solute transfer between compartments is by diffusion and convection. For convection, the rate of mass transfer (flux) is the flow rate multiplied by concentration multiplied by sieving coefficient. For diffusion, flux is the concentration difference multiplied by a mass transfer area coefficient. Osmosis plays a significant role in mass transfer.

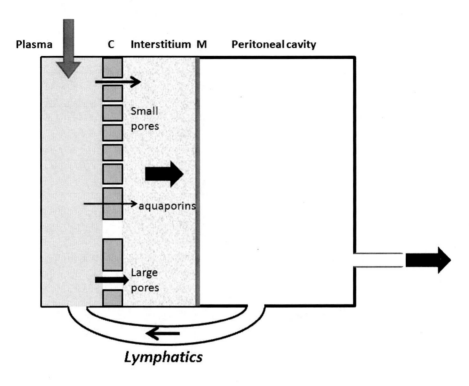

Figure 1. Model for peritoneal clearance. C=capillary wall. M=mesothelium.

The capillary cell wall is considered to be the most important barrier to diffusion. Its function can be predicted by the three-pore model which considers three channels for solute transfer. [23] The large and small channels are gaps between capillary epithelial cells. The aquaporins are trans-cellular channels which transmit only water. The aquaporins are important for osmotic transfer of fluid, under the influence of a low-molecular weight osmotic agent such as glucose. Solute transfer is via the large and small pores. The transfer of large solutes such as beta-2-microglobulin is mostly via large pores.

The diffusive mass transfer coefficients for various solutes are approximately in proportion to the reciprocal of the square root of their molecular weight. For a small solute such as urea, the diffusion is rapid enough to achieve almost complete equilibrium with the dialysate during a typical dwell of four hours. Therefore, urea clearance can be increased by increasing the frequency or volume of the dialysate exchanges.

In contrast to urea, a larger solute such as beta-2-microglobulin diffuses so slowly that the concentration in the dialysis is far from equilibrium during a typical dwell period. Therefore increasing the frequency of the dialysate exchange cycles will have minimal impact on clearance. By stretching and increasing the effective peritoneal surface area, increasing exchange volume may increase large solute clearance significantly.

The solute-specific peritoneal mass transfer area coefficient (MTAC) represent the absolute limits for the clearance rates of solutes by peritoneal dialysis. MTAC is around 20 ml/min for urea, 10 ml/min for creatinine and correspondingly lower for higher molecular weight solutes.

Even within the spectrum of small solutes, different diffusion rates for different solutes require a different strategy for their removal. Phosphate clearance is improved by increasing cycle volumes and reducing frequency of exchanges in patient with low mass transfer coefficients. [24]

Normalizing Factor – Volume or Surface Area?

In general, the concentration of solute in biological fluids has a similar range regardless of body size. This even holds true to a great extent between species, for example the normal range for BUN is identical in cats, humans, horses and whales. This means that, in the absence of renal impairment, G/K is relatively constant, regardless size. G is related to dietary intake and/or metabolic rate and is generally considered to vary in proportion to body surface area. Therefore, K is normally lower in smaller individuals, in proportion to surface area.

For this reason, in order to identify abnormal values of K, body surface area is taken into account by normalizing to $1.73m^2$. This is achieved by multiplying K by 1.73 and dividing by surface area estimated from height and weight using a prediction equation.

In theory, dialysis dose should also be normalized to body surface area. However, the dose of intermittent treatments is often normalized to urea distribution volume, related to body weight. This is because the urea distribution volume is a required parameter of the urea kinetic model, described below. By normalizing to volume, rather than surface area, there would be a tendency to overestimating dose in smaller patients and underestimating in larger patients. There is some evidence that this is really the case, since larger patients have better-than-expected outcome and smaller patients [25,26] especially females, benefit from a higher dialysis dose, compared to larger patients. If the amount (or dose) of dialysis is prescribed in proportion to volume instead of surface area, a larger dose should be prescribed to pediatric patients or patients with low body weight. This is to compensate for their higher surface area to volume ratio.

Surface area is usually estimated from height (Ht, in cm) and weight(Wt, in Kg) using the DuBois and DuBois method in Equation 12. Body water volume can be estimated from height, age (in years), sex and weight using the Watson method in equations Equation 13 and Equation 14;

Surface area (SA, m^2) height (Ht, cm) and weight (Wt, Kg)	Equation 12.	$SA = 0.007184 \times Ht^{0.725} \times Wt^{0.425}$
Women: Body water volume (V, liter)	Equation 13.	$V = -2.097 + 0.2466 \times Wt + 0.1069 \times Ht$
Men: Age in years	Equation 14.	$V = 2.447 + 0.3362 \times Wt + 0.1074 \times Ht - 0.09516 \times Age$

In dialysis patients, the Watson method is known to overestimate V, presumably because dialysis patients have a lower muscle mass in proportion to body weight compared to the subjects originally studied by Watson. Muscle has a relatively higher water content compared to other tissue. The overestimation of V by the Watson method is approximately 30% but there is considerable variation between individuals.

The gold-standard method for measuring body water volume involves dilution of a known mass of tracer (e.g. deuterium) which distributes in body water. These methods are time-consuming and the tracer measurements can be expensive.

Body water volume can now be accurately, non-invasively and cheaply measured using bioimpedance. [27] The method analyses the electrical conducting properties of the body to determine its fluid content. A bioimpedance measurement takes about 5 minutes and there is good agreement between bioimpedance and tracer dilution methods.

Variable-volume Single-pool Urea Kinetic Model

A kinetic model is required to handle intermittent dialysis techniques where steady state is not achieved (especially hemodialysis, hemofiltration and hemodiafiltration). The term kinetic (from Greek kinētikos, from kinein to move) refers to the changing concentrations and clearance rates which occur during intermittent treatments. A kinetic model is a mathematical representation of the dialysis process, and adds two additional parameters, the solute distribution volume (V, in units of volume, e.g. ml) and time (e.g. minutes) to the clearance parameters C, G and K. The model allows for the fact that the parameters change over time and that any one of the parameters can be calculated if the others are known.

The variable volume single-pool model was first described by Gotch and Sargent [28] This model considers a urea to be evenly distributed in the total body water of volume V. The model allows for changing V due to ultrafiltration during dialysis and accumulation of fluid during the period between dialysis sessions. The coefficient 'a' is the rate of change of V and will usually be negative during dialysis due to ultrafiltration and positive during the period between dialysis sessions. This value is calculated from measurements of pre-and post-dialysis weight, assuming that changes in weight are due only to changes in V over a period of 2-3 days.

Equation 15. $C_t = C_0 \times \left(\frac{V}{V+a\times t}\right)^{\frac{K+a}{a}} + \frac{G}{K+a} \times \left[1 - \left(\frac{V}{V+a\times t}\right)^{\frac{K+a}{a}}\right]$

This variable volume single-pool equation is typically rearranged to yield two equations, one calculating G, the other calculating V.

As the two equations are inter-dependent, they are primed with an approximate value for G, then solved sequentially and repeatedly, updating values for G and V each time until there are no further changes in G and V. In practice 10 iterations are generally sufficient. In this method, K can be determined by direct measurement (e.g. conductivity clearance) or, more commonly estimated using Equation 5.

Adequacy of Dialysis

Where V has been calculated using an estimated K, calculated from manufacturer's data measured 'in-vivo' (Equation 5), the V will underestimate true V by about 30%. This is because 'in vitro' K is overestimates 'in-vivo' K by about 30%.

Calculation of V from measurements during a dialysis session. C0 and Ct are urea concentrations at the beginning and end of session. K=sum of renal and dialysis clearance, t=duration of session, a=rate of change in V (usually negative due to ultrafiltration).	Equation 16. $V = \dfrac{a \times t}{1 - \left[\frac{G - (K+a) \times C_0}{G - (K+a) \times C_t}\right]^{\frac{-a}{K+a}}}$
Calculation of G from measurements of the period between dialysis sessions. C0 and Ct are urea concentration at beginning and end of period, K=renal urea clearance, t=duration of period, a=rate of change in V (usually positive due to oral intake).	Equation 17. $G = (K+a) \times$ $\dfrac{C_t \times \left[1 + \frac{a \times t}{V}\right]^{\frac{K}{a}+1} - C_0}{\left[1 + \frac{a \times t}{V}\right]^{\frac{K}{a}+1} - 1}$

The single-pool model assumes that solute is distributed in a single, well-mixed pool represented by V. This is only approximately true. A double-pool model predicts changes in urea clearance much better (Figure 2). Fortunately, the immediate post-dialysis urea concentration predicted by the single-pool model is the same as for the two-pool model in a typical dialysis. For shorter treatments and those with lower Kt/V, the two-pool model predicts a lower post-dialysis urea than the single-pool model. In this case V will be underestimated by the single-pool model. For longer and higher-dose treatments, V will be overestimated. This error in V can be corrected using Equation 21.For solutes other than urea, kinetics cannot be predicted by the single-pool model. A two-pool model is required.

Single-pool Urea Kt/V (spKt/V)

The spKt/V is the hemodialysis dose measure derived from the single-pool urea kinetic model. K, t and V are the same as used in Equation 16. Since Equation 16 uses an estimate of K, usually an overestimate based on 'in vivo' clearance, the V will be an overestimate. These errors largely cancel each other out in the so that spKt/V is accurate, despite errors in K.

In practice, V is divided into a number of compartments, only one of which (the plasma water in the fistula) is cleared directly by dialysis. The boundaries separating the compartments may impede the transfer of solute from more peripheral compartments into the fistula, so that solute is retained to some extent in these peripheral compartments during dialysis. This compartmentalization of V has the effect of reducing the effectiveness of dialysis below that predicted by a single-pool model. Also, at the end of dialysis, the concentration of solute in the post-dialysis blood (sampled from the fistula blood flow) will be significantly lower than in body water elsewhere and there will be a post-dialysis urea rebound as shown in Figure 4.

These limitations of the single-pool model cause spKt/V to overestimate hemodialysis dose, especially in short treatments. The overestimation is approximately 17% for a 4-hour treatment and 23% for a 3hour treatment.

Kt/V Pitfalls: Importance of Dialysis Time

The simplicity and intellectual elegance of Kt/V caused it to be enthusiastically adopted as a marker of dialysis adequacy. Official guidelines established minimum levels of Kt/V for adequacy. The current KDOQI guidelines (2006) recommend a minimum spKt/V of 1.2 without mentioning dialysis time in the recommendation. This implies that it is possible to offset shorter dialysis time by increasing K as long as Kt/V is maintained. It also implies that dialysis dose should be prescribed in proportion to V. Both these implications are problematic.

Shorter dialysis is less effective at removing all solutes compared to a longer dialysis with the same spKt/V. This reduction in solute removal is relatively greater for phosphate and for larger solutes. It is also more difficult to remove excess fluid with shorter treatments as there is a limit to the ultrafiltration rate which can be tolerated by the patient. With shorter treatments, any failure to achieve the prescribed treatment time e.g. late start, early termination) will have a relatively greater effect on dialysis dose.

By prescribing dialysis in proportion to V, smaller patients, particularly those with low muscle mass, will be prescribed relatively lower doses of dialysis. Uremic patients may become malnourished, lose muscle mass and their V falls. This results in a tendency for Kt/V to increase, prompting a reduction in prescribed K or t, and leading to increased uremia. It may be possible to deliver dialysis safely in a shorter time, but all relevant factors must be taken into account, not just Kt/V. Steps must be taken to ensure adequate phosphate and large solute removal, and removal of all excess fluid. Unless the patient has significant renal function, this becomes progressively more difficult as dialysis time is decreased. It is worth emphasizing that a low Kt/V in an anuric patient always indicates inadequate dialysis and is associated with worse outcome. However, the reverse is not necessarily true. *A high or 'adequate' Kt/V on its own is not evidence of adequate dialysis.*

Two Pool Model

The body can be considered as a large number of compartments representing the intra- and extra-cellular volumes of the various tissues and organs. Solute transfer (flux) across membranes (e.g. cell membranes or vascular basement membrane) is considered to be driven by diffusion. Flux between tissues or organs is by convection due to plasma water flow. This distinction is important because flux by convection is the same for all solutes, whereas flux by diffusion will vary between solutes. Solutes with higher molecular weight diffuse more slowly.

In practice, the solute kinetics of dialysis can be described adequately by a model with only two virtual compartment volumes (V1 and V2). Only V1 is cleared by dialysis. Solute generation (G) occurs in V2 only. Solute flux between V2 and V1 depends on a clearance term (Ki), which combines diffusion and flow. In this case, the two compartments are representative of all compartments in which the solute is distributed and do not correspond to actual body structures. Similarly, Ki does not correspond to a measurable physiological property. The values of V1, V2 and Ki will be different for each solute.

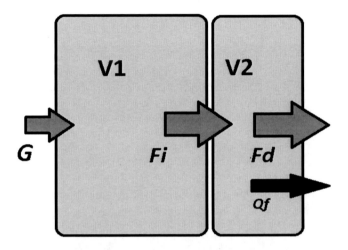

Figure 2. The two-pool model. The grey arrows indicate transfer of solute (e.g. mg/min) G is the generation rate, Fi is the transfer between compartments, Fd is the transfer out of the body due to dialysis and renal function. Vi and V2 are the compartment (pool) volumes (e.g. liters). The black arrow represents ultrafiltration.

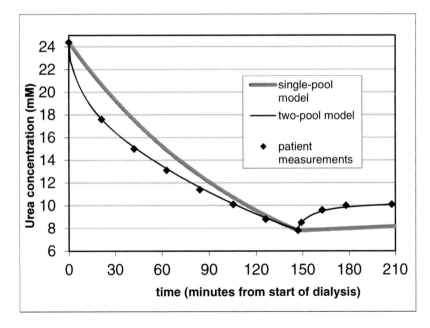

Figure 3. Measured blood levels match closely to a two-pool model but not the single-pool model. A short, intensive dialysis (as shown here) is shown to emphasize the difference between the single-pool and two-pool models.

For urea, which diffuses easily across cell membranes (due to specific urea channels), V1 and V2 are mainly representative of tissue with high and low blood flow respectively.

Creatinine transfer across cell membranes is limited by a much slower rate of diffusion than urea. So V1 and V2 are mainly representative of extra- and intra-cellular water. B2-microglobulin is distributed in the extracellular fluid only. V1 and V2 are considered to be mainly plasma and interstitial water. 0 lists approximate values for the parameters of a two-pool model for various solutes.

The model is described by Equation 18 and Equation 19.

Concentration in compartment 1 (C1)	Equation 18.	$C1_{t+\Delta t} = C1_t + \frac{Ki \times (C1_t - C2_t) - Kd \times C1_t}{V1 - Qf \times t} \times \Delta t$
Concentration in compartment 2(C2)	Equation 19.	$C2_{t+\Delta t} = C2_t + \frac{G - Ki \times (C1_t - C1_t)}{V2} \times \Delta t$

The model is initiated by providing values of $C1_0$ and $C2_0$ equal to the pre-dialysis concentration in plasma water. New values for $C1_0$ and $C2_0$ are computed iteratively by repeatedly solving Equation 18 and Equation 19 using a small increment in t (e.g. 1 minute) until t = 10080 (the number of minutes in a week). The cycle is repeated after automatically guided adjustments in G and either K or V until steady state is achieved and C1 matches the post-dialysis concentration at the appropriate time point. If both values for K and V supplied to the model are approximate (e.g. V from the Watson equation and K from Michael's equation), then the model will calculate accurate values for Kt/V, nPCR (a function of G/V), equilibrated solute concentrations, TAC and TAD. If an accurate value for either K (e.g. from online clearance) or V (e.g. from bioimpedance) is supplied, then the other can be calculated accurately by the model.

The two-pool model assumes that mass transfer between compartments is driven by flow or diffusion. This is not true for solutes which are actively transported across the cell membrane (e.g. phosphate).

Table 4. Typical solute-specific variables for two-pool model

	V/body water	V1/V	V2/V	Ki/V2 (min-1)
urea	1	0.2	0.8	0.044
Creatinine	1	0.33	0.67	0.022
Beta-2-microglobulin	0.33	0.25	0.75	0.011

Equilibrated Kt/V (eKt/V)

The eKt/V is calculated using the single pool model but with the equilibrated or post-rebound concentration instead of the immediate post-dialysis concentration. The eKt/V accounts for the delayed transfer between body compartments in the calculation of Kt/V. It can be calculated using pre and post-dialysis blood samples, but the post dialysis sample is drawn some time after the end of dialysis to allow for re-equilibration. For urea this time should be at least 30 minutes. Alternatively, the equilibrated, post-dialysis concentration can be calculated using the appropriate 2-pool model as the (C1 x V1 + C2 x V2) /(V1+V2).

For urea, the single-pool Kt/V (spKt/V) overestimates eKt/V by about 20%. This overestimation is relatively greater in shorter treatments and in those where a lower dose of dialysis is prescribed (e.g. to take account of renal function or more frequent dialysis).

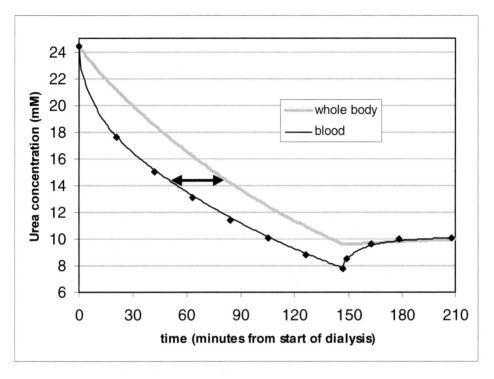

Figure 4. The fall in urea concentration in the whole body lags behind the blood during intermittent hemodialysis dialysis by around 35 minutes (arrows).

Practical Use of Two-pool Model

The two-pool model is used to calculate the concentration of solute at each time point (e.g. every minute) during a week. This can then be used to calculate the post-rebound (equilibrated), time averaged (TAC) and peak concentrations and time averaged deviation (TAD).

An abbreviated version of the two-pool model uses a single parameter, the solute-specific patient clearance time (tp), to quantify the time required for solute to transfer from all parts of the body into the fistula. [29] The tp is, in effect, the sum effect of Ki/V for all body compartments. The tp can be used to calculate the equilibrated post-dialysis concentration and, therefore eKt/V.

The 35 minute patient clearance time can be used to correct errors in V resulting from use of a single-pool model (Equation 21).

To calculate the post-rebound or equilibrated concentration (Reb) from dialysis time (td), tp, pre and post-dialysis concentrations.	Equation 20. $Reb = pre \times \left(\frac{post}{pre}\right)^{\left(\frac{td}{td+tp}\right)}$
To correct V calculated from the single-pool model (Vsp)	Equation 21. $V = Vsp \times \dfrac{td+tp}{td+tp \times ln\left(\frac{pre}{post}\right)}$

Table 5. Suggested tp values for various solutes

Solute	Tp (minutes)
Urea	35
Creatinine	70
Beta-2-microglobulin	110

Mechanism of Transfer of Solute between Compartments

Solute transfers from one compartment to another by convection or diffusion. Convection is driven by flow (e.g. blood flow, Q) form one compartment to another. Flux by convection is the same for any solute and is equal to the difference in concentration multiplied by flow rate between compartments.

Diffusion occurs between compartments separated by a membrane (e.g. cell membrane, dialyzer membrane or vascular basement membrane). Flux by diffusion is equal to the concentration difference between compartments multiplied by a solute-specific mass transfer area coefficient (MTAC). The MTAC is influenced by the geometric configuration of the compartment (e.g. ratio of surface area to volume), membrane surface area, the ease at which solute can diffuse through the compartment's fluid volume and the ease at which the solute can pass through the membrane. The MTAC value varies between solutes and is lower for higher molecular weight solutes which diffuse more slowly. For solutes small enough to pass through the membrane pores unimpeded, MTAC is inversely proportional to the Stokes-Einstein radius and, therefore, also inversely proportional to the square root of the solute's molecular weight. [30]

Since MTAC for all compartments within the body is difficult or impossible to determine, a simpler, combined solute-specific diffusion term (Ks) has been proposed [36] Ks is equal to the MTAC divided by compartment volume. This assumes that the ratio of surface area to volume is similar for all cells (i.e. cells have generally similar size) and that the membrane permeability is similar for all cells. The value for Ks can be measured relatively easily for erythrocytes. In this way, MTAC for any compartment can be estimated by multiplying Ks with the compartment's volume.

Diffusion across the capillary basement membrane is described by another solute-specific diffusion term (Kv). For small solutes such a urea and creatinine, Kv is relatively large (compared to Ks or Q and does not inhibit inter-compartment transfer significantly. Kv for larger solutes such as albumin and dextrans of various molecular weights has been well studied in the peritoneal membrane.

The Diffusion-adjusted Regional Blood Flow Model

The diffusion-adjusted regional blood flow model is the most realistic kinetic model described so far. [31] It considers four main compartments as shown in Figure 5.

The model considers the solute distribution volume (V) divided into four compartments (Le, Li, He, Hi). Le and He are extracellular fluid, Li and Hi are intracellular fluid. Le and Li represent tissue which is perfused by low blood flow (e.g. resting muscles), He and Hi represent tissue perfused by high blood flow (e.g. brain). Flux between He and Le is equal to the concentration difference multiplied by blood water flow (Ql). Flux between intra and extracellular compartments is equal to concentration difference multiplied by the solute-specific diffusion term (KS) multiplied by the intracellular compartment volume. Flux across the capillary wall may be an important limiting factor for larger solutes and is equal to the concentration difference multiplied by Kv x extracellular compartment volume.

The model adds additional steps to Equation 18 and Equation 19 to calculate the concentrations in the additional compartments. Additionally, the effects of cardio-pulmonary recirculation (using cardiac output and dialyzer clearance Kid) and the diffusion across erythrocyte membranes in the dialyzer (using Ks) are accounted.

The advantage of this model is that the various compartments and solute transfer terms can be related to actual physiological entities and can be measured independently. The model has been validated for urea and creatinine.

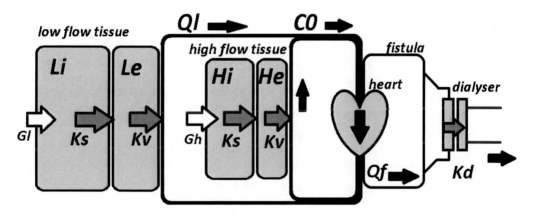

Figure 5.

Online Conductivity Clearance

Clearance in hemodialysis can be measured frequently and accurately by the dialysis machine using the conductivity clearance method. [32] This method makes use of the fact that the electrical conductivity of the dialysis fluid is proportional to the concentration of ionic components, mainly sodium. The dialysis machine measures the conductivity and flow in the dialysis fluid entering and leaving the dialyzer. From these measurements, the flux of ionic components is calculated. By analyzing changes in flux after step changes in dialysate conductivity (resulting from temporary changes in the concentrate mixing ratio), the clearance can be calculated. The ionic clearance has been shown to be very close to urea clearance due to the similar molecular weight of sodium and urea.

Due to the timing of the measurements, conductivity clearance includes the effect of any access recirculation but not cardiopulmonary or multi-compartment effects.

By making repeated measurements of conductivity clearance during dialysis, Kt can be calculated accurately for the dialysis session. An accurate value for V is required to calculate Kt/V. This can be obtained by urea kinetic modeling using Equation 16 and Equation 17 or by bioimpedance.

With Kt from conductivity clearance and V from bioimpedance, Kt/V can be calculated without blood samples. Using the two-pool model with K from conductivity clearance and V from bioimpedance, eKt/V can be calculated.

If V calculated by the Watson equations are used (Equation 13 and Equation 14), the Kt/V calculated by online clearance will be about 36% less than spKt/V calculated by UKM. This difference is due to the Watson method overestimating V in dialysis patients. [33]

With a measurement of pre-dialysis concentration, Kt from conductivity clearance and V from bioimpedance the post-dialysis concentration, G and nPCR can be calculated using the 2-pool model. In this way the troublesome post-dialysis sample is avoided.

On-line UV Clearance

Certain solutes in dialysate absorb ultraviolet (UV) light. These include creatinine, uric acid, bile acids, amino acids and peptides (but not urea). Fresh dialysate has negligible UV absorbance. Any increase of UV absorbance in spent dialysate (compared to fresh dialysate) can be assumed to be due to the presence of solutes which have passed through the dialyzer membrane from the blood. UV absorbance is proportional to the concentration of a UV absorbing solute. By incorporating a UV source and detector in the dialysate circuit, the UV absorbance of spent dialysate can be continuously monitored.

Since the identity of the UV absorbing solute in the dialysate is unknown and will vary between patients, it is not possible for UV to quantify concentration or flux absolutely. However, relative changes in UV absorbance over a period of dialysis will reflect the relative changes in concentration in the dialysate and also the relative change in transmembrane flux. [34]

As long as the blood flow, dialysate flow and membrane diffusion characteristics remain constant, relative changes in concentration of a solute in dialysate will be the same as the change in the relative concentration of the same solute on the blood side of the membrane. The Kt/V can be calculated from the log of this relative change $\frac{C0}{Ct}$ using a simplified kinetic equation, which ignores the effects of generation and ultrafiltration (Equation 22).

Equation 22. $\frac{Kt}{V} = \ln\frac{C0}{Ct}$

In practice, blood flow, dialysate flow or dialyzer membrane diffusion characteristics may change during dialysis. If flows are reduced, or a the dialyzer membrane becomes fouled by protein or clot, the flux of UV-absorbing solute will fall due to reduced clearance and this fall will add to the fall due to falling concentrations in blood, resulting in an overestimation in Kt/V. This potential error can be reduced by dividing the dialysis session into a number of periods and calculating Kt/V separately for each period. Flow and membrane permeability is more likely to be constant during an individual period. The overall Kt/V for the dialysis session is calculated as the sum of the Kt/V for each period. Ideally a new period should be started each time the blood or dialysate flow changes.

While the identity of UV-absorbing dialyzed solute is unknown, it is considered to represent solutes with molecular weight 113 (creatinine) or greater. These solutes may be more typical of dialyzable uremic toxins than urea. It is likely that the Kt/V calculated by UV absorbance will be influenced by any atypical distribution of UV-absorbing solute in plasma (e.g. the high bilirubin level in liver disease).

Direct Calculation of Kid

Kid can be calculated from a measurement of concentration at the dialyzer blood inlet (Cb_{in}), blood outlet (Cb_{out}) ultrafiltration and inlet blood flow (Qb) using Equation 23

$$\text{Equation 23. } Kd = Qb \times \frac{Cb_{in} - Cb_{out} \times \left(1 - \frac{Qf}{Qb}\right)}{Cb_{in}}$$

Qb depends on the rotational speed of the blood pump, pressure loading (particularly the below-atmospheric pump inlet pressure), pump insert dimensions, elastic recoil of the pump insert. The blood flow rate displayed on the front panel of the dialysis machine may not be sufficiently accurate. Blood flow can be measured independently by an ultrasound flow monitor if required.

In theory, Qb should be plasma water flow, not blood flow. Similarly Cb_{in} and Cb_{out} should be concentrations in plasma water. Most laboratories report concentrations in plasma, so Cb_{in} and Cb_{out} are underestimated by about 7%. This effectively cancels out the opposite error resulting from using Qb as whole blood flow instead of plasma water flow.

For solutes other than urea, Cb_{in} Cb_{out} will be subject to changing concentrations as solute diffuses out of erythrocytes. If whole blood flow is used as Qb, the blood samples should be allowed to stand for sufficient time to allow for re-equilibration. For creatinine, this time is about 4 hours.

K can be calculated from dialysate inlet flow (Qd), CB_{in} and the concentrations at dialysate inlet and outlet (CD_{in}, CD_{out}) using Equation 24. In this case Cb_{in} should be the concentration in plasma water. For urea, this can be calculated from the concentration in whole blood using Equation 9. For other solutes, the plasma should be separated from erythrocytes immediately on sampling to avoid any diffusion of solute out or erythrocytes. The concentration in plasma should be corrected to allow for the presence of plasma proteins using Equation 8.

$$\text{Equation 24. } Kd = (Qd + Qf) \times \frac{CD_{out} - CD_{in} \times \left(1 - \frac{Qf}{Qd}\right)}{CB_{in}}$$

In many dialysis machines, Qd is driven by a volumetric pump and its rate is known accurately. For solutes other than sodium, potassium, glucose, calcium, bicarbonate, lactate and magnesium, CD_{in} can be assumed to be zero and the measurement of CD_{in} can be omitted. CB_{in} must be adjusted for blood water content.

Measuring Concentration in Blood: Problems and Pitfalls

Most laboratories report concentration in whole plasma. This will underestimate concentrations in plasma water by about 7% due to the presence of plasma protein. [35] The mass of solute removed by diffusion and convection depend on the concentration in water. Where clearance is calculated from a ratio of concentrations in blood (e.g. Kt/V from pre- and post- dialysis blood samples or blood-side direct clearance measurement), the errors cancel out. However, clearance is calculated from the ratio of concentration in blood and urine or blood and dialysis fluid, will be overestimated by about 7%.

The majority of dialyzable solutes are distributed between plasma and erythrocyte water. Dialysis only clears the plasma water. During hemodialysis, there is a difference in concentration between plasma and erythrocyte water. This difference depends on the intensity of dialysis and the solute-specific diffusion constant as described in the diffusion-adjusted flow model.

For solutes other than urea, blood samples should be allowed to stand for a period of time before separation to allow solute to re-equilibrate. The required time depends on the specific diffusion constant. For creatinine, it is at least 4 hours. [36]

The post-hemodialysis sample is particularly problematic. After dialysis, the solute concentration remains stable for about 1 minute, then rises rapidly due to re-equilibration. Post-dialysis samples should be taken when concentration is stable, immediately after dialysis or when re-equilibration is complete (30-120 minutes after dialysis, depending on solute).

The post-dialysis sample may be diluted by washback fluid or by dialyzed blood re-circulated from the dialyzer when the needles are incorrectly placed or the vascular access is failing. This will cause the concentration to be underestimated and clearance overestimated. Post dialysis samples should be taken before the washback. Precautions should be taken to exclude or account for the effect of any access recirculation (e.g. by slowing the blood pump for 30 seconds before sampling).

Evidence

The National Cooperative dialysis study (NCDS), completing in 1981 provided the first RCT evidence that the dialysis prescription and dose could influence outcome. Patients were randomized to long (4.5h) and short (3.5h) dialysis treatments. Within each group the patients were further randomized to intensive dialysis, targeting a time-averaged BUN 50 mg/dl and a low intensity dialysis allowing BUN to rise to 100 mg/dl. The dialysis prescription was guided by a urea kinetic model. The results were that high intensity treatments had the best outcome. Longer dialyses had marginally improved outcome. Later analysis showed that the low intensity groups had Kt/V < 0.8. Within the high intensity group, Kt/V varied between 0.9 and 1.5 and there was no significant association between Kt/V and outcome within the group. The NCDS study and its urea kinetic analysis established the adequate level of dialysis at around a Kt/V of around 1 (perhaps a bit higher to allow a safety margin). In the decades since then, no RCT results have emerged to contradict these results.

Table 6. Major randomized controlled trials considering the impact of increased dialysis dose

Study	modality	Intervention (control)	outcome	result
NCDS 1981 [28]	HD	Intense dialysis lowering TAC to 50 g/dl (100 g/dl)	Admission or death	Lower TAC better (if adequately nourished)
		4.5hr (3.5hr)	Admission or death	>4.5h better
HEMO 2002 [15]	HD	eqKt/V > 1.45 (1.05)	Survival	no benefit
		High flux (low flux)	Survival	no benefit
ADEMEX 2002 [37]	PD	Increase Kt/V	Survival	no benefit
Hong Kong PD 2003 [38]	PD	Kt/V > 2.0 (1.5-1.7, 1.7-2.0)	Survival	no benefit
		Kt/V > 1.7 (<1.7)	ESA dose	Kt/V>1.7 better
Frequent nocturnal 2007 [39]	HD	6x/week nocturnal (3x/week 3.5-4h)	Left ventricular mass Quality of life	6x/week nocturnal better
MPO 2009 [17]	HD	High-flux (low flux)	Survival	High flux better (only in high risk group)
Frequent Dialysis 2010 [40]	HD	6x/week (3x/week)	Physical function score	6x/week better
			Left ventricular mass	6x/week better
CONTRAST study 2010 [41]	HD	HDF (low flux HD)	Serum phosphate	HDF better
			Serum beta-2-microglobulin	HDF better (only in patients without renal function)
			Survival	No benefit*
Long dialysis study 2011 [42]	HD	8hr 3x/week(4hr 3x/week)	Survival	8hr better
Turkish HDF study 2011 [43]	HD	HDF (High-flux HD)	Survival	No benefit*

*Preliminary findings published in abstract form 2011.

There is now a second RCT testing the effect of increasing hemodialysis intensity: the HEMO study [15] failed to show any benefit from increasing eqKt/V from 1.05 to 1.35.

The CANUSA study was a prospective observational study of incident CAPD patients and the first to report on association between Kt/V and outcome in PD. Subsequent reanalysis of CANUSA indicated that the dialysis component of Kt/V was relatively fixed and most of the variation was due to differences in renal function. Renal function but not dialysis Kt/V was associated with outcome. [13] Subsequently, two RCTs have failed to show any effect of increasing PD dose on outcome.

In the last few years, RCTs have been set up to examine the impact of increasing dialysis duration, frequency, membrane flux and convection. Of these, only the MPO study has demonstrated an improved survival with high-flux (compared to low-flux) membranes, but only in a prospectively declared sub-group of high-risk patients. The Turkish long dialysis study has demonstrated improved survival in patients treated with 8 hour hemodialysis (compared to 4 hour). Other RCTs have failed to prove survival advantage. Some of the RCTs demonstrated improvement in survival on secondary analysis. Improvements in surrogate outcomes (e.g. cardiac measurements, serum phosphate) have been demonstrated in the majority of the RCTs.

At present, it seems that the potential to improve survival using the dialysis methods currently available is rather limited. It may be better to concentrate on improving the quality of life of the dialysis patients, by making the dialysis less obtrusive and more convenient for the patient.

Table 6 lists the outcome from RCTs in dialysis.

Increasing Dialysis Dose

If we hope to improve the outcome for dialysis patients by providing a more complete replacement of renal function, we have to start by addressing the most significant limitations of our current techniques. Currently, it seems that small solute clearance is not the main limitation and increasing small solute clearance in isolation does not improve outcome. We should be increasing the clearance of larger solutes and addressing the known causes of cardiovascular mortality which can be prevented by dialysis, namely fluid overload, hypertension and phosphate retention.

The best way to achieve these goals is to preserve renal function. Where this is not possible, enhanced dialysis techniques may be required. These enhanced techniques are likely to be more costly and inconvenient to the patients so it makes sense to target these to anuric patients.

The accurate assessment of fluid status (e.g. by bioimpedance) together with blood pressure and physical assessment must be another important measure of dialysis adequacy. Bioimpedance also helps by providing an accurate value for the body water volume and nutritional state. A patient with evidence of fluid overload should be considered at risk and not adequately dialyzed. Conversely, dehydration places the patient at risk of thrombotic events and loss of renal function.

To increase large-solute clearance by hemodialysis requires increasing dialyzer membrane surface area and permeability and increasing weekly dialysis time. Adding convection can increase large solute clearance by up to 20%. These techniques will also increase phosphate clearance. Increasing the frequency of dialysis without increasing total weekly dialysis time increases small-solute clearance and reduces fluid accumulation between sessions but has minimal effect on phosphate and larger solutes.

If dialysis time is to be reduced below 12hours per week in anuric patients, additional care must be taken to ensure adequate dialysis. Increasing blood flow to maintain single-pool Kt/V is not sufficient on its own. An increase in dialyzer surface area in proportion to the increases in dialysate and blood flow is required to ensure that the clearance of larger solutes are increased in proportion. Additional tests (e.g. serum beta-2-microglobulin and phosphate level) may be required to monitor clearance. The control of fluid overload is more difficult in short dialysis and its assessment more important.

Fluid overload can be caused by excessive fluid intake, excessive salt intake, intolerance to ultrafiltration or errors in the assessment of dry weight. Each requires a specific strategy to reverse. Dietary salt restriction, which reduces thirst and fluid weight gain, stopping vasodilator drugs, which improves tolerance to ultrafiltration and modifying the ultrafiltration strategy can eliminate the fluid overload without any increased cost or inconvenience to the patient. When these measures are insufficient or ineffective, the ultrafiltration rate can be reduced by increasing total weekly treatment time.

In peritoneal dialysis, large solute clearance is increased by increasing exchange volume, which stretches and increases peritoneal surface area. [44] High volumes have disadvantages to the patient. Cytokine appearance is increased, [45] ultrafiltration is reduced and the patient may experience discomfort. High volumes are tolerated better when the patient is lying during the night. Periods when there is no dialysis (i.e. a 'dry' period) should be avoided. Increasing the frequency of exchanges may improve small solute clearance, but may decrease large solute clearance by reducing effective dwell time.

Fluid management is particularly difficult in the anuric peritoneal dialysis patient. A strategy to reduce exposure to glucose, and especially glucose degradation products, is required to prevent peritoneal inflammation and loss of osmotic ultrafiltration function. On the other hand, the use of glucose polymer is limited to the long dwell period.

References

[1]   Morton RL, Tong A, Webster AC, Snelling P, Howard K. Characteristics of dialysis important to patients and family caregivers: a mixed methods approach. Nephrol Dial Transplant. (2011) first published online April 11, 2011 doi:10.1093/ndt/gfr177.

[2]   Seldin DW. The development of the clearance concept. J Nephrol. 2004 Jan-Feb;17(1):166-71.

[3]   Gotch FA. The current place of urea kinetic modelling with respect to different dialysis modalities. Nephrol Dial Transplant. 1998;13[Suppl 6]:10–145.

[4]   Keshaviah P. The solute removal index – A unified basis for comparing disparate therapies. Perit Dial Int. 1995;15:101–104.

[5]   Casino FG, Lopez T. The equivalent renal urea clearance: a new parameter to assess dialysis dose. Nephrol Dial Transplant. 1996 Aug;11(8):1574-81.

[6]   Lopot F, Nejedlý B, Sulková S. Physiology in daily hemodialysis in terms of the time average concentration/time average deviation concept. Hemodial Int. 2004 Jan 1;8(1):39-44.

[7]   Waniewski J, Debowska M, Lindholm B. Can the diverse family of dialysis adequacy indices be understood as one integrated system? Blood Purif. 2010;30(4):257-65. Epub 2010 Nov 12.

[8]   Leypoldt JK, Jaber BL, Zimmerman DL. Predicting treatment dose for novel therapies using urea standard Kt/V. Semin Dial. 2004 Mar-Apr;17(2):142-5.

[9]   Daugirdas JT, Tattersall J. Effect of treatment spacing and frequency on three measures of equivalent clearance, including standard Kt/V. Nephrol Dial Transplant. 2010 Feb;25(2):558-61.

[10] Vilar E, Wellsted D, Chandna SM, Greenwood RN, Farrington K. Residual renal function improves outcome in incremental haemodialysis despite reduced dialysis dose. Nephrol Dial Transplant. 2009 Aug;24(8):2502-10.

[11] Termorshuizen F, Dekker FW, Van Manen JG, et al. Relative contribution of residual renal function and different measures of adequacy to survival in hemodialysis patients: an analysis of the Netherlands Cooperative Study on the Adequacy of Dialysis (NECOSAD)-2. J Am Soc Nephrol. 2004;15:1061-1070.

[12] Termorshuizen F, Korevaar JC, Dekker FW, et al. The relative importance of residual renal function compared with peritoneal clearance for patient survival and quality of life: an analysis of the Netherlands Cooperative Study on the Adequacy of Dialysis (NECOSAD)-2. Am J Kidney Dis. 2003;41:1293-1302.

[13] Bargman JM, Thorpe KE, Churchill DN. Relative contribution of residual renal function and peritoneal clearance to adequacy of dialysis: a reanalysis of the CANUSA study. J Am Soc Nephrol. 2001 Oct;12(10):2158-62.

[14] Bammens B, Evenepoel P, Verbeke K, Vanrenterghem Y. Removal of middle molecules and protein-bound solutes by peritoneal dialysis and relation with uremic symptoms. Kidney Int. 2003;64:2238–2243.

[15] Eknoyan G, Beck GJ, Cheung AK, et al. Effect of dialysis dose and membrane flux in maintenance hemodialysis. New Engl J Med. 2002;347:2010–2019.

[16] Okuno S, Ishimura E, Kohno K, Fujino-Katoh Y, Maeno Y, Yamakawa T, Inaba M, Nishizawa Y. Serum beta2-microglobulin level is a significant predictor of mortality in maintenance haemodialysis patients. Nephrol Dial Transplant. 2009 Feb;24(2):571-7.

[17] Locatelli F, Martin-Malo A, Hannedouche T, Loureiro A, Papadimitriou M, Wizemann V, Jacobson SH, Czekalski S, Ronco C, Vanholder R; Membrane Permeability Outcome (MPO) Study Group. Effect of membrane permeability on survival of hemodialysis patients. J Am Soc Nephrol. 2009 Mar;20(3):645-54.

[18] Patzer JF 2nd, Bane SE. Bound solute dialysis. ASAIO J. 2003 May-Jun;49(3):271-81.

[19] Wabel P, Chamney P, Moissl U, Jirka T. Importance of whole-body bioimpedance spectroscopy for the management of fluid balance. Blood Purif. 2009;27(1):75-80.

[20] Michaels AS. Operating parameters and performance criteria for hemodialyzers and other membrane-separation devices. Trans Am Soc Artif Intern Organs. 1966;12:387-92.

[21] Ficheux A, Argilés A, Mion H, Mion CM. Influence of convection on small molecule clearances in online hemodiafiltration. Kidney Int. 2000 Apr;57(4):1755-63.

[22] Galach M, Ciechanowska A, Sabalińska S, Waniewski J, Wójcicki J, Weryńskis A. Impact of convective transport on dialyzer clearance. J Artif Organs. 2003;6(1):42-8.

[23] Rippe B. A three-pore model of peritoneal transport. Perit Dial Int. 1993;13 Suppl 2:S35-8.

[24] Badve SV, Zimmerman DL, Knoll, GA, Burns, K, McCormick, B. Peritoneal Phosphate Clearance is Influenced by Peritoneal Dialysis Modality, Independent of Peritoneal Transport Characteristics. Clin J Am Soc Nephrol. 2008;3:1711–1717.

[25] Lowrie EG, Li Z, Ofsthun N, Lazarus JM. The online measurement of hemodialysis dose (Kt): clinical outcome as a function of body surface area. Kidney Int. 2005 Sep;68(3):1344-54.

[26] Daugirdas JT, Greene T, Chertow GM, Depner TA. Can rescaling dose of dialysis to body surface area in the HEMO study explain the different responses to dose in women versus men? Clin J Am Soc Nephrol. 2010 Sep;5(9):1628-36.

[27] Matthie J, Zarowitz B, De Lorenzo A, Andreoli A, Katzarski K, Pan G, Withers P. Analytic assessment of the various bioimpedance methods used to estimate body water. J Appl Physiol. 1998 May;84(5):1801-16.

[28] Gotch FA, Sargent JA. A mechanistic analysis of the National Cooperative Dialysis Study (NCDS). Kidney Int. 1985 Sep;28(3):526-34.

[29] Tattersall JE, DeTakats D, Chamney P, Greenwood RN, Farrington K. The post-hemodialysis rebound: predicting and quantifying its effect on Kt/V. Kidney Int. 1996 Dec;50(6):2094-102.

[30] Einstein, A On the Motion – Required by the Molecular Kinetic Theory of Heat – of Small Particles Suspended in a Stationary Liquid. Annalen der Physik. 1905;17(8): 549–560

[31] Schneditz D, Platzer D, Daugirdas JT. A diffusion-adjusted regional blood flow model to predict solute kinetics during haemodialysis. Nephrol Dial Transplant. 2009 Jul;24(7):2218-24.

[32] Polaschegg HD. Automatic, noninvasive intradialytic clearance measurement. Int J Artif Organs. 1993 Apr;16(4):185-91.

[33] Lindley EJ, Chamney PW, Wuepper A, Ingles H, Tattersall JE, Will EJ. A comparison of methods for determining urea distribution volume for routine use in on-line monitoring of haemodialysis adequacy. Nephrol Dial Transplant. January 2009;24(1) 211-216.

[34] Castellarnau A, Werner M, Günthner R, Jakob M. Real-time Kt/V determination by ultraviolet absorbance in spent dialysate: technique validation. Kidney Int. 2010 Nov;78(9):920-5.

[35] Waniewski J, Heimbürger O, Werynski A, Lindholm B. Aqueous solute concentrations and evaluation of mass transport coefficients in peritoneal dialysis. Nephrol Dial Transplant. 1992;7(1):50-6.

[36] Schneditz D, Yang Y, Christopoulos G, Kellner J. Rate of creatinine equilibration in whole blood. Hemodial Int. 2009 Apr;13(2):215-21.

[37] Paniagua R, Amato D, Vonesh E, et al. Effects of increased peritoneal clearances on mortality rates in peritoneal dialysis: ADEMEX, a prospective, randomized, controlled trial. J Am Soc Nephrol. 2002;13:1307.

[38] Lo WK, Ho YW, Li CS, et al. Effect of Kt/V on survival and clinical outcome in CAPD patients in a randomized prospective study. Kidney Int. 2003;64:649.

[39] Culleton BF, Walsh M, Klarenbach SW, Mortis G, Scott-Douglas N, et al. Effect of frequent nocturnal hemodialysis vs conventional hemodialysis on left ventricular mass and quality of life: a randomized controlled trial. JAMA. 2007 Sep 19;298(11):1291-9.

[40] Chertow GM, Levin NW, Beck GJ, Depner TA, Eggers PW, Gassman JJ. In-center hemodialysis six times per week versus three times per week. N Engl J Med. 2010 Dec 9;363(24):2287-300.

[41] Penne EL, van der Weerd NC, van den Dorpel MA, Grooteman MP, Lévesque R. Short-term effects of online hemodiafiltration on phosphate control: a result from the randomized controlled Convective Transport Study (CONTRAST). Am J Kidney Dis. 2010 Jan;55(1):77-87.

[42] Ok E, Duman S, Asci G, Tumuklu M, Onen Sertoz O, Kayikcioglu M, Toz H, Adam SM, Yilmaz M, Tonbul HZ, Ozkahya M. Comparison of 4- and 8-h dialysis sessions in thrice-weekly in-centre haemodialysis: a prospective, case-controlled study. Nephrol Dial Transplant. 2011 Apr;26(4):1287-96.

[43] Ok E, Asci G, Ok ES,1 Kircelli F, Yilmaz M, Hur E, Demirci MS et. al. Comparison of postdilution on-line hemodiafiltration and Hemodialysis (Turkish HDF Study). Abstract Presented at ERA-EDTA meeting Prague 2011.

[44] Juergensen PH, Murphy AL, Kliger AS, Finkelstein FO. Increasing the dialysis volume and frequency in a fixed period of time in CPD patients: the effect on Kpt/V and creatinine clearance. Perit Dial Int. 2002 Nov-Dec;22(6):693-7.

[45] Paniagua R, Ventura Mde J, Rodríguez E, Sil J, Galindo T, Hurtado ME. Impact of fill volume on peritoneal clearances and cytokine appearance in peritoneal dialysis. Perit Dial Int. 2004 Mar-Apr;24(2):156-62.

In: Issues in Dialysis
Editor: Stephen Z. Fadem

ISBN: 978-1-62417-576-3
© 2013 Nova Science Publishers, Inc.

Chapter XVII

The AV Fistula

Fahad A. Syed and Eric K. Peden
The Methodist Hospital, Houston, Texas US

Abstract

The study of a fistula has not aged enough to answer all questions. However since the inception of the dialyzer in 1943 we have made significant progress in treating patients with end stage renal disease using dialysis. The function of dialysis has proven to perform best with a fistula. In our writing we have attempted to present in the best possible manner the approach that should be taken to create, maintain and treat the dysfunctional arteriovenous fistula. We have included scientific facts, standardized guidelines, our experience and the analysis of many research articles along with the brief description of the cutting technology that is or may soon be available to our aid in managing the "AV FISTULA".

Introduction

History of the AV Fistula

The surgical creation of the AV fistula started in 1930s with surgeons at Mayo Clinic creating collateral circulation in lower extremities of children with polio. [1] In 1961, this idea led to the formation of the veno-venous fistula, conceived by James E Cimino. [1] In 1966, Cimino, Brescia and Appel created the modern day "Radio-Cephalic Fistula" hence also known as the Brescia-Cimino-Appel fistula. [1] As per guidelines published by the National Kidney Foundation in 2006, which are still current, the radiocephalic fistula remains the preferred primary fistula. [2]

Patient Selection and Planning

Proper planning is paramount in dialysis access surgery. Ideally, planning for renal replacement therapy goes into effect as soon as the patient's GFR falls below 30 ml/min/1.73m, [3] CKD stage 4. The creation of a fistula requires significant lead time to ensure a successful access. Even though the number of patients transplanted every year is increasing, the number of ESRD patients that can be transplanted before they need hemodialysis is miniscule. Preparing the patient to have hemodialysis and allowing this to be as event free as possible, is quite a challenge. It demands meticulous preparation to ensure a functional access. Although selection and planning have significant overlap in practice we will attempt to expand on them separately hoping to make its easy to understand both. The following are important practices in preparing and managing surgical placement of access.

History and Physical Exam

A detailed history and thorough physical exam is crucial to creation of a good access and requires the following pertinent information:

1. Past medical history, including all major illnesses
2. Past surgical history including any previous coronary interventions, pacemaker/defibrillators and previous access procedures
3. Extremity Dominance and any symptoms of neuropathy
4. History of recent peripheral intravenous lines or previous central lines
5. Details of access procedures and their complications, including swelling or steal
6. Physical examination should look for other signs of vascular disease, including carotid bruits, a good pulse exam, and careful examination of the feet for ischemic changes
7. Documentation of an Allen test has also proven beneficial in planning the patient's access.
8. The neck and chest should be examined for prominent venous collaterals and edema, as these are common signs of central venous stenosis.

In some patients after the physical exam, the choice of access will be obvious. This is particularly true in young patients with good veins evident on physical exam with good pulses. The majority however will need vessel mapping to further interrogate their vasculature and chose the best access. Vessel mapping can be done with ultrasound or angiograms. Most commonly ultrasound is used because both arteries and veins can be evaluated in a safe, noninvasive, inexpensive manner with no pain for the patient.

Vessel Mapping

Venous Investigation
This should consist of:

i. Evaluating the size of the outflow vessels using ultrasound. This needs to be done along the entire extremity to ensure that a segment of the outflow vessel is not narrower distally to where the surgeon intends to make the anastamosis. As supported by Silva et al. the vein should at least be 2.5 mm to increase chances of successful access. [5]
ii. Visualizing the branching pattern. Recent studies have shown high percentage of variations in the venous system of the upper extremity. [48,49] Knowing these variations can prove to be of great value if identified at the time of planning.
iii. Sonographically evaluating the depth of the veins is necessary. This information is needed during planning of the surgery to ensure that the cannulation vein is kept within 6 mm of the skin. [2]
iv. Central venous system patency should also be assessed. Although not possible to directly image the brachiocephalic vein where stenoses commonly occur, waveforms in the axillary and subclavian veins commonly reflect evidence of central venous stenosis when present.

Arterial Investigation

Includes:

i. Measuring bilateral brachial artery pressures. Proximal arterial stenosis can be easily detected by this simple maneuver.
ii. Sizing of the inflow vessels, the brachial and radial arteries, is also necessary. The radial arterial diameter should be greater than or equal to 2 mm and a patent palmar arch should be present. [5]
iii. Duplex interrogation of the arteries detects luminal stenoses or occlusions accurately.
iv. Too small a vessel size or a severely calcified artery leads the selection of an alternative site or further evaluation with an arteriogram, which allows the surgeon to identify and possibly treat an arterial inflow stenosis.

In the absence of good vessel availability the next best choice is an AVG of synthetic or biological material. It is important to keep in mind that once a patient has received access in the form of an AVG reverting to a fistula is still possible. After every failed AV access the new attempt should always be to create a primary fistula. [2] Numerous studies have demonstrated that AVGs are inferior to AVF, as fistulae have the lowest rate of thrombosis, require fewer interventions and provide longer survival of access. [6-9]

The establishment of a fistula should ideally be done at least 6 months prior to initiating dialysis. [2] In the event the vessels are not satisfactory for an AVF, an AVG is preferable to continuing with catheter based dialysis. An AVG commonly needs at least 2-4 weeks before it can be accessed for dialysis to allow for resolution of edema and incorporation into the tissues. There are however some grafts which can be accessed earlier, as soon as 24 hours after insertion and additional vascular grafts are undergoing testing which would allow similar early access. These newer grafts should reduce the incidence of pseudoaneurysm which is one of the more common failure modes, following intimal hyperplastic response at the venous anastomosis.

Per current KDOQI guidelines, the fistulae most frequently created in order of preference are:

1. A Radiocephalic fistula
2. A Brachiocephalic fistula
3. A Basilic Vein Transposition fistula

The goal of fistula creation is to enable easy, reliable routine access of the fistula by dialysis staff personnel that will provide adequate flows for good clearance during dialysis. Maturation of the fistula is the process from creation of the fistula until it is ready to be utilized during dialysis. The maturation process involves dilation of the outflow vein with progressively increased flow. The vein remodels during this time with dilation and thickening due to increased flow and pressure in a complex biological process. There has historically been considerable debate on when a fistula is mature and ready for routine access. KDOQI has promoted the "rule of 6's" to standardize maturation criteria. The ideal state of a functional access is to have flow of approximately 600ml/min, be less than 6 mm in depth and have a minimal diameter of 6mm. [2] Maintaining a length of 10 cm of accessible vein is important to allow different cannulation sites. Sadly however, fistula outcomes are very mixed and in large reports, far from optimal. A recent multicenter prospective randomized controlled trial, published by Dember et al. explored the utility of clopidogrel to improve fistula outcomes. [40] The basis for the trial was that if clopidogrel could reduce AVF thrombosis, usability and maturation would be improved. Although fistula thrombosis was somewhat reduced in the clopidogrel group, the most striking finding was that approximately 60% of fistulas failed to meet criteria for maturation. This disappointing figure is a true challenge to the group of healthcare specialists devoted to the care of dialysis patients.

The challenge to create a functional fistula has led many investigators to explore what measures can be taken prior to placing a fistula and during its maturation phase to predict adequate maturation and to prolong its functionality. Through the 90s to the early part of this decade Silva, Robbin, Allon, Leblanc and Asif provided us with some evidence and confirmation of the benefits of pre-operative ultrasound based vessel mapping. [12-16] They all showed similar increases in the proportion of successful autogenous AVF. [12-16] By 2006 the NKF had also included this recommendation for vessel mapping in their KDOQI guidelines. [2]

Previously, presence of peripheral arterial disease and being African-American were suggested to be limiting factors in the success of functional access. [21,22] Formulas or equations to predict the outcome of access has only recently become an interesting topic of discussion. Lok has designed and validated a formula that predicted the "failure to mature" rate of the fistula in a given patient. [23] This formula was based on a scoring system developed using clinical variables. [23] The variables included age, gender, race, causes of renal failure, time on dialysis, comorbidities, anatomic configuration and side of access placement. [23] The data collected then underwent a univariate analysis. [23] Confidence intervals were calculated for these analyses and were provided as percentages of the odds ratio. [23] The scoring system for risk of failure to mature is based on the formula they created and scores patients between 0 and 10.5. This was translated into low risk starting at 0 to very high risk when the patient scored equal to or more than a 7. They categorized the risk as follows with their recommendations of clinical application which can be seen in figure 1.

These scores were based on points that were gathered from a clinical scoring system seen in figure 2.

An important issue in the planning of the fistula is enough lead time to ensure the availability of functional access at initiation of dialysis in the form of a fistula or graft, and not in the form of a catheter. The barriers to this goal were recently studied in Australia and New Zealand with some interesting results. [24] They prospectively studied the patient, physician and organizational issues to assess perceived barriers to the timely fistula placement. [24] Of their 319 patients that were started on hemodialysis, 59% were started on dialysis using a catheter. [24] They found factors as per patients, physicians and organizations that were perceived to have been the barriers leading to these outcomes. They are described in figure 3.The outcomes warrant a study done in the US to identify barriers in our practices. Identifying them can help overcome these barriers and improve our outcomes.

Even though the fistula first initiative has been successful in raising the bar, we have not yet met the 66% requirement set by the NKF. Most recent report on the fistula first website reports the national rate to have reached 58.3% in April of this year. As we are focused on ensuring that this target is met soon, we cannot overlook the importance of the planning that must go into surgically creating these fistulae. Creation of fistulas that do not mature leads to the patient's dependence on a catheter.

Careful planning, setting patient expectations for likely need of multiple procedures and careful following of the patient until the AVF is accessible are all crucial factors in creating successful fistulas. Allon wrote best by calling the sequence of planning for a fistula "akin to running a hurdle race". [73] The failure to do so often causes frustration on the part of the patient and likely prolongs the use of catheters. One of the criticisms the fistula first campaign received was the lack of goals set on fistula maturation. This lead to a series of studies showing worse AVF outcomes with higher numbers of fistulas but more dysfunctional AVFs that have failed to mature. [75] This lead to the greater appearance of catheters and with it came its complications. In 2008 Ash reported that over 70% of the patients starting chronic hemodialysis initiated their dialysis with central venous catheter. [74]

Post Operative Surveillance and Management of a Dysfunctional Fistula

The successful maturation of a fistula without requiring any interventions was reported to be as low as 39% by Barone et al. [50] Although thrombosis is the greatest cause of loss of access, it is failure to mature that plagues fistulas. It cannot be overemphasized that immature or unusable fistulas lead directly to increased and prolonged catheter dependence which cause catheter sepsis and central venous stenosis. Patients also get very used to catheter based dialysis during this time period and are more resistant to subsequent access procedures. Detecting access failure to mature and subsequent intervention are essential. [25,26] Creating fistulas is not enough. Fistulas must be carefully followed in the postoperative period for maturation and the attitude of "give it 6 more months" must be avoided for the health of our patients.

Two factors recognized as necessary for the AVF to be accessible by Beathard et al. were adequate blood flow and size large enough to allow cannulation. [28] Studies have been done proving, that those AVF that are going to mature, will do so within the first 2 to 4 wks. [30-34] Based on this Bethard et al. in their paper titled "Early Arteriovenous Fistula Failure: A Logical Proposal for When and How to Intervene" recommended the best way to approach this issue early on. To identify these failing fistulae and salvage them and to provide a functional access was well described. [29] A criterion was developed, by which the nursing staff was to evaluate the fistula. The criteria included:

1. An easily palpable superficial AVF
2. Adequate size for cannulation
3. A uniform thrill to palpation
4. Fistula which is relatively straight and at least 10 cm in length.

This evaluation was used to predict the outcome of the fistula with bedside examination by nurses with no high tech or expensive equipment. These examiners predicted accurately the outcome of 80% of the fistulae examined. [29]An exam to identify a dysfunctional fistula and interpret the exam to evaluate the need to intervene was very well described by Bethard et al. in the above mentioned paper. A prominent thrill should be present at the anatamosis and diminishes over the course of the fistula. The visible distention of the fistula should disappear as the fistula collapses when raising the arm overhead in the normal fistula. In the case of a juxta-anastomotic stenosis, the thrill is diminished and is much shorter in duration. [29] They recorded that a stenosis will produce a bounding pulse on the arterial side of the fistula with a thrill at the site of stenosis. The quality of the arterial inflow to the anastamosis can also be evaluated with the exam reported in this study. Complete digital occlusion of the vein several centimeters beyond the anatamosis will result in a normal AVF having a strong pulse. [29] Poor arterial inflow will present itself as a weak pulse as the occlusion is maintained in the vein distal to the anastamosis. [29] These simple steps can help differentiate the etiology of the early dysfunction between venous and arterial abnormalities. With this information in their study they were able to intervene and salvage 92% of the AVF, using percutaneous angioplasty and accessory vein obliteration. [29] This study emphasizes the importance of bedside evaluation of fistulas by nurses and nephrologists and the great impact it can have.

The concept of treating these "failing to mature" fistulae has also been studied at length. It has been concluded by Nassar et al., Bethard et al., Garcia et al., and many authors that balloon assisted maturation for failing to mature fistulae is an excellent idea and should be practiced. [35,36,37] They concluded with 83.2%, 92% and 85.4% success respectively in achieving functional access. [35,36,37] They all felt that a policy of continued observation, waiting for a failing fistula to mature will lead to disappointment. [35-37] The KDOQI guidelines suggest evaluating the fistula in 4 – 6 weeks and waiting 6 – 8 weeks to allow maturity. [2] If the AVF is felt to be inadequate intervention is recommended. [2] Based on the studies performed, addressing the matter of a failing fistula suggests, that early intervention will enable greater chances of attaining functional access. The long term outcomes of fistulae that require interventions to mature compared to those fistulas that mature without interventions has been studied and suggests that ongoing surveillance maybe beneficial. Lee et al. in a study of 173 patients, observed that 56% required no interventions, while 31% required one and 13% required two and more interventions to mature. [42] Of these, 75% of the fistula that required no interventions survived at 3 years compared to 57% of the single intervention maturations and 42% of multiple intervention maturations. [42]

Several studies have concluded that early surveillance and aggressive intervention help increase the number of fistula that can be salvaged. [17-19]

Subsequently, intervention for fistulas that fail to mature has gained favor rather quickly. In 2009 Miller et al. conducted a retrospective review of their approach to salvaging non-maturing fistula. [51] They reviewed 122 patients that were not maturing either due to lack of vessel diameter or too deep a vessel. [51] The rules of 6's presented by the KDOQI guidelines was used as markers in their study. [51] Patients underwent balloon assisted maturation (BAM) and they proved with a 2 year follow up that vessels too small i.e. <6mm in diameter or too deep i.e. >6mm deep should not be written off and that salvage attempts made using balloon angioplasty can help mature these fistula. [51] With a 24 month follow up they had secondary patencies of 61% and 53% for the fistulae too small or too deep, respectively. [51,52] The interesting concept of BAM is that many fistulas fail to develop due to diffusely small size, rather than a simple focal point of stenosis and that planned serial dilations can result in very functional fistulas. Previously, these small fistulas undoubtedly would have been abandoned.

Ongoing care of the fistula and its long term success depends at least in some part on the method of accessing the fistula. The traditional method is termed "rope ladder technique" and means moving puncture sites up and down the length of the fistula. The pioneers of the fistula suggested changing puncture sites at each dialysis. [61] Twardowski has been the leading voice in what he first described as the "constant site method" back in 1977. [62] A few years later he wrote the more extensive description of the "constant site method". [64] He concluded that insertion into a previously used site was quicker, cannulation was less painful, "bad stick" could be eliminated, hematoma formation could be reduced and infection rates were not significantly higher than with the former technique. [64] All his conclusions still stand firm. The practice has since been studied by many and is now referred to as the "button hole puncture" technique. [63]

At first, the button hole technique seems counterintuitive given that many feel it is repeat cannulations in the same area that can contribute to aneurysm formation. In general however, a fibrous tract develops at the access site and allows reliable cannulation with progression to a blunt needle. Figure 4 shows results from some recent comparative studies.

In the studies mentioned in figure 4, van Loon et al. also compared interventions required in the 2 groups. [67] They found statistical significance between the 2 groups, with the rope ladder group requiring more interventions. [67] Very recently, infections in patients using the button hole technique was studied by Labriola et al. [68] They interestingly saw that as they progressively shifted to the button hole technique for the rope ladder technique the rate of infections rose significantly. [68] With renewed education of the nurses through workshops drastic decline in the number of infections was noted. [68] van Loon et al. in their studies eluded to the same concern but did not elaborate. [68] As the above mini meta-analysis suggests van Loom's study noted a statistical significance in the rate of infections in their button hole cohort. Good technique is clearly paramount for good button hole outcomes. Our experience has mirrored that of the published literature, in that dialysis units with good button hole experience and standard practices in procedures have excellent outcomes and patient satisfaction whereas those dialysis units doing occasional button hole technique have disastrous problems that can lead to fistula abandonment, most commonly due to infection.

Thrombosed fistulas are a major challenge and treatment methods continue to evolve. Historically, thrombosed fistulas were thought to be less salvageable than thrombosed grafts and were commonly abandoned. An excellent review of the literature by Tordoir et al. looked at mechanical thrombectomy of thrombosed fistulae. From 1996 to 2009, endovascular and open surgical techniques were evaluated. [45] Clearly, a greater number of studies were reviewed explaining the outcomes post endovascular treatment of thrombosed fistulae. It was felt that a fair comparison might be difficult considering the numerous devices and drugs used in the endovascular approach. [45] However, the surgical thrombectomy proved to be the more successful long term therapy, with secondary patencies reaching 95% at 1 year. [45] It was noted that the more recent articles that supported the endovascular approach for thrombosed fistulae, showed much better rates of patency. [45] This could be attributed to the improving catheter skills of todays vascular surgeon.

Future of the AV Fistula

Additional research is ongoing to improve access maturation and patency in dialysis patients. A search of www.clinicaltrials.gov shows many ongoing dialysis access trials. The trend has been to focus on preventing the development of the neointimal hyperplasia. Fistula failure to mature along and grafts propensity for thrombosis seems largely related to intimal hyperplasia near the anastomosis to the vein. Although reports of different anastomotic techniques have questioned fistula outcomes, most research currently focuses on adding biologically active components to induce a more functional fistula maturation.

Trials are ongoing using elastase to try to improve access outcomes. A compound has been developed, using Recombinant Human Type I Pancreatic enzyme. In an ongoing study, it is applied onto the vessels surface, after creating fistulas and grafts. The primary outcomes measured include acute increase in vessel diameter and blood flow with secondary measurements of access maturation and patency. The studies are titled PRT-201, sponsored by Proteon Therapeutics. [77]

Another attempt to influence fistula maturation involves use of allogenic human endothelial cells. The has been to use tissue cultured human aortic endothelial cells to naturally induce better vascular healing after access surgery, hopefully decreasing intimal hyperplasia. One early report described use of a biodegradeable delivery system, that is wrapped around the anastomosis in both fistulas and grafts. [76] The initial study was powered only for safety and thus no clear patency benefit was reported and unfortunately, the treatment group had increased antibody levels compared to the control group, which would clearly be an issue in patients seeking transplant. Further studies are needed.

A fascinating approach to the issue of dialysis access has gone from inception to implementation. Tissue engineered blood vessels, are the new frontier. The ability to use autologous cells, grow them in vitro and use them in vivo is intuitively attractive. [46] This should decrease the immune response to this native implant and allow better control of infections. An early report of a phase I clinical was done in 9 patients as proof of concept. [46] As exciting as this new concept is, cost of this technology maybe prohibitive.

Conclusion

The advent of Dr. Willem Kolff's dialyzer and the invention of the fistula, both have been a lifeline for patients with end stage renal disease. The number of patients with ESRD is rising steadily. It is imperative that all physicians stay actively involved in the treatment of these patients and access remains one of the most costly and biggest challenges for these patients. As per KDOQI guidelines, early referral for fistula creation can have substantial impact on outcomes. Careful planning of access surgery with thorough preoperative evaluation is crucial, as is close monitoring of fistulas in the early postoperative period. This requires involvement of the dialysis unit staff, the nephrologist, and the surgeon. Very simple physical examination of the access can be very informative to identify problems and avoid unnecessary delays in fistula maturation. Without involvement of the dialysis staff and nephrologists, a proliferation of inadequate fistulas is likely to result. Fistula creation and access techniques at the dialysis units have several similarities; dedicated programs with standardized protocols lead to better outcomes and patient satisfaction. Ongoing monitoring of the fistula once being accessed is a controversial subject with several options existing. Overall, an experienced person physically examining the fistula and tracking of volume flows seem to be the most helpful. We look forward to new and ongoing research to improve dialysis access and outcomes, which increasingly is incorporating biological approaches to reducing access failure. Arteriovenous fistulas and their complexities highlight that dialysis patients benefit from a systematic approach and the concentrated effort of dedicated specialists.

References

[1] Gupta NE. A Milestone in Hemodialysis: James E. Cimino, MD, and the Development of the AV Fistula. Renal & Urology News. 2006 Oct; [cited 2011 Nov 23]. Available from: http://www.renalandurologynews.com/a-milestone-in-hemodialysis-james-e-cimino-md-and-the-development-of-the-av-fistula/article/99130/

[2] National Kidney Foundation. Updates; Clinical Practice Guidelines and Recommendations. 2006; [cited 2011 Nov 23]. Available from: http://www.kidney.org/+professionals/KDOQI/guideline_upHD_PD_VA/index.htm

[3] National Kidney Foundation. Clinical Practice Guidelines and Recommendations. 2002; [cited 2011 Nov 23]. Available from: http://www.kidney.org/+professionals/kdoqi/guidelines_ckd/toc.htm

[4] Sidawy AN, Gray R, Besarab A, et al. Recommended standards for reports dealing with arteriovenous hemodialysis accesses. J Vasc Surg. 2002 March;3(35):603-610.

[5] Silva MB, Hobson RW, Pappas PJ, et al. A strategy for increasing use of autogenous hemodialysis access procedures: impact of preoperative noninvasive evaluation. J Vasc Surg. 1998 Feb;27(2):302- 307.

[6] Pisoni RL, Young EW, Dykstra DM, et al. Vascular access use in Europe and the United States: Results from the DOPPS. Kidney Int. 2002;61:305–316.

[7] Mehta S. Statistical summary of clinical results of vascular access procedures for haemodialysis, in Sommer BG, Henry ML (eds). Vascular Access for Hemodialysis-II (ed 2). Chicago, IL, Gore, 1991, pp 145–157.

[8] Perera GB, Mueller MP, Kubaska SM, Wilson SE, Lawrence PF, Fujitani RM. Superiority of autogenous arteriovenous hemodialysis access: Maintenance of function with fewer secondary interventions. Ann Vasc Surg. 2004;18:66–73.

[9] Huber TS, Carter JW, Carter RL, Seeger JM. Patency of autogenous and polytetrafluoroethylene upper extremity arteriovenous hemodialysis accesses: A systematic review. J Vasc Surg. 2003;38:1005–1011.

[10] Dhingra RK, Young EW, Hulbert-Shearon TE, Leavey SF, Port FK. Type of vascular access and mortality in U.S. hemodialysis patients. Kidney Int. 2001;60:1443–1451.

[11] Ives CL, Akoh JA, George J, Vaughan-Huxley E, Lawson H. Pre-operative vessel mapping and early post-operative surveillance duplex scanning of arteriovenous fistulae. J Vasc Access. 2009 Jan-Mar;10(1):37-42.

[12] Silva MB Jr, Hobson RW 2nd, Pappas PJ, et al. A strategy for increasing use of autogenous hemodialysis access procedures: impact of preoperative noninvasive evaluation. J Vasc Surg. 1998;27:302-7.

[13] Robbin ML, Gallichio MH, Deierhoi MH, Young CJ, Weber TM, Allon M. US vascular mapping before hemodialysis access placement. Radiology. 2000;217:83-8.

[14] Allon M, Lockhart ME, Lilly RZ, et al. Effect of preoperative sonographic mapping on vascular access outcomes in hemodialysis patients. Kidney Int. 2001;60:2013-20.

[15] Leblanc M, Saint-Sauveur E, Pichette V. Native arteriovenous fistula for hemodialysis: what to expect early after creation? J Vasc Access. 2003;4:39-44.

[16] Asif A, Ravani P, Roy-Chaudhury P, Spergel LM, Besarab A. Vascular mapping techniques: advantages and disadvantages. J Nephrol. 2007;20:299-303.

[17] Mendes RR, Farber MA, Marston WA, Dinwiddie LC, Keagy BA, Burnham SJ. Prediction of wrist arteriovenous fistula maturation with preoperative vein mapping with ultrasonography. J Vasc Surg. 2002;36:460-3.

[18] Parmar J, Aslam M, Standfield N. Pre-operative radial arterial diameter predicts early failure of arteriovenous fistula (AVF) for haemodialysis. Eur J Vasc Endovasc Surg. 2007;33:113-5.

[19] Robbin ML, Chamberlain NE, Lockhart ME, et al. Hemodialysis arteriovenous fistula maturity: US evaluation. Radiology. 2002;225:59-64.

[20] United States Renal Data System. [cited 23 Nov 2011]. Available from: http://www.usrds.org/qtr/default.html

[21] Woods JD, Turenne MN, Strawderman RL, Young EW, Hirth RA, Port FK, Held PJ. Vascular access survival among incident hemodialysis patients in the United States. Am J Kidney Dis. 1997;30:50–57.

[22] Obialo CI, Tagoe AT, Martin PC, Asche-Crowe PE. Adequacy and survival of autogenous arteriovenous fistula in African American hemodialysis patients. ASAIO J. 2003;49:435– 439.

[23] Lok CE, Allon M, Moist L, Oliver MJ, Shah H, Zimmerman D. Risk equation determining unsuccessful cannulation events and failure to maturation in arteriovenous fistulas. J Am Soc Nephrol. 2006 Nov;17(11):3204-12.

[24] Lopez-Vargas PA, Craig JC, Gallagher MP, Walker RG, Snelling PL, Pedagogos E, Gray NA, Divi MD, Gillies AH, Suranyi MG, Thein H, McDonald SP, Russell C, Polkinghorne KR. Barriers to Timely Arteriovenous Fistula Creation: A Study of Providers and Patients. Am J Kidney Dis. 2011 Mar 14. [Epub ahead of print]

[25] Hakim RM, Breyer J, Ismail N, Schulman G. Effects of dose of dialysis on morbidity and mortality. Am J Kidney Dis. 1994;23:661–669.

[26] Centers for Medicare & Medicaid Services. 2003 Annual Report. End Stage Renal Disease Clinical Performance Measures Project. Baltimore, MD, Department of Health and Human Services, Centers for Medicare & Medicaid Services, Center for Beneficiary Choices, 2003.

[27] Sehgal AR, Snow RJ, Singer ME, et al. Barriers to adequate delivery of hemodialysis. Am J Kidney Dis. 1998;31:593–601.

[28] Beathard GA, Settle SM, Shields MW. Salvage of the nonfunctioning arteriovenous fistula. Am J Kidney Dis. 1999 May;33(5):910-6.

[29] Asif A, Roy-Chaudhury P, Beathard GA. Early arteriovenous fistula failure: a logical proposal for when and how to intervene. Clin J Am Soc Nephrol. 2006 Mar;1(2):332-9.

[30] Tordoir JH, Rooyens P, Dammers R, van der Sande FM, de Haan M, Yo TI. Prospective evaluation of failure modes in autogenous radiocephalic wrist access for haemodialysis. Nephrol Dial Transplant. 2003;18:378–383.

[31] Yerdel MA, Kesenci M, Yazicioglu KM, Doseyen Z, Turkcapar AG, Anadol E. Effect of haemodynamic variables on surgically created arteriovenous fistula flow. Nephrol Dial Transplant. 1997;12:1684–1688.

[32] Lin SL, Huang CH, Chen HS, Hsu WA, Yen CJ, Yen TS. Effects of age and diabetes on blood flow rate and primary outcome of newly created hemodialysis arteriovenous fistulas. Am J Nephrol. 1998;18:96–100.

[33] Lin SL, Chen HS, Huang CH, Yen TS. Predicting the outcome of hemodialysis arteriovenous fistulae using duplex ultrasonography. J Formos Med Assoc. 1997;96:864–868.

[34] Wong V, Ward R, Taylor J, Selvakumar S, How TV, Bakran A: Factors associated with early failure of arteriovenous fistulae for haemodialysis access. Eur J Vasc Endovasc Surg. 1996;12:207–213.

[35] Nassar GM, Nguyen B, Rhee E, Achkar K. Endovascular treatment of the "failing to mature" arteriovenous fistula. Clin J Am Soc Nephrol. 2006 Mar;1(2):275-80.

[36] Beathard GA, Arnold P, Jackson J, Litchfield T. Aggressive treatment of early fistula failure. Kidney Int. 2003;64:1487–1494.

[37] De Marco Garcia LP, Davila-Santini LR, Feng Q, Calderin J, Krishnasastry KV, Panetta TF. Primary balloon angioplasty plus balloon angioplasty maturation to upgrade small-caliber veins (<3 mm) for arteriovenous fistulas. J Vasc Surg. 2010 Jul;52(1):139-44.

[38] Dixon BS, Beck GJ, Dember LM, Vazquez MA, Greenberg A, Delmez JA, Allon M, Himmelfarb J, Hu B, Greene T, Radeva MK, Davidson IJ, Ikizler TA, Braden GL, Lawson JH, Cotton JR Jr, Kusek JW, Feldman HI; for the Dialysis Access Consortium (DAC) Study Group. Use of Aspirin Associates with Longer Primary Patency of Hemodialysis Grafts. J Am Soc Nephrol. 2011 Apr;22(4):773-781.

[39] Dixon BS, Beck GJ, Vazquez MA, Greenberg A, Delmez JA, Allon M, Dember LM, Himmelfarb J, Gassman JJ, Greene T, Radeva MK, Davidson IJ, Ikizler TA, Braden GL, Fenves AZ, Kaufman JS, Cotton JR Jr, Martin KJ, McNeil JW, Rahman A, Lawson JH, Whiting JF, Hu B, Meyers CM, Kusek JW, Feldman HI, Group, DACS: Effect of dipyridamole plus aspirin on hemodialysis graft patency. N Engl J Med. 2009;360:2191–2201.

[40] Dember LM, Beck GJ, Allon M, Delmez JA, Dixon BS, Greenberg A, Himmelfarb J, Vazquez MA, Gassman JJ, Greene T, Radeva MK, Braden GL, Ikizler TA, Rocco MV, Davidson IJ, Kaufman JS, Meyers CM, Kusek JW, Feldman HI; Dialysis Access Consortium Study Group. Effect of clopidogrel on early failure of arteriovenous fistulas for hemodialysis: a randomized controlled trial. JAMA. 2008 May 14;299(18):2164-71.

[41] Capodanno D, Patel A, Dharmashankar K, Ferreiro JL, Ueno M, Kodali M, Tomasello SD, Capranzano P, Seecheran N, Darlington A, Tello-Montoliu A, Desai B, Bass TA, Angiolillo DJ. Pharmacodynamic effects of different aspirin dosing regimens in type 2 diabetes mellitus patients with coronary artery disease. Circ Cardiovasc Interv. 2011 Apr 1;4(2):180-7.

[42] Lee T, Ullah A, Allon M, Succop P, El-Khatib M, Munda R, Roy-Chaudhury P. Decreased cumulative access survival in arteriovenous fistulas requiring interventions to promote maturation. Clin J Am Soc Nephrol. 2011 Mar;6(3):575-81.

[43] Chan MR, Bedi S, Sanchez RJ, Young HN, Becker YT, Kellerman PS, Yevzlin AS. Stent placement versus angioplasty improves patency of arteriovenous grafts and blood flow of arteriovenous fistulae. Clin J Am Soc Nephrol. 2008 May;3(3):699-705.

[44] Salman L, Asif A. Stent graft for nephrologists: concerns and consensus. Clin J Am Soc Nephrol. 2010 Jul;5(7):1347-52.

[45] Tordoir JH, Bode AS, Peppelenbosch N, van der Sande FM, de Haan MW. Surgical or endovascular repair of thrombosed dialysis vascular access: is there any evidence? J Vasc Surg. 2009 Oct;50(4):953-6.

[46] McAllister TN, Maruszewski M, Garrido SA, Wystrychowski W, Dusserre N, Marini A, Zagalski K, Fiorillo A, Avila H, Manglano X, Antonelli J, Kocher A, Zembala M, Cierpka L, de la Fuente LM, L'heureux N. Effectiveness of haemodialysis access with an autologous tissue-engineered vascular graft: a multicentre cohort study. Lancet. 2009 Apr 5;373(9673):1440-6.

[47] Aihara K, Azuma H, Akaike M, Sata M, Matsumoto T. Heparin cofactor II as a novel vascular protective factor against atherosclerosis. J Atheroscler. 2009 Oct;16(5):523-31

[48] Anaya-Ayala JE, Younes HK, Kaiser CL, Syed O, Ismail N, Naoum JJ, Davies MG, Peden EK. Prevalence of variant brachial-basilic vein anatomy and implications for vascular access planning. J Vasc Surg. 2011 Mar;53(3):720-4.

[49] Hyland K, Cohen RM, Kwak A, Shlansky-Goldberg RD, Soulen MC, Patel AA, Mondschein JI, Solomon JA, Stavropoulos SW, Itkin M, Yeh H, Markmann J, Trerotola SO. Preoperative mapping venography in patients who require hemodialysis access: imaging findings and contribution to management. J Vasc Interv Radiol, 2008 Jul;19(7):1027-33.

[50] Barone GW, Wright CF, Krause MW, Brosnahan GM, Portilla D, Banerjee S, McCowan TC, Culp WC, Yousaf M. Hemodialysis access success: beyond the operating room. Am J Surg. 2007;194:668-71.

[51] Miller GA, Goel N, Khariton A, Friedman A, Savransky Y, Trusov I, Jotwani K, Savransky E, Preddie D, Arnold WP. Aggressive approach to salvage non-maturing arteriovenous fistulae: a retrospective study with follow-up. J Vasc Access. 2009 Jul-Sep;10(3):183-91.

[52] Samett EJ, Hastie J, Chopra P, Pradhan S, Ahmed I, Chiramel T, Joseph R. Augmented balloon-assisted maturation (aBAM) for non-maturing dialysis arteriovenous fistula. J Vasc Access. 2011;12(1):9-12.

[53] Lumsden AB, MacDonald MJ, Kikeri D, Cotsonis GA, Harker LA, Martin LG. Prophylactic balloon angioplasty fails to prolong the patency of expanded polytetrafluoroethylene arteriovenous grafts: Results of a prospective randomized study. J Vasc Surg. 1997 Sep;26(3):382-90; discussion 390-2.

[54] Palder SB, Kirkman RL, Whittemore AD, Hakim RM, Lazarus JM, Tilney NL. Vascular Access for hemodialysis. Ann Surg. 1986;202:235-9.

[55] Imparato AM, Baracco A, Kim GE, Zeff R. Intimal and neointimal fibrous proliferation causing failure of arterial reconstruction. Surgery. 1972;72:1007-17.

[56] Bell DD, Rosental JJ. Arteriovenous graft life in chronic hemodialysis. Arch Surg. 1988;123:1169-72.

[57] MacDonald MJ, Martin LG, Hughes JD, Kikeri D, Stout DC, Harker LA, Lumsden AB. Distribution and severity of stenoses in functioning arteriovenous grafts: duplex and angiographic study. J Vasc Technol. 1996;20(3);131-6.

[58] Lumsden AB, Chen C, Ku DN. Neovascularization in the venous neointimal hyperplastic lesions of arteriovenous grafts. J Am Soc Nephrol. 1994;5:421.

[59] Davidson CJ, Newman GE, Sheikh KH, Kisslo K, Stack RS, Schwab SJ. Mechanisms of angioplasty in hemodialysis fistula. Kidney Int. 1991:4091-5.

[60] Brescia MJ, Cimino JE, Appel K, Hurwich BJ. Chronic Hemodialysis Using Venipuncture and a Surgically Created Arteriovenous Fistula. N Engl J Med. 1966;275:1089-1092.

[61] Twardowski Z. Buttonhole method for needle insertion into A-V fistula. Nephrol Dial Pol. 2006;10:156-158.

[62] Twardowski Z, Lebek R, Kubara H. [Sze.cioletnie kliniczne do.wiadczenie z wytwarzaniem i u¿ytkowaniem wewnêtrznych przetok têtniczo-¿ylnych u chorych leczonych powtarzanymi hemodializami]. Pol Arch Med Wewn. 1977;57:205.

[63] Kronung G. Plastic deformation of Cimino fistula by repeated puncture. Dial Transpl. 1984;13:635-638.

[64] Twardowski Z. Kubara H. Different sites versus constant sites of needle insertion into arteriovenous fistulas for treatment by repeated dialysis. Dial Transpl. 1979;8:978-980.

[65] Struthers J, Allan A, Peel RK, Lambie SH. Buttonhole Needling of Ateriovenous Fistulae: A Randomized Controlled Trial. ASAIO J. 2010 Jul-Aug;56(4):319-22.

[66] Hashmi A, Cheema MQ, Moss AH. Hemodialysis patients' experience with and attitudes toward the buttonhole technique for arteriovenous fistula cannulation. Clin Nephrol. 2010 Nov;74(5):346-50.

[67] van Loon MM, Goovaerts T, Kessels AG, van der Sande FM, Tordoir JH. Buttonhole needling of haemodialysis arteriovenous fistulae results in less complications and interventions compared to the rope-ladder technique. Nephrol Dial Transplant. 2010;25:225–230

[68] Labriola L, Crott R, Desmet C, André G, Jadoul M. Infectious Complications Following Conversion to Buttonhole Cannulation of Native Arteriovenous Fistulas: A Quality Improvement Report. Am J Kidney Dis. 2011 Mar;57(3):442-8.

[69] Lin PH, Bush RL, Yao Q, Lumsden AB, Chen C. Evaluation of platelet deposition and neointimal hyperplasia of heparin-coated small-caliber ePTFE grafts in a canine femoral artery bypass model. J Surg Res. 2004 May 1;118(1):45-52.

[70] Davidson I, Hackerman C, Kapadia A, Minhajuddin A. Heparin bonded hemodialysis e-PTFE grafts result in 20% clot free survival benefit. J Vasc Access. 2009 Jul-Sep;10(3):153-6.

[71] Peeters P, Verbist J, Deloose K, et al. Results with heparinbonded polytetra-fluoroethylene grafts for femoral bypasses. J Cardiovasc Surg. 2006;47:407-13.

[72] Bosiers M, Deloose K, Verbist J, et al. Heparin-bonded expanded polytetra-fluoroehylene vascular graft for femoropopliteal and femorocrural bypass grafting: 1-year results. J Vasc Surg. 2006;43:313-9.

[73] Allon M. Current management of vascular access. Clin J Am Soc Nephrol. 2007 Jul;2(4):786-800.

[74] Ash SR. Advances in tunneled central venous catheters for dialysis: design and performance. Semin Dial. 2008 Nov-Dec;21(6):504-15.

[75] Allon M, Lok CE. Dialysis fistula or graft: the role for randomized clinical trials. Clin J Am Soc Nephrol. 2010 Dec;5(12):2348-54.

[76] Conte MS, Nugent HM, Gaccione P, Guleria I, Roy-Chaudhury P, Lawson JH. Multicenter phase I/II trial of the safety of allogeneic endothelial cell implants after the creation of arteriovenous access for hemodialysis use: the V-HEALTH study. J Vasc Surg. 2009 Dec;50(6):1359-68.e1.

[77] Clinical trials. [cited 23 Nov 2011]. Available from: http://www.clinicaltrials.gov.

In: Issues in Dialysis
Editor: Stephen Z. Fadem

ISBN: 978-1-62417-576-3
© 2013 Nova Science Publishers, Inc.

Chapter XVIII

Cardiac Surgery in the End-Stage Renal Disease Population: General Considerations, Risk Factors and Clinical Outcomes

Javier E. Anaya-Ayala[1], Mark G. Davies[2] and Michael J. Reardon[3],*
Department of Cardiovascular Surgery, Methodist DeBakey Heart & Vascular Center,
The Methodist Hospital, Houston, Texas, US
[1]Department of Cardiovascular Surgery, Methodist DeBakey Heart & Vascular Center,
Houston, TX, US
[2]Weill Medical College at Cornell University, New York, NY; Department of
Cardiovascular Surgery, Methodist DeBakey Heart & Vascular Center, Houston, TX, US
[3]Weill Medical College at Cornell University, New York, New York; Department of
Cardiovascular Surgery, Methodist DeBakey Heart & Vascular Center, Houston, TX, US

Abstract

End-stage renal disease (ESRD) continues to be an important health care problem in the United States due to the aging population and increase in the incidence of risk factors. Despite the new and evolving technologies, as well as advances in renal replacement therapies and kidney transplantation, the prognosis of this population remains unfavorable. Approximately 50% of deaths are caused by cardiovascular events; hence, cardiovascular disease is the single best predictor of death. The high prevalence of cardiovascular disease is attributable to the presence of multiple factors such as advanced age and the improvements in survival. In recent years, cardiovascular disease has led to a significant increase in the number of referrals of ESRD and dialysis-dependent patients

---

* Correspondence: Michael J. Reardon, MD Professor of Cardiothoracic Surgery, Department of Cardiovascular Surgery, Methodist DeBakey Heart & Vascular Center, 6550 Fannin Street, Suite 1401 Houston, TX 77030 Email: MReardon@tmhs.org

for cardiac surgery, including coronary revascularization and heart valve surgery. Several clinical studies have shown that the outcomes of this population are worse compared to those without ESRD, with an increased morbidity and mortality following surgery.

Indeed, a better understanding of the cause of deterioration and morbidity and mortality among patients with ESRD may help to improve the poor surgical outcomes in this challenging population. However, the most effective treatment for cardiovascular events among the ESRD population is still prevention.

Keywords: Cardiovascular disease, End-Stage Renal Disease, Dialysis, Surgical intervention

Cardiovascular Risk Factors in ESRD Patients

The risk of cardiovascular disease in end-stage renal disease (ESRD) patients has been estimated to be 20 times higher than the general population and it remains five-fold higher after renal transplantation. [1,2] The high prevalence of cardiovascular disease is attributable to the presence of multiple factors such as: advanced age (average age of dialysis initiation is 66 years), gender (male), elevated low density lipoprotein cholesterol (LDL), decreased high-density lipoprotein (HDL) cholesterol, history of diabetes mellitus (DM), smoking, lack of physical activity, psychosocial stress, menopause, and family history of early cardiovascular disease. [2]

Other factors related to the presence of chronic kidney disease (CKD) that do not represent an increased risk by themselves, but play an important role, are the elevated activity of the renin–angiotensin–aldosterone system, the abnormal calcium and phosphate metabolism (leading to vascular calcification), dyslipidemia, inflammation, thrombogenic factors, increased oxidative stress, and possibly hyper-homocysteinemia. [1,3] Inflammation and oxidative stress are risk factors in the development of atherosclerosis that also increase the progression of CKD. The chronic inflammatory process may predispose patients to both malnutrition and atherosclerosis; in addition Interleukin (IL)-6 predicts hypercholesterolemia, malnutrition, and atherosclerosis in ESRD patients on renal replacement therapy. [4] Tumor necrosis factor (TNF)-α and IL-1 have been associated with anorexia, rapid weight loss, and decline in body protein. Protein-energy malnutrition (PEM) and inflammation continue to be critical candidates for the high rate of hospitalization and mortality in *maintenance* dialysis patients. Epidemiological studies have repeatedly shown a very important association between clinical outcome and measures of both malnutrition [4-6] and inflammation in ESRD, particularly in dialysis patients. [7,8] Furthermore, some studies have demonstrated that these 2 conditions tend to occur concurrently and coexist in individuals with ESRD; many factors that engender one of these conditions may also lead to the other. [9,10] Therefore, the term malnutrition-inflammation complex syndrome (MICS) [11] was proposed to indicate the combination of these 2 conditions in these patients. This "syndrome" has recently become the main focus of attention for outcome research concerning maintenance dialysis patients. In addition, low weight for height, hypercholesterolemia, and hypocreatininemia contribute to the deterioration of the general status of the patient.

Ischemic Heart Disease in the ESRD Population

The prevalence of coronary artery disease (CAD) among patients with ESRD ranges from 25% to 60%, with the prognosis being significantly worse in ESRD dialysis patients than in the general population. [12] Acute myocardial infarction (MI) is frequently underdiagnosed, and accounts for approximately 20% of deaths. Diagnostic tests, such as dobutamine stress echocardiography, stress myocardial perfusion imaging, and the measurement of cardiac troponin T and *Creatine kinase-MB* (CK-MB), have proven to be useful by noninvasively providing valuable information regarding ischemic load. One study reported by Ohtake et al. [13] found that 53.3% of asymptomatic patients beginning dialysis had more than 50% stenosis of at least one major coronary artery during coronary angiography. These results clearly demonstrated that despite the absence of cardiac events, stage 5 CKD patients are already at a very high risk for CAD at the initiation of renal replacement therapy (RRT).

Coronary artery disease is underdiagnosed in patients with ESRD because they have atypical manifestations (dyspnea, silent MI related to diabetic neuropathy, baseline ST and T wave abnormalities that can be confused with left ventricular hypertrophy (LVH) or pericarditis, and decreased specificity of biomarkers, such as troponins and CK-MB). Coronary artery disease has a mortality rate of the 30% compared with 2% mortality in patients with Kidney Disease Outcomes Quality Initiative (KDOQI) stage 1 disease, 6% in patients with mild CKD, and 20% in those with severe CKD. [1] The long-term mortality is about 26% at the time of the coronary event, 59% at 1 year, 73% at 2 years, and 70% at 5 years. In most of the cases the cardiac troponin (cTn) remains elevated in patients with ESRD.

The indications for coronary revascularization in dialysis patients are the same as those in other patients, [14] that is:

1. Failure of medical therapy to control symptoms
2. Left main CAD
3. Triple-vessel CAD associated with left ventricle (LV) dysfunction or easily inducible ischemia

Heart Valve Disease in the ESRD Population

Dialysis patients are associated with a higher risk for the development of heart valve diseases; especially calcified degeneration of cardiac valves. [15] Aortic valve stenosis is common in patients who experience long-term dialysis. Therefore, it is expected that the incidence of aortic valve stenosis or insufficiency requiring surgical intervention will increase as the life expectancy of ESRD and dialysis-dependent patients is extended. Essentially, the surgical management of dialysis patients is associated with specific problems. For example, in patients with calcified cardiac valves the aortic wall is also calcified. Therefore, ascending aortic perfusion and cross-clamping are sometimes hazardous. These technical difficulties in surgical management have increased the mortality and morbidity after operations, and surgical indications are generally determined based on a balance between the surgical benefit and early outcomes.

The indications for aortic valve replacement (AVR) are one of the major concerns for dialysis-dependent patients. Selection of the type of prosthetic valve is another major subject of debate. Although there have been several recommendations for mechanical or bioprosthetic valves, the protocol for valve selection for dialysis patients has not been well clarified, as the description of the valve selection for dialysis patients is not available from the current American College of Cardiology/American Heart Association (ACC/AHA) Task force on 2006 practices guidelines. [15,16] The risk with the use of mechanical heart valves is the lifelong necessity of Warfarin use in the dialysis patient. The risk with bioprosthetic valve use is the potential for early calcification and structural valve deterioration in the dialysis patient. This must be carefully balanced based on the patient's risk for bleeding, potential length of remaining life, and patient wishes.

Cardiac Surgery in the ESRD Population

The number of patients with ESRD requiring cardiac surgery has steadily increased over the last 2 decades. In 2000, Liu et al. [17] published the outcomes of a large multicenter series that included more than 15,000 patients. The authors reported a 1.8% incidence of ESRD among this patient cohort. Also, a review article analyzing the Society of Thoracic Surgeons national database entries for patients undergoing coronary artery bypass graft (CABG) between 1990 and 1999 reported an increasing rate of patients with renal failure (creatinine > 2 mg/dL or dialysis-dependent). [18] Similarly, Rahmanian et al. [19] observed a significant increase in the prevalence of patients with ESRD having heart surgery from January 1998 to September 2006 (3% in 1998 vs. 5.1% in 2006, P=0.008). The demographic profile of this patient population was similar to that reported in other previous articles. [17,20]

A) Preoperative Medical Optimization for Cardiac Surgery

ESRD affects multiple systems and organs in the human body. The high rate of associated multisystem comorbidity and clinical effects of ESRD mandate a systematic and careful approach to preoperative preparation for surgery. [21] The main objectives of the preoperative evaluation and medical optimization include:

1. The dialytic correction of metabolic status, as this becomes critical during the perioperative period and should not be assumed simply from the patient's biochemical test results during the preoperative blood work. Dialysis dose can be determined using an estimation of the volume of blood cleared during a treatment, the so-called Kt/V. National and international standards exist to define the target values for these measures. It remains unclear whether achieving dialysis adequacy above the normal target level improves surgical outcomes. [22]
2. Management and correction of anemia, blood pressure, heart failure, glucose, calcium phosphate and parathyroid hormone, fluid and electrolytes, and nutritional statues are very important during the preoperative evaluation. Under-dialysis may bring a patient to major heart surgery with pre-existing metabolic imbalance and

fluid overload. Both of these conditions will likely be made worse by the procedure, especially if it involves the use of the cardiopulmonary bypass machine. Over-dialysis usually brings the patient to surgery in a volume-depleted state, which is not difficult to manage.

3. With respect to vascular access, the nephrologist has to communicate with other involved clinicians to discuss how the hemodialysis access should be maintained, cared for, and used, and discuss possible access problems and logistical issues relating to perioperative provision of hemodialysis, as well as infection control issues.

4. Bleeding and adequate hemostasis are a principle concern. Hemodialysis-dependent patients are at increased risk of perioperative bleeding due to chronic uremia associated with defective platelet granule release of serotonin and thromboxane A2 (activation defect), reduced activity of platelet surface receptor (aggregation defect), and reduced von Willebrand factor (adhesion defect). [23] Also, anemia may alter the normal pattern of flow in vessels, in which red blood cells are found predominantly centrally and platelets are thrust outward towards the vessel wall.

Preoperative Anesthetic Assessment

The key role of preoperative assessment is to identify correctable problems and institute therapy that optimizes the patient's organ function prior to the surgical and anesthetic challenge. Scores such as the Revised Cardiac Risk Index (RCRI) [24] can assist in identifying risks.

B) Intraoperative Management

There are a number of general perioperative care aspects to be considered in the dialysis population. [21] Intravenous access and blood pressure monitoring should avoid the extremity where the AV fistula or graft is located, as compression of the access must not occur. With respect to central venous access, the subclavian approach has been associated with an increase in the rate of subclavian vein stenosis. This can become severe enough to prevent both the future use of this vessel, as well as the successful placement of an AV access in the ipsilateral arm due to inadequate venous outflow.

Anesthetic Drugs

Propofol is an intravenous induction agent that can also be administered by continuous infusion to maintain anesthesia or sedation. The pharmacokinetics of bolus administration and maintenance infusion do not seem to be markedly altered in ESRD patients. [25] Sevoflurane has been used in renal disease and dialysis-dependent ESRD patients and it appears to be safe, with serum inorganic fluoride levels and elimination rates no different than in healthy controls. [26,27] ESRD patients have below normal levels of plasma cholinesterase. This results in prolonged action of the depolarizing muscle relaxant suxamethonium and the non-depolarizing relaxant mivacurium. [28,29] A significant hyperkalemic response to suxamethonium is not observed in chronic renal failure provided the preoperative potassium levels are within normal limits. [30] The non-depolarizing muscle relaxant drug atracurium and its stereoisomer cis-atracurium undergo Hoffmann elimination (exhaustive methylation), which is a process independent of renal and hepatic function, making these agents useful neuromuscular blockers for kidney disease patients. [31]

Analgesics

When using perioperative opioid analgesic requirements for hemodialysis patients, it is important to recognize the effect of renal failure both on the clearance of the parent drug and its metabolites. Dialysis will also play an important role in deciding which opioid, if any, to utilize. [32] Remifentanil, a potent µ receptor agonist with a constant context-sensitive half-life, is metabolized by plasma non-specific esterases, making it safely and reliably provided through infusion for intraoperative analgesia and prevention of hemodymic response in dialysis-dependent ESRD patients. [33] Although ESRD prolongs the elimination half-life and reduces the central clearance of remifentanil, the clinical significance of these findings appears to be minimal. [34] Naturally, intraoperative use of such an agent requires additional techniques for providing postoperative analgesia. Non-steroidal anti-inflammatory drugs (NSAIDs) are often used in hemodialysis patients either to reduce cardiovascular risk or to help control chronic pain. A careful risk/benefit decision needs to be made on an individual patient basis before prescribing NSAIDs to this group, both during and after surgery.

Intravenous Fluids

Careful management and consideration should be given to the type and quantity of fluid administered during surgery. [21] This will be determined by the preoperative hydration status of the patient, the duration of surgery, and the estimated fluid losses along with dynamic preload measures. Large volumes of 0.9% saline solution may lead to hypernatremia and significant hyperchloremic acidosis, although this can be corrected by dialysis. Ringer's solution contains less sodium and chloride, but some advocate avoidance because it contains potassium. There is a wide range of colloid fluids on the market, broadly breaking down into dextrans, gelatins, and starches. Compared to higher molecular weight versions, lower molecular weight starches have been shown to reduce the incidence of delayed graft function after renal transplantation and are increasingly used as first-line colloids. [21]

C) Postoperative Care

Hemodialysis should ideally be delayed until the risk of fluid shifts and major bleeding has decreased. Some authors suggest dialysis be re-established at 24 hours postoperatively, depending on the nature of the surgery. Anticoagulation may need to be reduced or discontinued. [35] The re-establishment of postoperative dialysis will require close liaison with a nephrologist. A specific plan for dialysis should be in place preoperatively. The immediate postoperative period will require close attention to fluid and electrolyte balance. As with intraoperative fluids, during the postoperative period a low background maintenance fluid infusion is administered (taking into account native urine output and insensible losses), and supplemented by bolus doses of crystalloid or colloid to maintain hemodynamic stability and help reduce the likelihood of fluid overload. Electrolytes, urea, and creatinine levels should be checked in the early postoperative period and as indicated thereafter. The management of hypertension, ischemic heart disease, and heart failure should be re-established the as soon as it is feasible in the postoperative period.

Outcomes of Cardiac Surgery in Dialysis-Dependent Patients

Morbidity

Numerous studies have reported the association of ESRD with major postoperative complications, such as reoperations for bleeding and coagulation disorders, and stroke related to the burden of atherosclerotic disease, which predisposes ESRD patients to thromboembolic events and ischemic injury due to low perfusion pressure during cardiopulmonary bypass. Other complications observed in this patient population during the postoperative period are failure to wean from ventilator settings resulting in prolonged respiratory failure, sternal wound infection, mediastinitis, and sepsis. [36,37] Rahmanian et al. identified ESRD as an independent predictor of respiratory failure (OR 2.9; 95% CI, 1.4-2.8; P<0.001) and sepsis (OR 2.7; 95% CI, 1.6-4.3; P<0.001). In this study, gastrointestinal complications showed an association with ESRD in univariate analysis, but this association disappeared in multivariate analysis. [19] The immune-compromised states caused by uremia, frequent dialysis, diabetes, and corticosteroid therapy for autoimmune disease associated with that of kidney disease may increase the risk for perioperative infections in patients with ESRD. [38]

Some studies have demonstrated an important association between ESRD and postoperative stroke, with reports of 6% to 7%. However, this association was not found in the Rahmanian [19] study, which included 245 patients with a relatively low stroke rate of 3.3%. The risk of stroke in patients on dialysis undergoing cardiac surgery is related to the burden of atherosclerotic disease, which predisposes patients with ESRD to thromboembolic events and ischemic injury from low perfusion pressure during cardiopulmonary bypass (CPB). [17,39]

Mortality

ESRD is a major risk factor for postoperative mortality. In 2000, Horst and colleagues published a review analyzing a total of 20 different studies that included 863 dialysis-dependent patients who underwent all types of cardiac procedures. [37] In this review the overall mortality was 12.5%. In a multicenter study from New England, patients undergoing CABG procedures reported an adjusted mortality rate that was 3 times higher in dialysis-dependent patients (9.6%) when compared with those with normal renal function (3.1%). [17] These findings were confirmed by the Rahmanian et al. study, in which the adjusted risk of hospital mortality was more than 3 times higher in patients with ESRD. [19] The hospital mortality rate was increased regardless of the underlying procedure. The highest mortality rate, however, was observed in patients undergoing valvular surgery and combined valve/CABG procedures. These findings support 2 small, previous studies that focused primarily on operative mortality in patients who underwent valve surgery. [37,38] In these studies, crude mortality was 3 to 4 times higher in patients undergoing valvular surgery compared with values in those who underwent isolated CABG. One possible explanation for the poorer outcome in these patients is a delay in surgical intervention because of an underestimation of valvular disease. In patients with ESRD, typical presentations of valvular heart disease caused by volume overload, such as shortness of breath, pleural effusions, and other symptomatology of congestive heart failure, can be concealed by dialysis, making accurate diagnosis difficult via physical examination. This is particularly difficult in the clinical assessment of murmurs. [37] Coexisting conditions, such as anemia and hypertension, also frequently exaggerate murmurs. In addition, because of the known high operative risk, some of these patients might be referred late for cardiac surgery with advanced valvular lesion, including extensive calcification and impaired left ventricular dysfunction. Another interesting finding reported in the study published by Rahmanian et al. is that dialysis dependent patients with peripheral arterial disease (PAD) were 2.5 times more likely to experience hospital mortality compared to patients with ESRD and without PAD. [19] This is probably a manifestation of the extent of atherosclerotic disease in these patients, affecting multiple organs. These findings suggest that earlier detection of cardiac disease, as well as other associated atherosclerotic diseases, might lead to an earlier referral and potentially improve operative outcome in this high-risk population.

Long-term Outcomes and Survival

Data related to long-term outcomes and survival in ESRD patients after cardiac surgery remains limited. In a systematic review of the literature by Frenken et al., 5 case series, comprising a total of 97 patients, reported a 5-year survival between 39% and 67%. [40] In the subgroup of patients undergoing valve procedures, the 5-year survival was only 39%. Franga et al., [41] in their series of 44 patients, reported a 3-year and 5-year survival of 64% and 32%, respectively. Jault and colleagues followed 99 patients who underwent cardiac surgery from 1980 to 1998 and observed a survival of 47% at 6 years. [42] In a study published by Rahmanian et al., which included 214 discharged patients, 1-year, 3-year, and 5-year survivals were 72.3% ± 3.3%, 53.3% ± 4.0%, and 39.0% ± 4.5%, respectively. [19] Late survival was not different when patients were stratified by underlying procedure. In this study, previous stroke and PAD were strong independent predictors of late mortality. Three-year survival was 14.1% ± 7.2% and 32.8% ± 7.8% for patients with previous stroke and PAD, respectively. These observations were confirmed when patients were stratified by predicted mortality by using the EuroSCORE. [19] These findings confirm that ESRD and associated atherosclerotic disease negatively affect late outcome after cardiac surgery. Systematic, preoperative work-up for detection of coexisting atherosclerotic disease is crucial in order to optimize patient selection and to improve early and late outcomes for patients with ESRD undergoing cardiac surgery.

Conclusion

End-stage renal disease requiring dialysis continues to be an important health care problem in the United States due to the aging population and increase in the incidence of risk factors. The improvements in survival of patients with ESRD in recent years have led to a substantial increase in the number of referrals of ESRD and dialysis-dependent patients for cardiac surgery, including coronary revascularization and heart valve surgery. The outcomes of this population are worse compared to those without ESRD, with an increased morbidity and mortality following surgery. A better understanding of the causes of deterioration and morbidity and mortality among patients with ESRD may help to improve the poor surgical outcome in this challenging population. Still, the most effective treatment for cardiovascular events among the ESRD population is prevention.

References

[1]   Sharma R, Gaze D, Mehta R, et al. Cardiac Structural and Functional abnormalities in end stage renal disease patients with elevated cardiac troponin T. Heart. 2006;92:804–809.

[2]   Shoji T, Emoto M, et al. Advanced atherosclerosis in predialysis patients with chronic renal failure. Kidney Intl. 2002;61:2187–2192.

[3]   United States Renal Data System. Data report 2009. [cited 2011 Jan 11]. Available from: http://www.usrds.org/2009/.

[4]   Kalantar-Zadeh K, Supasyndh O, Lehn RS, McAllister CJ, Koople JD. Normalized protein nitrogen appearance is correlated with hospitalization and mortality in hemodialysis with Kt/V greater than 1.20. J Ren Nutri. 2003;13:15-25.

[5]   Fung F, Sherrard DJ, Gillen DL, et al. Increased risk for cardiovascular mortality among malnourished end stage renal disease patients. Am J Kidney Dis. 2002;40:307-314.

[6]   Kalantar-Zadeh K, Kopple JD. Relative contributions of nutrition and inflammation to clinical outcome in dialysis patients. Am J Kidney Dis. 2001;38:1343-1350.

[7]   Qureshi AR, Alvestrand A, Divino-Filho JC, et al. Inflammation, malnutrition and cardiac disease as predictors of mortality in dialysis patients. J Am Soc Nephrol. 2002;13(Suppl 1):S28-S36.

[8]   Zimmermann J, Herrlinger S, Pruy A, Metzger T, Wanner C. Inflammation enhances cardiovascular risk and mortality in hemodialysis patients. Kidney Int. 1999;55:648-658.

[9]   Stenvinkel P, Heimburger O, Pultre F, et al. Strong association between malnutrition, inflammation and atherosclerosis in chronic renal failure. Kidney Int. 1999;55:1899-1911.

[10]   Bergstrom J. Inflammation, malnutrition, cardiovascular disease and mortality in end-stage renal disease. Pol Arch Med Wewn. 2000;104:641-643.

[11] Kalantar-Zadeh K, Kopple JD, Block G, Humphreys MH. A malnutrition-inflammation score is correlated with morbidity and mortality in maintenance hemodialysis patients. Am J Kidney Dis. 2001;38:251-1263.

[12] Hojs R, Ekart R. Cardiac Troponin T (cTnT) in Hemodialysis Patients with Asymptomatic and Symptomatic Atherosclerosis. Arch Med Res. 2005;36:367-371.

[13] Ohtake T, Kobayashi S, Moriya H, et al. High prevalence of occult coronary artery stenosis in patients with chronic kidney disease at the initiation of renal replacement therapy: an angiographic examination. J Am Soc Nephrol. 2005;16:1141–1148.

[14] Murphy SW. Management of heart failure and coronary artery disease in patients with chronic kidney disease. Semin Dial. 2003;16(2):165-72.

[15] Tanaka K, Tajima K, Takami Y, Okada N, Terazawa S, Usui A, Ueda Y. Early and late outcomes of aortic valve replacement in dialysis patients. Ann Thorac Surg. 2010 Jan;89(1):65-70.

[16] Carabello BA, Lytle BW, Chatterjee K, et al. ACC/AHA 2006 Guidelines for the management of patients with valvular heart disease: A report of the American College of Cardiology/American Heart Association Task Force on Practice Guidelines. JACC. 2006;48:e1-148.

[17] Liu JY, Birkmeyer NJ, Sanders JH, Morton JR, Henriques HF, Lahey SJ, et al. Risk of morbidity and mortality in dialysis patients undergoing coronary artery bypass surgery. Northern New England Cardiovascular Disease study group. Circulation. 2000;102:2973-7.

[18] Ferguson TB Jr, Hammill BG, Peterson ED, DeLong ER, Grover FL. A decade of change- risk of profiles and outcomes for isolated coronary artery bypass grafting procedures, 1990-1999: a report from the STS National Database Committee and Duke Clinical Research Institute. Society of Thoracic Surgeons. Ann Thorac Surg. 2002;73:480-90.

[19] Rahmanian PB, Adams DH, Castillo JG, Vassalotti J, Filsoufi F. Early and late outcome of cardiac surgery in dialysis-dependent patients: single-center experience with 245 consecutive patients. J Thorac Cardiovasc Surg. 2008;135(4):915-22.

[20] Zimmet AD, Almeida A, Goldstein J, Shardey GC, Pick AW, Lowe CE, et al. The outcome of cardiac surgery in dialysis-dependent patient. Heart Lung Circ. 2005;14:187-90.

[21] Trainor D, Borthwick E, Ferguson A. Perioperative Management of the Hemodialysis Patient. Semin Dial. 2011;24(3):314-326.

[22] Hemodialysis adequacy 2006 work group: Clinical practice guidelines for hemodialysis adequacy, update 2006. Am J Kidney Dis. 2006;48(Suppl.1):S2-S90.

[23] Galbuseera M, Remuzzi G, Boccardo P. Treatment of bleeding in dialysis patients. Semin Dial. 2009;22:279-286.

[24] Lee TH, Marcantonio ER, Mangione CM, Thomas EJ, Polancsyk CA, Cook EF, Sugarbaker DJ, Donaldson MC, Poss R, Ho KK, Ludwing LE, Peda A, Goldman L. Derivation and prospective validation of simple index for prediction of cardiac risk of major noncardiac surgery. Circulation. 1999;100:1043-1049.

[25] Kirvela M, Olkkola KT, Rosenberg PH, Yli-Hankala A, Salmeka K, Lindgren L. Pharmacokinetics of Propofol and haemodynamic changes during induction of anesthesia in patients with end-stage renal disease. Br J Anaesth. 1998;81:854-860.

[26] Mazze RI, Callan CM, Galvez ST, Delgado-Herrar L, Mayer DB. The effects of Sevoflurane on serum creatinine and blood urea nitrogen concentrations: a retrospective, twenty-two center, comparative evaluation of renal function in adult surgical patients. Anesth Analg. 2000;90:683-688.

[27] Nishiyama T, Abiki M, Hanaoka K. Inorganic fluoride kinetics and renal tubular function after Sevoflurane anesthesia in chronic renal failure patient receiving hemodialysis. Anesth Analg. 1996;83:574-577.

[28] Ryan DW. Preoperative serum cholinesterase concentration in chronic renal failure patients receiving hemodialysis. Anesth Analg. 1996;83:574-577.

[29] Ryan DW. Preoperative serum cholinesterase concentration in chronic renal failure. Clinical experience of suxamethonium in 81 patients undergoing renal transplant. Br J Anaesth. 1977;49:945-949.

[30] Thapa S, Brull SJ. Succinylcholine–induced hyperkalemia in patients with renal failure: an old question revisited. Anesth Analg. 2000;91:237-241.

[31] Boyd AH, Eastwood NB, Parker CJ, Hunter JM. Pharmacodynamics of the 1R cis-1R cis isomer of atracurium (51W89) in health and chronic renal failure. Br J Anaesth. 1995;74:400-404.

[32] Dean M. Opioid in renal failure and dialysis patients. J Pain Manage. 2004;28:497-504.

[33] Westmoreland CL, Hoke JF, Sebel PS, Hug CCJ, Muir KT. Pharmacokinetics of remifentanil (GI 87084B) and its major metabolite (GI90291) in patients undergoing elective inpatient surgery. Anesthesiology. 1993;79:893-903.

[34] Dahaba AA, Oettl K, Von Klobucar F, Reibnegger G, List WF. End-stage renal failure reduces central clearance and prolongs the elimination half-life of remifentanil. Can J Anaesth. 2002;49:39-374.

[35] Palevky PM. Perioperative management of patients with chronic kidney disease of ESRD. Best Pract Res Clin Anaesth. 2004;18:129-144.

[36] Horst M, Melhorn U, Hoerstrup SP, Suedkamp M, de Vivie ER. Cardiac Surgery in patients with end stage renal disease: 10 year experience. Ann Thorac Surg. 2000;69:96-101.

[37] Charytan DM, Kuntz RE. Risks of coronary artery bypass surgery in dialysis-dependent patients: analysis of the 2001 National Inpatient Sample. Nephrol Dial Tranplant. 2007;22:16665-71.

[38] The Parisian Mediastinitis study group. Risk factors for deep sternal wound infection after sternotomy: a prospective, multicenter study. J Thorac Cardiovasc Surg. 1996;111:12000-7.

[39] John R, Choudhri AF, Weinberg AD, Ting W, Rose EA, Smith CR, et al. Multicenter review of preoperative risk factors for stroke after coronary artery grafting. Ann Thorac Surg. 2000;69:30-6.

[40] Frenken M, Krian A. Cardiovascular Operations in patients with dialysis dependent renal failure. Ann Thorac Surg. 1999;68:887-93.

[41] Franga DL, Kratz JM, Crumbley AJ, Zellner JL, Stroud MR, Crawford FA. Early and long-term results of coronary artery bypass grafting in dialysis patients. Ann Thorac Surg. 2000;70:813-9.

[42] Jault F, Rama A, Bonnet N, Reagan M, Nectoux M, Peticlerc T, et al. Cardiac Surgery in patients receiving long term hemodialysis. Short and long term results. J Cardiovasc Surg. 2003;44:725-30.

In: Issues in Dialysis
Editor: Stephen Z. Fadem

ISBN: 978-1-62417-576-3
© 2013 Nova Science Publishers, Inc.

Chapter XIX

Assessing Health-Related Quality of Life with the KDQOL-36

Dori Schatell
Executive Director, Medical Education Institute, Inc.
Madison, Wisconsin, US

Abstract

Health-related quality of life (HRQOL) is patients' perceptions of their own mental health, physical health, and the degree to which their lives are burdened by kidney disease. HRQOL is measured in ESRD because it is a unique outcome in its own right that reflects patients' experiences, because low scores or a drop in scores predict morbidity and mortality in the ESRD population, and because Medicare requires it in both the Conditions for Coverage for Dialysis Facilities and as a Clinical Performance Measure. Medicare specifies use of the KDQOL-36 instrument to measure HRQOL. The 36-item paper and pencil tool takes about 10-15 minutes for patients to complete, and can be scored using a free Excel spreadsheet that is case-mix adjusted for age and gender, or with the KDQOL COMPLETE online tool that offers multiple languages and is case mix adjusted for age, gender, and diabetes status, with an annual licensing fee. KDQOL-36 scores provide valuable information to the interdisciplinary team for use in developing patient care plans. A variety of interventions, from longer and/or more frequent hemodialysis to exercise training to management of bone mineral metabolism have been found to improve health-related quality of life in patients on dialysis.

Background

The impact of end-stage renal disease (ESRD) and its treatment on patients is both profound and multidimensional. Patients' functioning and choices are disrupted in the areas of diet, schedule, sleep, vocational or volunteer activities, energy level, sexuality and fertility, body image, and physical and mental functioning. Health-related quality of life (HRQOL) is a way to assess patients in a global way that reflects the complexity of the disease and its impact on patients' day-to-day lives.

Healthy People 2020 defines *health-related quality of life* as "a multidimensional concept that includes domains related to physical, mental, emotional and social functioning. It goes beyond direct measures of population health, life expectancy and causes of death, and focuses on the impact health status has on quality of life." (U. S. Department of Health and Human Services, 2011)According to the Centers for Disease Control and Prevention (2011), these domains constitute important components of a construct of "health" that have become key elements of health surveillance and indicators of service needs. The subjective nature of patient HRQOL self-ratings is precisely the point: *only* the patient knows what it feels like to have ESRD. Commonly used biochemical markers such as Kt/V, serum albumin or phosphorus levels, or hemoglobin values do not reflect that experience.

We measure health-related quality of life in ESRD patients for three reasons. First, it is a unique outcome in its own right. Second, because HRQOL results independently predict morbidity and mortality in this population. And, third, because the prior two reasons were sufficiently compelling that the Centers for Medicare and Medicaid Services (CMS) now requires HRQOL measurement annually for most ESRD patients. As CMS requires use of the KDQOL-36 survey, this chapter will focus on the KDQOL-36, though there are other measures of HRQOL and depression that are also of value.

Generic HRQOL Measurement

Health-related quality of life was first formally measured and published for the 1986 RAND Medical Outcomes Study (MOS), an ambitious 2-year look at the behaviors of 523 randomly-selected clinicians and 22,462 patients with a variety of chronic physical and mental diseases. The purposes of the MOS were to "*(1) determine whether variations in patient outcomes were explained by differences in system of care, clinician specialty, and clinicians' technical and interpersonal styles, and (2) develop more practical tools for the routine monitoring of patient outcomes in medical practice.*" In addition to clinical endpoints, patients' perceptions of their own health and well-being, including social and role functioning in day-to-day life were assessed for the MOS. [1]

MOS researchers developed and validated the MOS health status scales for the study. The MOS tools were intentionally *generic*—able to assess HRQOL status across an array of chronic diseases; not specific to any particular disease. The initial 149 MOS items were refined into a 26-page, 116-item "Core Survey, which was designed to be self-administered to reduce costs and enhance respondent privacy. The tool measured eight health concepts: physical functioning, role limitations due to physical health problems, role limitations due to emotional health problems, social functioning, pain, energy/fatigue, emotional well-being, and general health perceptions. [2]

A 20-item "short-form-20" (SF-20) was used to screen large numbers of patients to identify those with chronic conditions that would qualify them for study participation. As the SF-20 exhibited floor effects and was thus unable to detect differences in very low levels of functioning, a longer version was subsequently developed which remains the best-known and most-used of the MOS survey family: the SF-36. Assessing the same eight health concepts as the Core Survey, the SF-36 could be administered by patients themselves or given over the phone or in person by a trained interviewer, fulfilling the need for a (relatively) brief yet psychometrically sound HRQOL survey. [3] In the absence of agreed-upon criteria for constructing and validating health scale items, the developer's strategy was to duplicate the full length MOS survey insofar as was possible with a limited item set. The SF-36 items cover more role limitations, are more applicable to older or retired people, and can distinguish between role limitations due to physical vs. mental health problems. Unlike the SF-20, floor effects with the SF-36 are rare. [3]

The MOS physical and mental component summary scales alone capture about 85% of the reliable variance of the full SF-36. The SF-12 contains just 12 items that reflect at least 90% of the variance in the SF-36. This 5-minute survey reduces response burden and permits group comparisons. [4] Most importantly for ESRD purposes, the SF-12 generates a summary of physical and mental functioning—and it is these two dimensions of HRQOL measurement that have proven to predict other important outcomes for people with ESRD.

Linking Generic HRQOL with Dialysis Patient Outcomes

In 1994, Kutner suggested that measurement of HRQOL could provide valuable clinical data that are sensitive to disease severity and treatment effects. [5] Just 3 years later, DeOreo first reported that among 1,000 dialysis patients studied prospectively for 2 years, two scales of the SF-36 did, in fact, predict key outcomes: morbidity, and mortality. [6] Mental component summary (MCS) scores below 42 were associated with a 25% prevalence of depression; low MCS scores were also associated with a greater likelihood of hospitalization. The physical component summary (PCS) score *predicted mortality as strongly as the normalized protein catabolic rate or delivered Kt/V*. Those whose PCS score was below the median for this group of patients (<34) were 1.5 times more likely to be hospitalized and twice as likely to die as those who scored at or above the median. Overall, dialysis patients exhibited MCS scores that were similar or slightly lower than those of the general population, but PCS scores that were substantially lower.

For several years, results of analyses conducted on a large HRQOL data set from Fresenius Medical Care's use of the SF-36 circulated in the renal community in memo form. These data were finally published in 2003. [7] Among 13,952 prevalent dialysis patients followed for 6 months, PCS and MCS scores were again significantly associated with morbidity and mortality. In a logistic regression model of factors related to the odds of hospitalization, significant predictors included diabetes; levels of albumin, creatinine, bicarbonate, phosphorus, hemoglobin, white blood cells, URR, and SGOT; and PCS scores. Age, sex, race, potassium level, iron and ferritin levels, and systolic blood pressure were not significant. A comparable hospitalization model found MCS scores to be significant as well. Both PCS *and* MCS significantly predicted the odds of death, along with age, sex, race, diabetes, and levels of albumin, creatinine, phosphorus, hemoglobin, ferritin, white blood cells, and systolic blood pressure. In fact, *each 1 point increase in PCS score was associated with a 2% reduction in the mortality rate*. The authors noted that "PCS was more closely linked to the odds of death than most of the other relevant variables included in the model:

only serum albumin, serum creatinine, and age were *more* predictive of mortality than PCS." Each 1 point increase in MCS was associated with a 1% reduction in the odds of hospitalization—and MCS scores <51 were associated with a progressive increase in the odds of death, after controlling for other factors in the model.

Renal-Specific HRQOL Measurement

Generic health-related quality of life tools have demonstrated value in ESRD clinical practice. But they don't provide any insight into the special challenges of life with kidney failure, and the survey items themselves are repetitive (e.g., "During the past 4 weeks, have you had any of the following problems with your work or other regular daily activities *as a result of your physical health*: A) Cut down on the *amount of time* you spent on work or other activities. B) *Accomplished less* than you would like. C) Were limited in the *kind* of work or other activities. D) Had *difficulty* performing the work or other activities (for example, it took extra effort)." [3] Anecdotally, renal social workers have reported a great deal of difficulty obtaining patient cooperation to complete the SF-36—at least beyond an initial administration of the survey—making its use challenging for ongoing clinical assessment.

The Kidney Disease Quality of Life Working Group at RAND, which developed the MOS family of HRQOL surveys, combined the SF-36 with renal-specific items to create the *Kidney Disease Quality of Life (KDQOL)* survey in 1994. [8] Its 97 renal-specific items were gleaned from a list generated by three focus groups conducted with small groups of ESRD patients who had experienced hemodialysis, peritoneal dialysis, and transplant; dialysis staff; and a review of the literature; and were constructed with 5-point Likert response scales ranging from "Not at all bothered" to "extremely bothered". Renal-specific domains included Symptoms/Problems (34 items), Effects of Kidney Disease on Daily Life (20 items), Burden of Kidney Disease (4 items), Work Status (4 items), Cognitive Function (6 items), Quality of Social Interaction (4 items), Sexual Function (4 items), Sleep (9 items), Social Support (4 items), Dialysis Staff Encouragement (6 items), and Patient Satisfaction (2 items). The completed survey was validated with a sample of 165 patients who had experienced a variety of treatments for end-stage renal disease, and found to have acceptable internal consistency (exceeding 0.70 for all scales except Quality of Social Interaction) and reliability. All scale scores were transformed such that each ranged from 0-100 points, with higher values indicating better functioning. In 1997, the KDQOL was reduced to a short form (KDQOL-SF, with the SF-36 plus 43 kidney disease-specific items and one overall health rating item, for a total of 80 items (version 1.3 differed from version 1.2 with the addition of one item about sexual activity). [9]

The *KDQOL-36*, developed in 2002, contains the MOS SF-12, which measures physical and mental functioning, plus 24 kidney-specific items in three domains: Burden of Kidney Disease, Symptoms/Problems, and Effects of Kidney Disease on Daily Life. The Dialysis Outcomes and Practice Patterns Study (DOPPS), a prospective observational study of lab values, demographics, co-morbidities, dialysis parameters, and HRQOL, found that among 10,030 patients in Europe, Canada, the U.S., New Zealand, and Japan, low HRQOL scores measured by the KDQOL-36 were linked with higher risks of death and hospitalization— independent of demographic factors and co-morbidities. As PCS and MCS scores fell, the risks of death and hospitalization rose significantly. Patients with PCS scores in the lowest quintile had a 56% higher risk of hospital stays and a 93% higher risk of death than those in the highest quintile. Researchers concluded that low PCS and MCS scores were as powerful an independent predictor of hospitalization and death as serum albumin. [10]

CMS Requirements for Health-Related Quality of Life Measurement

When the *Conditions for Coverage of Dialysis Facilities* were updated in 2008, they included a requirement for health-related quality of life measurement in section 494.90 Condition: Patient Plan of Care:

> *(6) Psychosocial status.* The interdisciplinary team must provide the necessary monitoring and social work interventions. These include counseling services and referrals for other social services, to assist the patient in achieving and sustaining an appropriate psychosocial status *as measured by a standardized mental and physical assessment tool* chosen by the social worker, at regular intervals, or more frequently on an as-needed basis. [11]

Following a recommendation from the National Quality Forum, the Centers for Medicare and Medicaid adopted use of the KDQOL-36 in April, 2008 to measure health-related quality of life as a *Clinical Performance Measure* (CPM)—one of a set of benchmarks of ESRD-related care developed under Section 4558 (b) of the (1998) Balanced Budget Act to measure and report the quality of dialysis services. [11]

The CPM for HRQOL requires clinics to report the number of patients in a clinic who complete a KDQOL-36 annually (as a percent of the number of eligible prevalent dialysis patients, including peritoneal dialysis, in-center hemodialysis, home hemodialysis) 1, with exclusions for:

- Patients under age 18 (a different survey that is standardized and age appropriate should be used with those under age 18);
- Those who cannot complete a KDQOL-36 due to cognitive impairment, dementia, active psychosis;
- Non-English speakers/readers (for whom there is no native language translation or interpreter);
- Patients on dialysis less than 3 months; or
- Patients who refuse to complete the KDQOL-36.

Ultimately, the plan is for CROWNWeb to collect data for this CPM. Because the CPM specified a health-related quality of life measurement tool, the ESRD state surveyors who enforce the Conditions for Coverage have been trained to expect the dialysis interdisciplinary team to use KDQOL-36 results when they develop a plan of care, and their survey materials and *Measures Assessment Tool* (MAT) reflect this CMS priority.

Scoring the KDQOL-36

The KDQOL-36 is too complex to be scored manually. Some items map onto multiple domains with different weighting for each domain. And, case mix adjustment is necessary to make the scores meaningful. There are two main options for scoring. The KDQOL Working Group maintains a website that offers the research version of the KDQOL-36 survey in multiple languages, a free Excel spreadsheet for data entry and scoring and includes DOPPS norms that allow case mix adjustment by age and gender. No patient or staff reports are available.

The Medical Education Institute offers a low-cost, license-based scoring service called KDQOL-COMPLETE. Arbor Research Collaborative for Health collected KDQOL-36 data from 1,282 U.S. prevalent in-center hemodialysis (HD) patients. Arbor statisticians determined that gender (M/F), diabetes (Y/N), and age (<45, 45-64, 65-74, 75+) were the demographic characteristics associated with the greatest variability in KDQOL-36 scores, so these case mix adjusters were built into KDQOL-COMPLETE. (NOTE: Race was examined, but did not contribute as much variation as the others.)

KDQOL-COMPLETE offers a clinical version of the KDQOL-36 survey (with a new introduction appropriate for ongoing monitoring use) in English, Spanish, French, French Creole, German, Italian, Polish, Simplified Chinese, Tagalog, and Korean, generates a one-page medical record summary for staff and a personalized patient report, securely stores and can track data over time, and permits owners of multiple clinics to assess each clinic's performance against the group's. (Discounts are offered for groups of two or more clinics.) A PDF manual, video tutorials, and telephone support are available, and the service is continually updated based on user input. Patients can complete the survey on paper for staff to enter, complete it online to eliminate data entry, or surveys can be mailed to the Medical Education Institute for data entry for a small additional fee.

Some developers of dialysis clinic management software also include a KDQOL-36 scoring tool.

Administering the KDQOL-36 to Patients

Typically, a social worker will administer the survey, which takes about 10-15 minutes. He or she should explain the purpose of the survey, and ask patients to complete it. The KDQOL-36 is optional; patients can refuse.

When possible, in-center patients should complete the survey independently during the first 2 hours of dialysis. Home dialysis patients may complete the survey during a clinic visit. If patients are not sure how to answer, they should be told that there are no "right or wrong" answers—just how they think or feel, and to choose the first answer that comes to mind. If patients are permitted to take the survey outside of the clinic, there is no way to know how involved they were in completing the survey or they may not return the survey. In-center hemodialysis patients who were interviewed for HRQOL in the HEMO study had higher PCS scores (despite multiple and more severe co-morbidities) than those who self-administered. [12] This suggests that response bias may occur when the survey is not self-administered.

Prior to scoring, it is important to verify that all items—or at least the first 12—have been completed. No scoring tool can provide a PCS or MCS score if any of these items are missing. Once scored, the social worker should discuss the scores and individual responses as soon as possible and provide the Patient Report if KDQOL COMPLETE is used. Rapid feedback may improve the rate of future KDQOL-36 participation.

If the social worker must complete a KDQOL-36 with a patient for any reason, he or she should:

- Speak clearly and confirm that the patient can hear.
- Avoid interpreting any item. Ask the patient to respond to what he or she believes the question asks.
- Repeat response options as often as needed, avoiding any sign of frustration.
- Consider using a visual aid to help patients track the questions and possible answers.
- Be sure the patient knows the time frame for each question. Some ask for the past 4 weeks; others have no time frame.
- Be sure the patient knows which questions ask about general health (Questions 1-12 and 17-28) and which ask about kidney disease (13-16 and 29-36).

Interpreting KDQOL-36 Scores and Using Them in Clinical Practice

PCS and MCS scores from the KDQOL-36 or other HRQOL surveys are associated with aggregate hospitalization and mortality for groups—not individuals. However, scores more than one standard deviation below the mean, or a drop of 10 points in a PCS or MCS score may signify a degree of health risk that could perhaps be preventable with intervention from the interdisciplinary team. [10]

Social workers can discuss results with patients, using language such as, "Research has shown that low scores are linked to higher risk of hospitalizations and even death. We want to help you avoid those things."

Certain interventions have been found to improve HRQOL scores among people with chronic kidney disease (most often on dialysis). These include:

- *Automated (vs. manual) peritoneal dialysis.* After 6 months, APD patients had higher SF-36 scores than those using CAPD, perhaps because the ability to do treatments while sleeping allowed more time for work, family, and social life. [13]
- *Icodextrin peritoneal dialysis fluid.* After a 13 week trial, patients using icodextrin had fewer dialysis symptoms and higher mean change scores on the KDQOL than those who received standard PD solution. [14]
- *Longer and/or more frequent hemodialysis.* Short daily or long nocturnal HD reduced cramping, headaches, hypotension, shortness of breath and other common dialysis symptoms and improved SF-36 scores in patients who switched from standard in-center HD. [15, 16]

- *Help with coping.* Adaptation training to help patients cope with the stresses of ESRD significantly improved SF-36 scores vs. usual care, [17] as did group psychosocial counseling. [18]
- *Exercise training.* Exercise programs have significantly improved exercise duration and peak workload, reduced depression, and improved both PCS and MCS on the KDQOL-36 in people on standard in-center HD [19-23] and peritoneal dialysis. [24]
- *Echocardiogram adjustment of dry weight.* Reaching ideal dry weight as measured by the size of the inferior vena cava was associated with SF-36 score improvements compared to usual care. [25] Presumably, other means of establishing dry weight definitively would produce similar benefits.
- *Improving bone mineral metabolism.* Compared to placebo, use of cinacalcet to reduce parathyroid hormone levels was associated with significantly lower risk of parathyroidectomy, cardiac-related hospitalization, fracture, and significantly higher PCS scores on the KDQOL. [26]
- *Treatment of restless legs syndrome.* Use of gabapentin significantly relieved RLS symptoms and improved several subscales of the SF-36. [27]

The interdisciplinary team can, for each patient, examine the KDQOL-36 scores. Domain scores that fall more than one standard deviation below the mean, particularly for PCS and MCS, should be addressed, as should pain or other symptoms that cause the patient physical and/or emotional distress. Using the scores, the team can design an individualized plan of care, as per the Conditions for Coverage. KDQOL-36 scores can also be used to generate quality assessment and performance improvement (QAPI) projects across one or more dialysis clinics.

Conclusion

Health-related quality of life (HRQOL) using the Kidney Disease Quality of Life survey is a valid, reliable method to assess patients' own perceptions of the impact of kidney failure and dialysis, and can be used to identify ways for the interdisciplinary team to intervene to improve patient outcomes.

References

[1] Tarlov AR, Ware JE Jr, Greenfield S, Nelson EC, Perrin E, Zubkoff M. The Medical Outcomes Study. An application of methods for monitoring the results of medical care. JAMA. 1989 Aug 18;262(7):925-30.

[2] Hays RD, Wells KB, Sherbourne CD, Rogers W, Spritzer K. Functioning and well-being outcomes of patients with depression compared with chronic general medical illnesses. Arch Gen Psychiatry 1995 Jan;52(1):11-9.

[3]   Sherbourne CD, Meredith LS, Rogers W, Ware JE Jr. Social support and stressful life events: age differences in their effects on health-related quality of life among the chronically ill. Qual Life Res. 1992 Aug;1(4):235-46.

[4]   12-Item Short Form Survey and the RAND Medical Outcomes Study. RAND Corporation 2011. [cited 23 Nov 2011]. Available from: http://www.rand.+ org/health/surveys_tools/mos/mos_core_12item.html.

[5]   Kutner NG. Assessing end-stage renal disease patients' functioning and well-being: measurement approaches and implications for clinical practice. Am J Kidney Dis. 1994 Aug;24(2):321-33.

[6]   DeOreo PB. Hemodialysis patient-assessed functional health status predicts continued survival, hospitalization, and dialysis-attendance compliance. Am J Kidney Dis. 1997 Aug;30(2):204-12.

[7]   Lowrie EG, Laird NM, Parker TF, Sargent JA. Effect of the hemodialysis prescription of patient morbidity: report from the National Cooperative Dialysis Study. N Engl J Med. 1981 Nov 12;305(20):1176-81.

[8]   Hays RD, Kallich JD, Mapes DL, Coons SJ, Carter WB. Development of the kidney disease quality of life (KDQOL) instrument. Qual Life Res. 1994 Oct;3(5):329-38.

[9]   Hays RD, Kallich J, Mapes D, Coons S, Amin N, Carter W. Kidney disease quality of life short form (KDQOL-SF TM), Version 1.3: A manual for use and scoring, 1997. [cited 2011 Aug 1] . Available from: http://www.rand.org/pubs/papers/P7994.html.

[10] Mapes DL, Lopes AA, Satayathum S, McCullough KP, Goodkin DA, Locatelli F, et al. Health-related quality of life as a predictor of mortality and hospitalization: the Dialysis Outcomes and Practice Patterns Study (DOPPS). Kidney Int. 2003 Jul;64(1):339-49.

[11] 42 CFR Parts 405, 410, 413 et al. Medicare and Medicaid Programs; Conditions for Coverage for End-Stage Renal Disease Facilities; Final Rule. Federal Register, Vol 73, No. 73. 2008 [cited 2011 Aug 1]. Available from: https://www.cms.gov/CFCs AndCoPs/downloads/ESRDfinalrule0415.pdf.

[12] Unruh M, Yan G, Radeva M, Hays RD, Benz R, Athienites NV, et al. Bias in assessment of health-related quality of life in a hemodialysis population: a comparison of self-administered and interviewer-administered surveys in the HEMO study. J Am Soc Nephrol. 2003 Aug;14(8):2132-41.

[13] Bro S, Bjorner JB, Tofte-Jensen P, Klem S, Almtoft B, Danielsen H, et al. A prospective, randomized multicenter study comparing APD and CAPD treatment. Perit Dial Int. 1999 Nov-Dec;19(6):526-33.

[14] Guo A, Wolfson M, Holt R. Early quality of life benefits of icodextrin in peritoneal dialysis. Kidney Int. Suppl 2002 Oct;(81):S72-9.

[15] Heidenheim AP, Muirhead N, Moist L, Lindsay RM. Patient quality of life on quotidian hemodialysis. Am J Kidney Dis. 2003 Jul;42(1 Suppl):36-41.

[16] Ting GO, Kjellstrand C, Freitas T, Carrie BJ, Zarghamee S. Long-term study of high-comorbidity ESRD patients converted from conventional to short daily hemodialysis. Am J Kidney Dis. 2003 Nov;42(5):1020-35.

[17] Tsay SL, Lee YC. Effects of an adaptation training programme for patients with end-stage renal disease. J Adv Nurs. 2005 Apr;50(1):39-46.

[18] Lii YC, Tsay SL, Wang TJ. Group intervention to improve quality of life in haemodialysis patients. J Clin Nurs. 2007 Nov;16(11C):268-75.

[19] Levendoglu F, Altintepe L, Okudan N, Ugurlu H, Gokbel H, Tonbul Z, et al. A twelve week exercise program improves the psychological status, quality of life and work capacity in hemodialysis patients. J Nephrol. 2004 Nov-Dec;17(6):826-32.

[20] Painter P, Moore G, Carlson L, Paul S, Myll J, Phillips W, et al. Effects of exercise training plus normalization of hematocrit on exercise capacity and health-related quality of life. Am J Kidney Dis. 2002 Feb;39(2):257-65.

[21] Painter P, Carlson L, Carey S, Paul SM, Myll J. Low-functioning hemodialysis patients improve with exercise training. Am J Kidney Dis. 2000 Sep;36(3):600-8.

[22] Molsted S, Eidemak I, Sorensen HT, Kristensen JH. Five months of physical exercise in hemodialysis patients: effects on aerobic capacity, physical function and self-rated health. Nephron Clin Pract. 2004;96(3):c76-81.

[23] Tawney KW, Tawney PJ, Hladik G, Hogan SL, Falk RJ, Weaver C, et al. The life readiness program: a physical rehabilitation program for patients on hemodialysis. Am J Kidney Dis. 2000 Sep;36(3):581-91.

[24] Lo CY, Li L, Lo WK, Chan ML, So E, Tang S, et al. Benefits of exercise training in patients on continuous ambulatory peritoneal dialysis. Am J Kidney Dis. 1998 Dec;32(6):1011-8.

[25] Chang ST, Chen CL, Chen CC, Lin FC, Wu D. Enhancement of quality of life with adjustment of dry weight by echocardiographic measurement of inferior vena cava diameter in patients undergoing chronic hemodialysis. Nephron Clin Pract 2004;97(3):c90-7.

[26] Cunningham J, Danese M, Olson K, Klassen P, Chertow GM. Effects of the calcimimetic cinacalcet HCl on cardiovascular disease, fracture, and health-related quality of life in secondary hyperparathyroidism. Kidney Int. 2005 Oct;68(4):1793-800.

[27] Micozkadioglu H, Ozdemir FN, Kut A, Sezer S, Saatci U, Haberal M. Gabapentin versus levodopa for the treatment of Restless Legs Syndrome in hemodialysis patients: an open-label study. Ren Fail. 2004 Jul;26(4):393-7.

In: Issues in Dialysis
Editor: Stephen Z. Fadem

ISBN: 978-1-62417-576-3
© 2013 Nova Science Publishers, Inc.

Chapter XX

Integrated Renal Disease Care

Franklin W. Maddux

Fresenius Medical CareWaltham, Massachusetts, US

Abstract

Health delivery systems are changing. Such changes represent a fundamental shift from the traditional payment systems for healthcare. Fee-for-service models of care that have dominated the delivery system landscape for decades are transforming into concepts of performance based reimbursement and Value Based Purchasing. These core changes to the health delivery model are driving a change in the way nephrologists approach delivering renal disease care. This change is both in the recognition of how to identify the patient within the continuum of renal disease and how to approach the unique conditions at each stage of the disease with a group of interventions based on evidence and best practices.

Introduction

It is the intention of the US Department of Health and Human Services to develop a concept of patient centered care that encompasses many of the targets defined by the Institute of Medicine's *Crossing the Quality Chasm* document from 2001. [1] This chapter outlines concepts of quality care, patient safety, and cost efficiency through eleven core characteristics of a changing healthcare delivery system:

- Patient safety
- Effectiveness
- Patient centered care
- Timeliness of care
- Efficiency

- Equity
- No needless deaths
- No needless pain
- No helplessness
- No waiting
- No waste

These concepts of quality, safety and cost efficiency are driven by reform efforts that are rooted in the financial realities of healthcare delivery in the United States. The Patient Protection and Affordable Care Act includes policies that are based on the tenet that improving patient safety and quality of care will reduce hospitalizations and make health care more affordable. [2] The Federal government, as the largest payer for healthcare in the United States through the Center for Medicare and Medicaid Services (CMS), has made a distinct and identifiable effort to migrate away from a strict fee-for-service provider payment structure for the delivery of healthcare services to what has been labeled "Value-Based Purchasing." Concepts of Value-Based Purchasing move the traditional fee-for-service system, which is substantially volume driven, toward a system of payment and reward focused on outcomes based measurements. In Value-Based Purchasing healthcare systems the payers expect both cost-effective and quality care for the dollars spent. [3] Medicare will not only pay for patient care based on clinical processes that result in improved patient outcomes, but will also include Patient Satisfaction and experience of care as measurable outcomes. This results in payment for desired processes of care and achievements as a result of that care.

The transition from fee-for-service, a riskless model, to performance risk models has stimulated the development of delivery systems that support global and bundled payment systems, pay for performance, shared savings & gain-sharing arrangements. Performance risk models of care have led to a migration toward partial and fully capitated payment systems for populations of beneficiaries. This movement to Value-Based Purchasing has also impacted private health plans, Medicare Advantage plans, chronic Special Needs Plans (cSNP), state Medicaid programs and the delivery of care in highly integrated health systems.

In addition, the existing costs of care have included a substantial proportion of deemed unnecessary hospitalizations. The Federal Government reported that "adverse" hospital events may impact as many as 1 in 7 hospitalized patients and early re-admission to the hospital occurs very frequently. These adverse events and readmissions are costly to Medicare and the healthcare system. In 2002 the first list of "Never Events" or "Serious Reportable Events" was published by the National Quality Forum. This list is updated every year and is generated from a consensus group of healthcare representatives. These serious events are reportable and measurable. Since 2009 CMS has ceased payment to hospitals and physicians for certain "Never Events" and commercial payers have joined this practice. [4] This constraint in payment for preventable complications has been part of the healthcare reform efforts to hold healthcare providers accountable for patient outcomes. While termination of payment for adverse events has been the "stick" in accountability, Pay for Performance incentives from CMS and commercial payers has been the "carrot." Payers are developing performance-sensitive payment methods to reward healthcare institutions and providers when clinical processes result in improved quality in measurable clinical outcomes. [5]

The care of patients with both chronic kidney disease (CKD) as well as end-stage renal disease (ESRD) in the United States is associated with substantial cost. [6] In both publically and privately insured populations chronic kidney disease not requiring dialysis and renal transplantation have been associated with a higher per capita medical cost. Since 1972 ESRD has been universally covered under the public payer system by Medicare as an entitled benefit. Patients with chronic kidney disease have a disproportionately high cost of care compared to the general beneficiary population. It has been estimated that over 33 million patients in the United States have chronic kidney disease and that the CKD population represents 1.5% of the Medicare beneficiaries and approximately 9% of the total Federal healthcare dollar spent. In 2008 Medicare expenditures for the end-stage renal disease portion of the population approached 27 billion dollars and it was approximately 6.6% of the overall Medicare expenditures. This expense of healthcare dollars for CKD and ESRD has created the context for and broad interest in developing a payment system that incorporates performance risk and highlights the characteristics of quality, safety and cost efficiency such that the development of integrated renal disease care is now being seriously considered in 2011.

Identifying the Patient Population

Kidney disease is one of the sentinel chronic diseases in which patients may be undiagnosed for many years unless specific screenings with certain blood or urine tests alert a physician to the presence of kidney disease. The NKF sponsored Kidney Disease Outcome Quality Initiative (KDOQI) and others have published guidelines for screening the population at risk for CKD. [7] The relentless and silent nature of the disease is frequently not recognized by the patient until substantial progression results in late stage disease and associated medical complications. Early diagnosis and intervention in CKD provide the opportunity to slow progression of disease and improve outcomes in CKD.

The KDOQI Guidelines and definition of CKD have provided an opportunity to assign patients to CKD stages, better define the clinical manifestations of complications at each stage, improve treatments to slow progression of disease and improve the preparation for renal transplantation or Renal Replacement Therapy in late stage disease. Guidelines for the evaluation and treatment of all stages of CKD have been published. These Guidelines include specific recommendations for Primary Care Providers to engage nephrologists in consultation and co-management of complicated patients in early CKD and all patient with a GFR of <30 ml/min/1.73 m2. In the continuum of care for renal disease primary care physicians account for the majority of care for patients with CKD Stages 1 and 2 and a gradual transition of care to the nephrology team occurs during CKD Stages 3 and 4. [8] CKD patient management and interventions change over this continuum of disease. In an effort to determine the impact that integrating renal care can have on the cost and quality of care the CKD population of patients may be divided into three primary cohorts:

1. Late Stage Chronic Kidney Disease
2. Incident End-Stage Renal Disease
3. Prevalent End-Stage Renal Disease

With each patient cohort there are specific interventions delivered that optimize care within these sub-categorized patient populations. These interventions are designed to have an impact on progression of renal disease, preparation for late stages of chronic kidney disease, incident outcomes for newly delivered renal replacement therapy, access to the broadest range of treatment options for patients with end-stage renal disease, success during the transition phase from CKD to ESRD, stabilization of the prevalent ESRD population and finally coordination of care for those patients whose illness and co-morbidities progress to the point of end of life. Each of these cohorts has separate and distinct outcomes, pathophysiology, and opportunities for improvement in the overall delivery model.

Principals for Care Coordination and Renal Disease

Coordinating care for chronic kidney disease and end-stage renal disease patients is a reasonable proposition based on the following realities for these patients: [9]

1. The majority of CKD patients have multiple co-morbidities with a high prevalence of diabetes, hypertension and cardiovascular disease in the renal disease patient population.
2. For patients with renal disease there is an unacceptably high rate of morbidity and mortality associated with the transition from chronic kidney disease to end-stage renal disease and renal replacement therapy.
3. There is ample evidence that supports high rates of hospitalization & mortality associated with transitions of care between the in-patient and out-patient venues of care.
4. Existing interventions and approaches have successfully demonstrated (through the CMS ESRD Demonstration Project) that improved clinical outcomes and reduce costs can be achieved.
5. The cost of care for kidney diseased patients is disproportionately high when compared with other chronic disease states and the general Medicare beneficiary population.

The interventions for conditions that exist in the three patient cohorts under an integrated care coordination program are designed to improve clinical outcomes, reduce cost and enhance the patient experience of care through better outcomes and more persistent attention from a multidisciplinary team. These activities can be divided into four categories that cross over one or more of the three patient cohorts including:

1. Education
2. Case management
3. Clinical care protocols and algorithms
4. Experience of care measurement tools

CKD Interventions

Assessing the interventions for the CKD population requires a focus on a number of primary drivers of improved outcomes. Programs in this area predominantly focus on education and case management including education of the patient on renal replacement therapy options, patient preparation for either transplantation or dialysis if and when the patient continues to progress, control of diabetes and high blood pressure in an effort to delay the progression of renal disease and identification of other co-morbidities, primarily cardiovascular, that can lead to increased morbidity and mortality. In addition, this group of patients requires appropriate counseling on issues of depression and end of life/palliative care. Interventions including an organized, structured, multi-disciplinary care team provide nutritional counseling, psychosocial counseling, medication counseling and medical attention to minimize the impact of co-morbid diseases, slow progression of CKD and prepare for Renal Replacement therapy should it become necessary are paramount to improving overall patient outcomes. [10]

Other specific results and goals include:

1. Timely referral from the primary care physician to the nephrology team which centers on co-management of the CKD patient with gradual transition of principal care from a primary care provider to the nephrologist as CKD progresses.
2. Reduction of high mortality rates in late stage CKD. A higher than expected proportion of patients die prior to having an opportunity for renal replacement therapy. CKD is an independent risk factor for early mortality. [11]
3. Early intervention in the complications of late stage CKD to improve patient outcomes and quality of life. These complications of CKD include symptomatic anemia, bone and mineral metabolism abnormalities, infection risk and nutritional challenges.
4. Improvement in the quality of life and patient experience in CKD. The psychosocial issues within the patient and family environment have an impact on the patient's functional status and quality of life as renal disease progresses.
5. Assuring a usable permanent dialysis access and a plan to avoid central venous catheters for patients who must start Renal Replacement Therapy.

Incident ESRD Interventions

Incident ESRD patients comprise those within the first 120 days of initiation of dialysis, are at the highest risk for hospitalization and death. Patients who have initiated dialysis without preparation such as CKD education and permanent access placement will benefit from intensive educational activities and case management at the start of dialysis. [12] Incident ESRD patient education and case management should help the patient and patient's family understand the complications of renal disease including anemia, bone and mineral metabolism, nutrition, infectious complications as well as, the need to address the psychosocial issues related to the impact that renal replacement therapy has on functional status and quality of life. Interventions during this period include education and case management to address catheter avoidance and vascular access care, nutritional supplementation in the event of a malnourished state, appropriate education on laboratory results and other metrics related to the core physiologic abnormalities of advanced renal disease, vaccinations for seasonal influenza, hepatitis and pneumococcal vaccine, appropriate care for co-morbid diseases especially highlighting the risks of cardiovascular disease, congestive heart failure, and fluid overload.

For Incident ESRD patients that receive renal replacement therapy through dialysis the specific performance objectives include:

1. Adequate preparation for renal replacement therapy to avoid beginning treatment in an unstable and unprepared situation known as "crashing" into dialysis. A crash into dialysis, an "unplanned" or "suboptimal start" to dialysis is associated with increased morbidity and mortality. [13]
2. Education on the primary modalities of care in an effort to enhance compliance, reduce depression and help patients make good choices for renal replacement therapy that fit within their lifestyle and capacities.
3. Clinical treatment and dialysis prescriptions associated with stabilization of the target weight, dialysis delivery, medication compliance and nutrition to avoid the extremely high early mortality and hospitalization.
4. The period of care up to 120 days from the start of dialysis defines the incident period. A directed effort to help achieve patient "graduation" to become a prevalent ESRD patient where the risk for hospitalization and mortality is reduced.

Prevalent ESRD Interventions

Prevalent dialysis patients, patients who are on dialysis and who are stable 120 days after initiation of dialysis therapy, as a group have improved outcomes compared to the incident dialysis population. [14] After 120 days ongoing supportive and educational activities should focus on the sustainability of the dialysis treatment modality enhanced by patient compliance with a properly prescribed dialysis regimen. The patient must partner with the dialysis care team to avoid decisions about activities and conditions that place them at additional risk.

Likewise the multi-disciplinary healthcare delivery team must provide coordinated care to protect patients from additional risk for adverse outcomes related to their co-morbidities. The healthcare team must be a resource to assist patients in making individual decisions about care.

For ESRD patients with multiple co-morbidities and for elderly patients with ESRD the healthcare team must continuously support the efforts of the patient, patient's family and caregivers to define goals of care. This ongoing assessment of goals of care can become critical at times when a patient becomes unstable or less functional. The healthcare team should be prepared to assist in decision making by the patient and their family regarding end of life care through a thoughtful and individualized approach. [15]

The healthcare team must develop a process of care to improve patient outcomes at times of transitions of care. Patients who move from one healthcare environment, such as the inpatient hospital setting, to another healthcare environment like the outpatient dialysis clinic requires special attention. Medication adjustment and reconciliation should be specifically addressed following an acute illness. After hospitalization erythropoietin dosing for anemia, dry-weight reassessment, and nutritional reassessment should occur as the patient re-enters the prevalent outpatient dialysis environment.

In the prevalent dialysis patient population the intervention opportunities fall into a number of categories that afford the renal disease patient an opportunity to minimize hospitalization and risk. These interventions include:

1. Educational activities regarding best practices and compliance with medical therapy
2. Specific therapy for complications related to co-morbid conditions
3. Vascular access maintenance and management
4. Frequent nutritional assessment and support particularly following hospitalization or acute illness
5. Clearly defined goals of care with attention to maintenance of functional capacity and quality of life
6. Mitigation of infection risk including recommended vaccination for Hepatitis B, Pneumococcus and seasonal influenza
7. Maintenance of circulation and aggressive avoidance of Peripheral Vascular Disease and the multiple risk of revascularization interventions
8. Aggressive shared decision-making and planning for end of life care if the patient's condition continues to progress and deteriorate

Accountable and Coordinated Renal Disease Care

As part of the Patient Protection and Affordable Care Act in 2010 the Department of Health and Human Services under the health reform initiatives developed a model of Value-Based purchasing that incorporates performance risk and shared savings into a payment platform for delivering accountable and coordinated care. This concept of Accountable Care Organizations (ACO) grew out of a variety of care coordination, disease management and patient-centered medical home initiatives that have been previously demonstrated by the Centers for Medicaid and Medicare Services (CMS). Further, CMS administrator, Dr. Donald Berwick, has articulated the concepts of a philosophy called the *Triple Aim* theory which includes the tri-fold goals of better health for patients, better health for communities and lower costs of care. [16]

Between 2005 and 2009 CMS performed an end-stage renal disease demonstration project that provided a capitation payment model for renal disease care with three disease management organizations. These entities each individually focused on specific areas of intervention. The results supported the concepts of care coordination for renal disease and were acknowledged as successful to varying degrees for each organization. The EndStage Renal Disease (ESRD) Disease Management Demonstration Evaluation Report produced by Arbor Research Collaborative for Health noted: [17]

...The results on patient-centered experiences and provider acceptance suggest the potential for Disease Management to improve patient satisfaction with their ESRD care, specifically through a patient's interaction with their NCM who coordinates health care services. Similarly, providers perceived that the Disease Management model of integrated care delivery also improved the quality of care delivered to their patients. It allowed providers to feel they had a greater impact on improving the quality of care and patient quality of life. ...-End Stage Renal Disease (ESRD) Disease Management Demonstration Evaluation Report

The proposed rule for the Accountable Care Organization was delivered to the medical community in the spring of 2011. This ACO rule offered an opportunity for primary care physicians and hospitals to develop legal entities that would take risk over a minimum of a three year period on at least 5,000 Medicare beneficiaries within a community and benefit in the Shared Savings achieved from a higher degree of coordination and reduction in hospitalizations that would be expected. During the period of assessment and comment on the accountable care proposed rule the renal community, including nephrologists, nephrology organizations and dialysis providers, highlighted the complex nature of CKD and ESRD care and suggested CMS consider a kidney disease centered care coordination effort for CKD and ESRD patients The benefits of a renal specific care coordination model for integrating renal disease care was appreciated by CMS, yet the path toward a renal specific ACO was complicated by the specific focus of the ACO model in primary care.

As part of the health reform activities, the Affordable Care Act also set in motion a sub-organization within CMS called The Center for Medicare and Medicaid Innovation (CMMI) to look at novel and innovative health delivery models. This "Innovation Center" offers a path for members of the dialysis and nephrology communities to come together to develop a set of principles for integrated kidney care that can be piloted on a large scale and ultimately achieve similar goals to those of the Shared Savings Program. These principles begin with the development of integrated kidney care models for end-stage renal disease patients receiving dialytic therapy. The participating organizations would be sponsored by nephrologists, nephrology groups, joint ventures between these medical groups and dialysis providers, and licensed dialysis facilities. The development of the principles for the pilot would include up to 50,000 patients over the three year period and the minimum five year agreement. Each integrated renal disease organization would be led by a sponsoring nephrologist medical director and shared governance among the nephrologist and other parties participating in the integrated care organization. As with the Primary Care driven ACO model, the goal would be a documented model of care that is patient centered, approved by the organization governing body and approved by CMS. In addition the renal care coordination organization would be primarily focused on quality improvement along with internal cost and quality reporting, ongoing analytic performance analysis and risk sharing on the cost of care for the renal disease patient requiring dialysis.

Because patients with end-stage renal disease can be identified and assigned relatively simply via the traditional CMS Form 2728 Medical Evidence Attestation, the ability to attribute a patient into the renal integrated care program would occur with initiation of dialysis. Patients would remain within the program until they either relocated out of the area of service where the pilot is occurring, the agreement ended, or the patient died.

As with Accountable Care Organizations a benchmark would be set for historical Part A and Part B spending. Outlier patients would be removed from the benchmark and their spending requirements adjusted for the co-morbid characteristics that lead to excessive costs in a predictable fashion. Within this shared savings and loss relationship the sponsors would have the opportunity to take risk on the overall cost of care as well as risk on quality performance within four domains including:

1. Experience of care
2. Preventative health
3. Renal disease process and outcomes
4. Coordination in co-morbidity management

As with the Primary Care ACOs there would need to be requirements for waivers from physician self-referral, anti-kickback and beneficiary inducement laws such that interventions and programs could be made operational within the integrated care organizations. The renal integrated care organizations would be allowed to receive shared savings, distributions and quality incentive bonuses while integrating interventions and technology without the impediment of the anti-kickback or inducement laws. These primary principles have been agreed upon such that both large and small providers of dialysis care and nephrology practices could participate in this shared savings model program. The degree of performance risk would accommodate a spectrum of risk from pay for performance incentives for appropriate process outcomes to full symmetric risk sharing on gains and losses on the cost of care for an individual patient against the benchmark.

Conclusion

In conclusion, the opportunity to identify and structure an integrated and coordinated approach to the care of patients with renal disease is desirable. Patient with renal disease represent a small number of beneficiaries with very high utilization and costs of care. There are specific health delivery models that have been shown to deliver improvements in measurable components of care while reducing the overall costs to the health system helping to support this population of patients with advance kidney disease. The efforts of the federal government to promote the ACO model and the demonstration that ESRD care under an integrated care program is well received by patients and can have positive results in quality and cost efficiency creates a compelling argument that renal disease care offers a good opportunity to align the interests of patients with the interests of the payers who support the programs that deliver care to those suffering from advanced stages of CKD.

References

[1] Institute of Medicine. Crossing the Quality Chasm, A New Health System for the 21st Century. Washington: National Academy Press; 2001.

[2]   healthcare.gov [www.healthcare.gov]. Washington DC: Department of Health and Human Resources. The Affordable Care Act One Year Later. 2011 [cited 2011 Jun 3]. Available from: http://www.healthcare.gov/law/introduction/index.html.

[3]   AHRQ [www.ahrq.gov].Value Based Purchasing 2011 [cited 2011 Jun 3]. Available from: http://www.ahrq.gov/qual/meyerrpt.htm.

[4]   AHRQ [www.ahrq.gov], Never Events Primer 2011 [cited 2011 Jun 3]. Available from: http://psnet.ahrq.gov/primer.aspx?primerID=3.

[5]   Milstein A, Ending Extra Payments for "Never Events" – Stronger Incentives for Patient Safety. NEJM. 2009;360(23):2388-2390.

[6]   USRDS ADR 2010, Chapter 9: Costs of Chronic Kidney Disease, 2010; pp 133-135.

[7]   Kidney Disease Outcomes Quality Initiative [www.kidney.org], New York: KDOQI Guidelines; [cited 2011 Jun 12]. Available from: http://www.kidney.org/+ professionals/kdoqi/guidelines_commentaries.cfm.

[8]   Internal Communications with Dr. Raymond M Hakim, Fresenius Medical Care North America, Continuum of Care for CKD, 2011.

[9]   USRDS ADR 2010, Chapter 1: CKD in the General Population, 2010; pp 44-46.

[10]   Levin A. The need for optimal and coordinated management of CKD. Kidney Int. Suppl 2005 Dec;(99):S7–S10.

[11]   Go A, Chertow G, Fan D, McCulloch C, Hsu C. Chronic kidney disease and the risks of death, cardiovascular events, and hospitalization. N Engl J Med. 2004 Sep 23;351(13):1296-305.

[12]   Wingard RL, Pupim LB, Krishnan M, Shintani A, Ikizler TA, Hakim RM. Early intervention improves mortality and hospitalization rates in incident hemodialysis patients: Right Start program. Clin J Am Soc Nephrol. 2007 Nov;2(6):1170-5.

[13]   Barrett BJ, Garg AX, Goeree R, Levin A, Molzahn A, Rigatto C, Singer J, Soltys G, Soroka S, Ayers D, Parfrey PS. A Nurse-coordinated Model of Care versus Usual Care for Stage 3/4 Chronic Kidney Disease in the Community: A Randomized Controlled Trial. Clin J Am Soc Nephrol. 2011 Jun;6(6):1241-7.

[14]   Internal Communication Dr. Kevin Chan, Fresenius Medical Care North America. 2011

[15]   Renal Physicians Association. Shared Decision Making in the Appropriate Initiation of and Withdrawal from Dialysis. Rockville MD: RPA Publication, 2nd edition, 2010.

[16]   Berwick D, Nolan T, Whittington J. The Triple Aim: Care, Health, And Cost. Health Affairs. 2008; 27(3):759-769.

[17]   Arbor Research Collaborative for Health. End Stage Renal Disease (ESRD) Disease Management Demonstration Evaluation Report. Ann Arbor MI, December 8, 2010, p. 8.

Index

A

access, xvii, 1, 7, 9, 16, 23, 26, 28, 29, 30, 33, 38, 39, 43, 45, 60, 61, 71, 75, 76, 82, 113, 115, 117, 126, 127, 136, 142, 178, 180, 190, 202, 247, 270, 275, 286, 288, 296, 297, 298, 299, 300, 301, 302, 303, 304, 305, 306, 308, 313, 334, 335, 337

access device, 76

accommodation, 70

accountability, 332

accounting, 19

acetic acid, 68

acid, 4, 68, 116, 150, 151, 164, 173, 174, 176, 182, 184, 189, 198, 200, 204, 210, 248, 253, 286

acidosis, 36, 51, 149, 151, 154, 155, 156, 162, 163, 164, 176, 195, 202, 203, 314

acquaintance, 9

acquired immunity, 174, 175, 185

acquisition of knowledge, 40

acute kidney injury, 1, 6, 23, 49, 56, 57, 124, 126

acute renal failure, 16, 28

adaptation(s), 136, 329

adhesion, 173, 175, 180, 188, 209, 313

adipocyte, 259, 263

adiponectin, 263

adipose, 141, 158, 213, 263

adipose tissue, 141, 158, 213, 263

adiposity, 136, 195

adjustment, 17, 25, 94, 139, 252, 255, 256, 326, 328, 330, 337

adolescents, 31, 32, 98, 104, 105, 107, 108, 111, 112

adults, 103, 105, 106, 107, 108, 109, 151, 182, 194, 215, 253, 259, 260, 262, 263

advancement(s), 1, 3, 5, 10, 11, 13, 17, 19, 27

adverse effects, 126, 129, 141, 265, 266

adverse event, 98, 177, 332

advocacy, 59

aerobic capacity, 330

African-American, 298

age, 9, 16, 17, 21, 26, 42, 43, 45, 46, 51, 52, 61, 67, 70, 71, 89, 90, 91, 94, 96, 97, 106, 119, 123, 124, 128, 135, 208, 219, 251, 253, 256, 266, 277, 298, 305, 309, 310, 321, 323, 325, 326, 329

aggregation, 313

aging population, 309, 317

agonist, 250, 314

AIDS, 159, 179

albumin, 21, 78, 137, 151, 162, 176, 178, 193, 194, 195, 197, 200, 201, 202, 203, 204, 205, 206, 247, 252, 255, 257, 272, 284, 322, 323, 325

albuminuria, 27

aldosterone, 36, 137, 138, 310

alertness, 131

algorithm, 245

allergic reaction, 129

alpha-tocopherol, 189

alters, 161, 176, 187

American culture, 124

American Heart Association, 312, 318

amino acid(s), 150, 152, 153, 176, 194, 198, 200, 204, 286

aminogram, 203

amyloidosis, 12, 184

anabolic steroids, 21

anabolism, 218

analgesic, 314

anastomosis, 297, 302

anatomy, 138, 306

anemia, xvii, 21, 22, 23, 31, 32, 138, 141, 174, 182, 186, 187, 243, 244, 245, 246, 247, 248, 249, 250, 256, 312, 313, 316, 335, 337
aneurysm, 301
angiography, 311
angioplasty, 300, 301, 305, 306, 307
angiotensin converting enzyme, 175, 188
angiotensin II, 149, 154, 156, 164, 166, 176, 255, 261
anorexia, 130, 176, 197, 204, 310
anorexia nervosa, 204
antibiotic, 75, 190
antibody, 59, 171, 174, 187, 302
anticoagulant, 4, 5
antigen, 56, 171, 173, 180, 184, 187, 188
antigenicity, 173
antihypertensive agents, 32, 103
antihypertensive drugs, 107, 108
anti-inflammatory drugs, 314
antioxidant, 189
anxiety, 130
aorta, 57, 215
aortic stenosis, 211
aortic valve, 211, 217, 311, 312, 318
APC, 171, 175
aplasia, 248, 250
apoptosis, 169, 171, 174, 177, 178, 179, 180, 183, 184, 190, 191, 192
apoptotic pathways, 180
appetite, 108, 176
arginine, 261
arrest, 57, 215
arteries, 210, 217, 296, 297
arteriogram, 297
arteriography, 38
arteriovenous shunt, 66
artery, 54, 55, 59, 89, 138, 175, 188, 215, 216, 217, 275, 297, 306, 308, 311, 312, 318, 319
arthritis, 178, 188
asbestos, 75
ascites, 138
ascorbic acid, 173, 248
aseptic, 117
assessment, 18, 25, 51, 52, 53, 59, 136, 141, 143, 144, 146, 147, 148, 249, 271, 273, 290, 291, 313, 316, 324, 325, 328, 329, 336, 337, 338
assets, 39
asymptomatic, 146, 311
atherogenesis, 170, 184
atherosclerosis, 21, 164, 170, 176, 177, 184, 186, 207, 208, 209, 213, 214, 218, 254, 256, 258, 261, 306, 310, 317
ATP, 138, 152, 163, 164

atria, 137
atrophy, 154, 159, 160, 161, 162, 163, 164, 165
audit, 91
authority, 25
autoantibodies, 186
autoimmunity, 175, 188
automation, 79
autonomy, 124, 126, 127, 128
autopsy, 262
autosomal dominant, 212
avoidance, 46, 144, 314, 336, 337
awareness, 35, 36, 125, 127

B

Bacillus subtilis, 68
bacteremia, 178
bacteria, 116, 180
bacterial infection, 174
bacterial pathogens, 190
bacterium, 117
balloon angioplasty, 301, 305, 307
barriers, 43, 47, 56, 63, 81, 129, 143, 199, 299
basal lamina, 158
base, 20, 23, 50, 116, 138, 164, 205, 206, 250, 253
basement membrane, 216, 280, 284
batteries, 116, 257
behaviors, 60, 322
benchmarks, 325
beneficial effect, 92, 181
beneficiaries, 113, 332, 333, 338, 339
benefits, 14, 16, 22, 36, 59, 70, 77, 119, 125, 127, 128, 131, 136, 143, 272, 298, 328, 329, 338
benign, 60
bias, 91, 97, 201, 326
bicarbonate, 116, 145, 155, 164, 165, 180, 288, 323
bile acids, 286
bilirubin, 194, 287
biochemistry, 153
biocompatibility, 12, 179, 180
biocompatible materials, 12
bioethics, 15
biological fluids, 277
biomarkers, 146, 168, 311
biopsy, 52, 63
biosynthesis, 203
bleeding, 312, 313, 314, 315, 318
blindness, 70
blood, 3, 4, 5, 11, 12, 21, 23, 36, 43, 51, 54, 56, 57, 60, 61, 67, 68, 69, 71, 76, 79, 80, 93, 100, 103, 106, 107, 111, 117, 135, 137, 138, 139,

142, 144, 145, 146, 147, 148, 151, 152, 173, 174, 175, 176, 177, 178, 179, 180, 184, 185, 186, 187, 189, 191, 246, 247, 249, 251, 252, 253, 254, 255, 256, 257, 258, 259, 260, 261, 262, 272, 273, 274, 275, 279, 281, 282, 283, 284, 285, 286, 287, 288, 290, 299, 302, 305, 306, 312, 313, 319, 323, 333, 335

blood circulation, 117

blood flow, 54, 57, 67, 272, 274, 275, 279, 281, 284, 285, 286, 287, 290, 299, 302, 305, 306

blood monocytes, 185

blood pressure, 21, 36, 51, 68, 69, 80, 93, 100, 103, 106, 107, 111, 135, 137, 138, 139, 142, 144, 145, 146, 147, 148, 175, 254, 255, 273, 290, 312, 313, 323, 335

blood transfusion(s), 5, 21, 23, 68, 76, 173, 174, 178, 179, 186

blood urea nitrogen, 176, 319

blood vessels, 57, 79, 302

blueprint, 16

body image, 321

body mass index (BMI), 141, 142, 150, 177, 195, 197, 198, 199, 200

body size, 269, 277

body weight, 139, 141, 151, 155, 160, 197, 201, 267, 277, 278

bone(s), xvii, 23, 24, 169, 197, 207, 208, 209, 210, 211, 212, 213, 214, 215, 216, 218, 219, 220, 248, 250, 251, 254, 257, 258, 259, 260, 264, 265, 321, 328, 335

bone cadmium content, 252

bone form, 208, 209, 210, 211, 212, 213, 214, 215

bone growth, 216

bone marrow, 169, 248

bone mass, 219

bone resorption, 210, 211, 212, 213, 214

bone volume, 213

bonuses, 339

brain, 31, 57, 63, 142, 285

branching, 297

brass, 252

breakdown, 19, 152, 153, 156, 159, 162, 165, 173

Britain, 29

burn, 149, 154

burnout, 45

buttons, 75

buyer, 18

bypass graft, 59, 308, 312, 318, 319

C

C reactive protein, 252

cachexia, 108, 140, 150, 151, 154, 159, 166, 261

cadmium, 251, 252, 256, 257, 258, 262, 263, 264

calcification, 2, 24, 109, 141, 177, 207, 208, 209, 210, 211, 212, 213, 214, 215, 216, 217, 218, 310, 312, 316

calcium, 24, 51, 107, 155, 162, 208, 210, 212, 213, 214, 216, 248, 253, 254, 264, 288, 310, 312

caliber, 305, 308

calorie, 101, 143, 204

calvaria, 218

cancer, 60, 150, 154, 155, 159, 160, 164, 181, 183, 185, 245, 257, 260, 262

candidates, 14, 15, 27, 50, 59, 60, 68, 72, 73, 123, 310

capillary, 12, 137, 275, 276, 284, 285

capital expenditure, 120

carcinoma, 60, 64, 159, 167, 168, 181, 262

cardiac catheterization, 56

cardiac muscle, 158

cardiac output, 275, 285

cardiac risk, 318

cardiac surgery, 181, 310, 312, 315, 316, 317, 318

cardiomyopathy, 31, 138, 140, 145, 146

cardiopulmonary bypass (CPB), 181, 313, 315

cardiovascular disease, 24, 52, 70, 76, 115, 120, 168, 177, 189, 215, 254, 257, 259, 260, 261, 262, 309, 310, 317, 330, 334, 336

cardiovascular function, 144

cardiovascular morbidity, 116, 207, 243

cardiovascular risk, 83, 177, 208, 216, 261, 314, 317

care model, 338

caregivers, 125, 127, 336

caregiving, 132

carotenoids, 173

carotid bruit, 296

cartilage, 210, 217

cartoon, 66

case study, 262

catabolism, 160, 168, 195, 203, 212

catheter, xviii, 8, 16, 26, 43, 75, 99, 117, 126, 190, 247, 275, 297, 299, 302, 336

cation, 145

cattle, 158, 165

causation, 208

CD8+, 174, 179, 187

CD95, 179

CDC, 60

cell culture, 175, 176, 187

cell death, 169

cell differentiation, 175, 187, 207, 209, 211

cell line, 175, 183, 208
cell membranes, 272, 280, 281
cell metabolism, 149
cell signaling, 163
cell surface, 259
cellulose, 4, 5, 11, 12, 180
cellulose triacetate, 180
central nervous system, 137
certification, 24, 44
ceruloplasmin, 151, 259
challenges, 1, 3, 7, 21, 27, 33, 96, 116, 120, 177, 303, 324, 335
chemical(s), 13, 66
chemokines, 169
chemotaxis, 173, 184
Chicago, 5, 66, 304
childhood, 103, 104, 105, 107, 109, 196
children, 14, 31, 76, 85, 97, 98, 101, 102, 104, 105, 107, 108, 109, 111, 112, 196, 260, 295
Chile, 69
China, 263
Chinese women, 262
chlorine, 13
cholecalciferol, 175
cholesterol, 151, 176, 177, 310
cholinesterase, 313, 319
chondrocyte, 210
chromium, 247, 251, 252, 259, 264
chronic diseases, 43, 150, 174, 249, 265, 322, 333
chronic illness, 79
chronic kidney disease, 1, 23, 32, 33, 36, 37, 46, 110, 114, 121, 132, 146, 149, 161, 165, 167, 183, 186, 188, 193, 205, 207, 208, 216, 217, 218, 219, 220, 243, 244, 245, 246, 247, 248, 249, 253, 254, 260, 261, 263, 310, 318, 319, 327, 333, 334
chronic kidney failure, 164
chronic renal failure, 18, 28, 31, 32, 66, 82, 109, 163, 181, 183, 186, 188, 203, 204, 205, 218, 246, 264, 313, 317, 319
circulation, 7, 57, 117, 138, 140, 180, 275, 295, 337
cirrhosis, 138
cities, 14, 17, 259
clarity, 57, 125
classes, 37, 38
classification, 23, 24, 33, 215
cleavage, 154, 155, 180
cleft palate, 215
clinical application, 298
clinical assessment, 273, 316, 324
clinical examination, 141, 145, 147

clinical interventions, 69
clinical symptoms, 191
clinical trials, 21, 22, 81, 308
clone, 21
closure, 46
clustering, 167
cognitive dysfunction, 253
cognitive function, 31
cognitive impairment, 128, 130, 325
cognitive skills, 40
coherence, 125
collaboration, 12, 15, 23, 98
collagen, 145, 188, 209
collateral, 295
colon, 159
colonization, 190
color, 129
commercial, 1, 5, 54, 198, 332
common signs, 296
communication, 9, 15, 16, 23, 36, 38, 46, 59, 70, 71
communication skills, 46
community(ies), xvii, xviii, 13, 14, 15, 23, 27, 36, 66, 79, 115, 116, 128, 193, 206, 323, 337, 338
comorbidity, 45, 94, 97, 312, 329
comparative analysis, 99
complement, 36, 170, 171, 179, 180
complexity, 43, 153, 156, 322
compliance, 24, 91, 111, 138, 141, 142, 143, 329, 336, 337
complications, 56, 64, 67, 68, 78, 99, 104, 108, 113, 115, 117, 118, 149, 150, 151, 152, 154, 156, 174, 249, 256, 265, 296, 299, 307, 315, 332, 333, 335, 337
composition, 136, 181, 191
compounds, 170, 252
comprehension, 39
compression, 313
computer, 245
conductivity, 76, 278, 285, 286
conference, xvii, 24
configuration, 284, 298
conflict, 126, 127, 128
confounders, 252, 255, 256
congestive heart failure, 21, 116, 121, 135, 138, 147, 316, 336
Congress, 15, 16, 20, 25, 68, 73, 121, 123, 142, 245
conjugation, 152, 153
consensus, 24, 59, 125, 126, 128, 306, 332
consent, 49, 57, 59, 60
consolidation, 25
constipation, 129

construction, 5
consulting, 38
consumption, 113, 136, 139, 193, 196, 200
contact time, 17, 19
containers, 17, 76
contamination, 178, 257
contingency, 127
continuous ambulatory peritoneal dialysis (CAPD), 77, 85, 86, 139
contour, 116, 117
control group, 253, 254, 302
controlled studies, 115
controlled trials, 20, 86, 97, 98, 266, 289
controversial, 52, 168, 170, 303
controversies, 15
convergence, xvii
cooperation, 66, 324
coordination, 20, 334, 337, 338
COPD, 43
copper, 251, 252, 259, 264
coronary artery bypass graft, 59, 312, 318, 319
coronary artery disease (CAD), 89, 138, 306, 311, 318
coronary heart disease, 146, 257
correlation, 255, 257
corrosion, 76
corticosteroid therapy, 315
corticosteroids, 7
cost, 1, 3, 13, 14, 15, 16, 17, 18, 19, 20, 25, 26, 50, 51, 54, 65, 66, 68, 69, 70, 72, 75, 76, 79, 80, 81, 85, 91, 92, 95, 98, 101, 111, 116, 125, 137, 143, 193, 201, 202, 246, 265, 266, 271, 291, 302, 326, 331, 332, 333, 334, 338, 339
cost saving, 26
costimulatory molecules, 173
cotton, 4, 11
counseling, 130, 143, 198, 205, 325, 328, 335
covering, 2, 15
craving, 139, 140
c-reactive protein (CRP), 168, 175, 176, 178, 180, 201
creatinine, 51, 67, 91, 92, 93, 94, 96, 99, 118, 119, 176, 177, 253, 254, 256, 257, 270, 271, 277, 284, 285, 286, 287, 288, 312, 314, 319, 323
creativity, 5
crises, 39
critical analysis, 146
criticism, 69
cross sectional study, 92, 93, 148, 183
crystals, 212
cultural differences, 128
culture, 79, 124, 128, 174, 175, 176, 209, 216

cure, 151
cycles, 67, 91, 92, 276
cycling, 75, 82, 99, 100, 247
cyclooxygenase, 189
cysteine, 155, 189, 258
cytochrome, 156
cytokines, 151, 159, 160, 168, 169, 170, 171, 173, 174, 175, 176, 177, 179, 180, 187, 189, 192, 209, 258, 263
cytoplasm, 152
cytoskeleton, 191
cytotoxicity, 169

D

daily living, 45
damages, 258
data set, 20, 51, 323
database, 88, 244, 312
death rate, 161, 205
deaths, xviii, 76, 86, 88, 159, 254, 309, 311, 332
decay, 3
defects, 150, 162, 163, 216
defence, 168, 181
deficiency(ies), 154, 158, 176, 204, 213, 214, 216, 247, 248, 249
degradation, 149, 150, 152, 153, 154, 155, 156, 159, 160, 162, 163, 164, 174, 194, 202, 203, 291
dehydration, 195, 290
delayed gastric emptying, 176
dementia, 26, 325
demographic characteristics, 70, 326
demographic factors, 324
dendritic cell, 171, 173, 174, 183
denial, 46, 59
deoxyribonucleic acid, 189
Department of Health and Human Services, 63, 64, 305, 322, 331, 337
dependent variable, 69
deposition, 216, 308
depression, 79, 126, 130, 322, 323, 328, 335, 336
deprivation, 174, 177
depth, 21, 27, 98, 126, 136, 297, 298
dermatitis, 196
detectable, 138
detection, 43, 192, 316
developing nations, 196
deviation, 268, 269, 283, 327, 328
diabetes, 21, 43, 45, 49, 51, 52, 59, 89, 90, 113, 115, 121, 124, 154, 156, 160, 178, 188, 189, 207, 208, 209, 213, 214, 215, 216, 219, 244,

346 Index

251, 253, 258, 260, 261, 263, 305, 306, 310, 315, 321, 323, 326, 334, 335
diabetic nephropathy, 212, 218, 253, 260
diabetic neuropathy, 311
diabetic patients, 251, 253, 254, 255, 258, 263, 264
diagnostic criteria, 161, 205
dialysis, xvii, xviii, 1, 3, 4, 5, 6, 7, 8, 9, 10, 11, 12, 13, 14, 15, 16, 17, 18, 19, 20, 21, 22, 23, 24, 25, 26, 27, 28, 29, 30, 31, 32, 35, 37, 38, 39, 40, 41, 42, 43, 44, 45, 46, 47, 49, 50, 51, 58, 59, 61, 65, 66, 67, 68, 69, 70, 71, 72, 73, 74, 75, 76, 77, 78, 79, 80, 81, 82, 83, 85, 86, 87, 90, 92, 93, 96, 97, 98, 99, 100, 101, 102, 103, 104, 105, 106, 107, 108, 109, 110, 111, 113, 114, 115, 116, 117, 118, 119, 120, 121, 123, 124, 125, 126, 127, 128, 129, 130, 131, 132, 133, 135, 136, 138, 139, 141, 142, 143, 144, 145, 146, 147, 148, 150, 152, 155, 161, 167, 168, 171, 176, 177, 178, 179, 180, 181, 182, 185, 187, 189, 190, 191, 192, 193, 195, 198, 199, 200, 201, 202, 203, 204, 205, 206, 208, 215, 218, 244, 247, 248, 249, 251, 252, 254, 256, 258, 259, 261, 262, 265, 266, 267, 268, 269, 270, 271, 272, 273, 275, 276, 277, 278, 279, 280, 281, 282, 283, 284, 285, 286, 287, 288, 289, 290, 291, 295, 296, 297, 298, 299, 301, 302, 303, 305, 306, 307, 308, 309, 310, 311, 312, 313, 314, 315, 317, 318, 319, 321, 323, 324, 325, 326, 327, 328, 329, 330, 333, 335, 336, 337, 338, 339
diastolic blood pressure, 254
dichotomy, 211
diet, 4, 10, 27, 38, 51, 105, 108, 136, 143, 150, 151, 152, 160, 196, 197, 198, 203, 204, 205, 209, 211, 257, 321
dietary intake, 136, 143, 277
differential diagnosis, 204
diffusion, 92, 140, 273, 274, 275, 276, 277, 280, 281, 282, 284, 285, 286, 287, 288
diffusion rates, 277
diffusivity, 272
dignity, 124, 129, 131
dilated cardiomyopathy, 138, 140
dilation, 298
diluent, 160
direct measure, 278, 322
directors, 25
disability, 16, 115, 119, 144, 154
disappointment, 3, 300
disaster, 24
discitis, 129
discomfort, 75, 119, 291

disease progression, 253
disease rate, 20
diseases, 43, 52, 150, 163, 167, 168, 174, 179, 190, 202, 249, 258, 260, 264, 265, 311, 316, 322, 333, 335, 336
disequilibrium, 270
disorder, 24, 167, 196, 207, 219, 220
disproportionate growth, 85, 86
dissatisfaction, 61
distress, 328
distribution, 19, 70, 80, 137, 152, 194, 202, 204, 212, 214, 267, 277, 278, 285, 287
diverticulitis, 202
dizziness, 142
DNA, 171, 180, 192, 256
DNA repair, 256
doctors, 124
dogs, 5, 158, 165
donors, 51, 53, 56, 57, 58, 59, 60, 61, 63, 64, 209, 212
dosage, 103, 106, 107, 211
dosing, 19, 25, 32, 245, 306, 337
double-blind trial, 204
down-regulation, 189
drainage, 71, 115
dream, 7
drugs, 50, 61, 107, 108, 115, 120, 135, 139, 173, 176, 178, 194, 291, 302, 314
due process, 128
dyslipidemia, 310
dyspnea, 311

E

economic problem, 81
economics, 3, 19, 121
edema, 3, 97, 137, 142, 145, 147, 151, 196, 296, 297
editors, 81, 144, 145, 161
education, 14, 15, 26, 33, 36, 37, 38, 39, 40, 42, 43, 44, 46, 47, 60, 61, 71, 143, 301, 335
effluent, 68
egg, 205
electrical conductivity, 285
electricity, 70, 71, 117
electrolyte, 66, 116, 119, 145, 314
electrolyte imbalance, 119
elucidation, 175
embolism, 4
emergency, 127
emotion, 9
emotional distress, 328
emotional health, 322

emotional stability, 68
emotional well-being, 322
emphysema, 263
employers, 39
employment, 16, 40, 120, 143
empowerment, 36, 46
encephalomyelitis, 175
encoding, 154, 155, 163
endocarditis, 178
endocrine, 208
endothelial cells, 261, 302
endothelial dysfunction, 188
endothelium, 147
endotoxemia, 178, 188
endotoxins, 171, 177
end-stage renal disease (ESRD), 3, 28, 29, 31, 32,
    33, 46, 81, 85, 87, 109, 111, 121, 126, 133,
    135, 136, 146, 161, 182, 185, 186, 188, 196,
    215, 243, 244, 247, 251, 252, 254, 256, 258,
    261, 262, 309, 310, 317, 318, 321, 324, 329,
    333, 334, 337, 338
endurance, 9, 154
energy, 21, 41, 51, 74, 116, 117, 151, 161, 176,
    194, 195, 197, 198, 203, 204, 205, 213, 244,
    254, 257, 258, 310, 321, 322
energy expenditure, 204
engineering, 1, 66, 77, 247
England, 13, 15, 18, 163, 164, 315, 318
environment, 24, 25, 35, 43, 44, 52, 105, 108,
    113, 115, 120, 136, 166, 216, 252, 262, 335,
    336
enzyme(s), 149, 152, 153, 156, 174, 175, 187,
    188, 194, 259, 302
enzyme inhibitors, 175, 187
epidemic, 255
epidemiology, 177, 190, 253, 261
epithelial cells, 189, 276
Epstein Barr, 60
equilibrium, 19, 77, 82, 276
equipment, 7, 9, 44, 68, 70, 71, 72, 75, 78, 115,
    116, 178, 300
erythrocyte membranes, 285
erythrocytes, 275, 284, 287
erythropoietin, 1, 21, 31, 32, 103, 181, 186, 187,
    190, 243, 246, 247, 248, 250, 337
ethical issues, 15, 64, 69
ethics, 3, 126
ethnicity, 124
ethyl alcohol, 4
ethylene, 7
etiology, 3, 248, 300
EU, 116, 180
Europe, 5, 22, 75, 106, 303, 324

Eurotransplant, 109
evidence, 20, 21, 23, 60, 72, 81, 89, 90, 91, 97,
    98, 100, 115, 137, 144, 145, 150, 151, 155,
    158, 174, 184, 201, 202, 208, 210, 214, 218,
    252, 254, 257, 277, 280, 288, 290, 297, 298,
    306, 331, 334
evolution, 13, 32, 39, 218
exchange transfusion, 5
exclusion, 53
excretion, 29, 51, 137, 168, 214, 262, 270
execution, 169
exercise, 31, 44, 71, 111, 154, 244, 321, 328, 330
Expanded Criteria Donor (ECD), 49
expenditures, 17, 25, 120, 333
experimental autoimmune encephalomyelitis, 175
expertise, 38, 45, 53
exploitation, 245
exposure, xvii, 60, 72, 169, 179, 180, 191, 251,
    252, 253, 254, 255, 256, 257, 258, 259, 260,
    261, 262, 263, 291
external validity, 86
extra-cellular fluid volume (ECFV), 135
extracellular matrix, 173, 208, 209
extracts, 163

F

fabrication, 28
factories, 256
families, 39, 46, 69, 115, 124, 125, 126, 127, 128
family environment, 335
family history, 310
family life, 70
family members, 38, 115, 125, 143, 158
family relationships, 37
fantasy, 63
fasting, 150, 164
fat, 139, 141, 151, 161, 177, 196, 197, 209, 211,
    212, 213
fatty acids, 173, 194
FDA, 9, 21, 22, 23, 32, 73, 142, 244
FDA approval, 73
fear, 42, 71, 129
fears, 71, 79
Federal Government, 29, 332, 339
federal mandate, 252
Federal Register, 33, 63, 329
feelings, 41
ferritin, 248, 249, 255, 323
fertility, 107, 321
fertilizers, 257
fetuin-A, 176, 207, 211, 212, 214, 218
fever, 177, 189

fiber(s), 1, 11, 12, 29, 158, 166, 275
fiber membranes, 12
fibrinogen, 203
fibroblasts, 208
fibrosis, xviii, 135, 138, 140, 145, 146, 248
filters, 75, 103, 105
filtration, 23, 42, 45, 135, 136, 139, 142, 144,
    165, 195, 253, 254, 257, 271, 274
financial, 13, 68, 78, 107, 115, 128, 130, 332
financial resources, 107, 115
fistulas, 219, 298, 299, 300, 301, 302, 303, 304,
    305, 306, 307
fixation, 115
flame, 11, 29
flexibility, 40, 86
flight(s), 54, 159, 166
fluctuations, 136
fluid, 11, 13, 17, 51, 75, 80, 86, 93, 104, 109,
    115, 116, 117, 118, 120, 135, 137, 138, 140,
    141, 142, 143, 144, 147, 148, 180, 265, 266,
    272, 273, 276, 278, 280, 282, 284, 285, 288,
    290, 291, 312, 314, 327, 336
fluid balance, 93, 104
focus groups, 324
folate, 248
food, 19, 113, 115, 143, 150, 176, 201
food intake, 176
force, xvii, 13, 18, 50, 136, 151, 179, 312
formation, 24, 59, 170, 173, 174, 208, 209, 210,
    211, 212, 213, 214, 215, 216, 218, 248, 295,
    301
formula, 19, 25, 298
fouling, 274
fractures, 24
fragments, 154, 180, 192
France, 105, 108, 139
free radicals, 157, 158, 170
freedom, 40, 113, 115, 120
funding, 1, 14, 15, 66, 124
funds, 14, 66, 68, 123
fusion, 250

G

gamma-tocopherol, 189
GAO, 25
gene expression, 156, 160, 163, 165, 174, 211,
    243, 250
gene pool, 177
gene promoter, 218
gene regulation, 250
genes, 154, 163, 164, 173, 179, 191, 209, 216
genetic factors, 170

genotype, 184
Germany, 103, 108, 167, 262
glomerulonephritis, 3, 23, 138, 187
glucocorticoid receptor, 165
glucose, 6, 96, 102, 139, 169, 219, 276, 288, 291,
    312
glutamic acid, 210
glutamine, 177, 189
glutathione, 248
glycosylated hemoglobin, 258
glycosylation, 170
God, 29
governance, 24, 338
grants, 215
granules, 198
gravity, 197
gross domestic product, 124
growth, 17, 18, 67, 68, 72, 75, 85, 86, 104, 108,
    111, 112, 120, 158, 162, 164, 165, 166, 174,
    209, 216, 217, 218, 260
growth factor, 158, 164, 165, 166, 209, 218
growth hormone, 108
guidance, 126
guidelines, xvii, 2, 21, 23, 24, 27, 30, 32, 33, 91,
    125, 205, 246, 247, 249, 280, 295, 298, 300,
    301, 303, 312, 318, 333, 340
guilt, 127
gunpowder, 5

H

hair, 71
half-life, 194, 314
harmful effects, 177
HBV, 174, 178
head trauma, 164
healing, 9, 167, 168, 181, 302
health, 4, 15, 16, 18, 19, 20, 25, 26, 31, 32, 35,
    39, 42, 46, 52, 55, 56, 58, 79, 85, 94, 101, 120,
    124, 128, 130, 135, 136, 194, 202, 265, 266,
    299, 309, 317, 319, 321, 322, 324, 325, 327,
    329, 330, 331, 332, 337, 338, 339
Health and Human Services, 63, 64, 305, 322,
    337
health care, 4, 15, 19, 26, 35, 39, 42, 79, 120,
    124, 130, 194, 309, 317, 332, 338
health care costs, 79, 120, 124
health care professionals, 130
health care system, 194
health expenditure, 124
health problems, 322, 323
health status, 322, 329
Health-related quality of life (HRQOL), 321, 328

heart disease, 21, 115, 146, 244, 257, 315, 316, 318

heart failure, 21, 31, 51, 116, 121, 135, 138, 147, 159, 166, 175, 188, 190, 312, 315, 316, 318, 336

heart valves, 312

heat shock protein, 185, 189

height, 6, 277, 310

helplessness, 70, 81, 332

hematocrit, 21, 22, 32, 142, 243, 275, 330

hematoma, 301

hemochromatosis, 174

hemodialysis, 6, 13, 16, 21, 23, 26, 28, 30, 31, 32, 33, 35, 38, 39, 40, 42, 45, 65, 66, 67, 68, 69, 70, 71, 72, 73, 76, 77, 78, 79, 80, 81, 82, 83, 85, 86, 89, 95, 99, 103, 104, 105, 106, 107, 108, 109, 110, 111, 112, 113, 115, 117, 121, 123, 126, 136, 139, 140, 141,143, 144, 145, 146, 147, 148, 150, 151, 161, 162, 168, 178, 181, 182, 183, 184, 185, 186, 187, 188, 189, 190, 191, 192, 200, 202, 204, 205, 206, 212, 215, 243, 244, 245, 247, 248, 249, 250, 251, 252, 254, 255, 257, 258, 259, 260, 261, 262, 263, 264, 266, 267, 268, 269, 270, 271, 272, 274, 276, 278, 279, 280, 283, 285, 288, 289, 290, 296, 299, 303, 304, 305, 306, 307, 308, 313, 314, 317, 318, 319, 321, 324, 325, 326, 327, 329, 330, 340

hemoglobin, 21, 22, 23, 32, 141, 152, 243, 244, 245, 246, 247, 249, 254, 258, 322, 323

hemophilia, 61

hemostasis, 313

hepatitis, 23, 64, 68, 174, 178, 181, 185, 187, 190, 336

hepatitis a, 68, 336

hepatocytes, 263

hepatotoxicity, 263

herpes virus, 179

heterozygote, 165

HHS, 24

high blood pressure, 335

high fat, 209, 211, 212, 213

high school, 67

historical reason, 270

history, 3, 27, 28, 29, 52, 60, 139, 147, 201, 253, 254, 296, 310

HIV/AIDS, 179

home hemodialysis, 16, 26, 35, 65, 66, 67, 68, 69, 70, 71, 72, 73, 76, 77, 78, 79, 80, 81, 82, 83, 104, 106, 111, 112, 115, 121, 269, 325

home peritoneal dialysis, 16, 35, 65, 73, 75, 76, 77, 82

homeostasis, 136, 145, 161, 203, 207, 212, 219

homicide, 56

homocysteine, 170, 177, 184

Hong Kong, 17, 289

hormone(s), 108, 159, 162, 194, 212, 213, 248, 254, 256, 328

hormone levels, 328

horses, 158, 277

hospice, 127, 128, 129

hospitalization, 22, 23, 26, 107, 108, 144, 150, 161, 168, 178, 181, 243, 266, 310, 317, 323, 324, 327, 328, 329, 334, 335, 336, 337, 340

host, 54, 56, 58, 168, 181, 202

House, xviii, 13

hub, 38

human, 1, 4, 21, 31, 49, 56, 60, 61, 62, 63, 108, 117, 118, 120, 136, 158, 159, 164, 165, 181, 183, 184, 185, 186, 187, 189, 191, 193, 195, 202, 203, 209, 211, 212, 213, 215, 216, 218, 219, 243, 245, 246, 247, 248, 250, 252, 302, 312

human behavior, 60

human body, 312

human immunodeficiency virus (HIV), 60, 61, 165, 179, 247

human leukocyte antigen, 56

human subjects, 120, 195

humoral immunity, 171

Hunter, 319

husband, 66, 75

hydroxyapatite, 207, 210, 211, 212, 216

hydroxyl, 174, 255, 261

hygiene, 91

hypercalcemia, 213

hypercholesterolemia, 177, 310

hyperglycemia, 36

hyperkalemia, 319

hyperlipidemia, 214

hypernatremia, 314

hyperparathyroidism, 141, 208, 212, 214, 251, 256, 260, 330

hyperphosphatemia, 213, 214

hyperplasia, 219, 302, 308

hypersensitivity, 174

hypertension, 6, 14, 21, 23, 32, 43, 50, 51, 52, 70, 78, 110, 113, 116, 124, 135, 138, 140, 141, 144, 145, 146, 214, 251, 253, 259, 261, 262, 265, 290, 315, 316, 334

hyperthermia, 189

hypertonic saline, 143

hypertrophy, 3, 21, 93, 100, 101, 106, 108, 110, 135, 138, 146, 158, 164, 165, 182, 248, 311

hypophosphatemia, 213

hypotension, 56, 142, 147, 327

I

hypothesis, 144, 150, 186, 259
hypovolemia, 141
hypoxia, 250
hypoxia-inducible factor, 250

iatrogenic, xviii
ice pack(s), 54
ideal, 6, 7, 9, 12, 17, 83, 116, 124, 141, 142, 144, 266, 298, 328
identical twins, 63
identification, 59, 61, 335
identity, 286, 287
IFN, 171, 187
IL-17, 178
IL-8, 175, 176, 178
image, 297, 321
imbalances, 119, 136
imitation, 170
immune activation, 167, 169, 190
immune function, 184
immune response, 56, 170, 174, 175, 176, 185, 187, 188, 302
immune system, 7, 167, 168, 169, 170, 171, 172, 174, 175, 176, 178, 179, 181, 186, 187
immunity, 170, 173, 174, 175, 178, 185, 189
immunization, 171, 178
immunobiology, 50
immunocompetent cells, 169
immunodeficiency, 168, 247
immunogenicity, 51
immunoglobulins, 175
immunomodulatory, 176
immunosuppression, 56, 177, 179
immunosuppressive agent, 16
implants, 308
imported products, 252
improvements, xvii, 56, 94, 97, 120, 151, 160, 265, 271, 309, 317, 328, 339
impurities, 76
in vitro, 3, 4, 174, 183, 184, 189, 192, 209, 211, 212, 218, 219, 258, 279, 302
in vivo, 164, 180, 184, 209, 250, 279, 302
incidence, 17, 20, 26, 31, 76, 90, 99, 167, 168, 181, 190, 209, 297, 309, 311, 312, 314, 317
independence, 44, 69, 70, 71
independent living, 42
India, 69, 198
individual characteristics, 35
individuals, 86, 98, 170, 174, 178, 179, 180, 202, 254, 257, 277, 278, 310, 327
induction, 174, 178, 179, 180, 192, 313, 318

industry(ies), 4, 5, 7, 12, 19
infarction, 311
infection, xviii, 16, 24, 40, 45, 60, 61, 70, 75, 91, 99, 102, 117, 170, 177, 179, 181, 184, 190, 191, 202, 247, 251, 255, 256, 258, 301, 313, 315, 319, 335, 337
inferior vena cava, 138, 142, 328, 330
infertility, 262
inflammation, 24, 93, 101, 106, 149, 151, 156, 159, 160, 161, 164, 165, 167, 168, 169, 170, 171, 173, 174, 176, 177, 178, 180, 182, 185, 186, 188, 189, 191, 192, 195, 197, 200, 201, 203, 204, 212, 214, 247, 251, 254, 255, 256, 257, 258, 261, 263, 291, 310, 317, 318
inflammatory mediators, 160, 173
inflation, 17, 18, 25
informed consent, 49, 57, 59, 60
infrastructure, 1, 14
inhibition, 155, 160, 163, 165, 168, 175, 185, 188, 213, 259, 263
inhibitor, 188, 210, 211, 213, 214, 218
initiation, 21, 26, 43, 55, 90, 126, 129, 173, 245, 299, 310, 311, 318, 335, 336, 338
injections, 160
injury, 1, 6, 23, 49, 54, 56, 57, 124, 126, 149, 154, 155, 158, 178, 187, 203, 209, 214, 315
innate immunity, 170, 178, 185
inoculation, 61
insertion, 75, 297, 301, 307
institutions, 42, 332
insulation, 9
insulin, 4, 149, 154, 155, 156, 160, 162, 163, 164, 165, 166, 176, 178, 185, 202, 213, 219, 247, 259
insulin resistance, 149, 163, 176, 185, 202, 247, 259
insulin signaling, 162
integration, 18
intelligence, 70
intelligence quotient, 70
interferon, 175, 185
interferon gamma, 185
interferon-γ, 175
internal consistency, 324
international standards, 312
internist(s), 14, 16
interpersonal relationships, 128
intervention, 40, 47, 124, 125, 126, 127, 128, 130, 199, 200, 253, 254, 299, 300, 301, 310, 311, 316, 327, 329, 333, 335, 337, 340
intestine, 4, 170
intima, 213
inventors, 28

investment, 58
iodine, 72, 247
ions, 194
ipsilateral, 60, 313
iron, 21, 22, 173, 174, 186, 246, 247, 248, 249, 264, 323
irradiation, 7
irrigation, 75
ischemia, 49, 54, 55, 57, 140, 173, 177, 187, 212, 311
isolation, 4, 71, 290
isotope, 141
issues, xviii, 2, 3, 15, 17, 18, 20, 27, 40, 54, 57, 59, 60, 64, 68, 69, 71, 72, 73, 118, 124, 126, 128, 130, 249, 251, 299, 313, 335
iteration, 23

J

Japan, 198, 249, 259, 324
joint ventures, 338

K

K^+, 136
kidney(s), 1, 3, 4, 5, 6, 7, 11, 16, 19, 23, 24, 26, 27, 28, 29, 32, 33, 35, 36, 37, 38, 39, 40, 41, 43, 45, 46, 49, 50, 51, 52, 53, 54, 55, 56, 57, 58, 59, 60, 61, 62, 63, 64, 66, 69, 78, 79, 82, 94, 100, 101, 103, 104, 110, 113, 114, 116, 120, 121, 123, 124, 126, 129, 132, 136, 137, 138, 146, 149, 150, 154, 161, 162, 164, 165, 167, 174, 175, 176, 181, 182, 183, 186, 187, 188, 193, 196, 200, 202, 205, 207, 208, 213, 215, 216, 217, 218, 219, 220, 243, 244, 245, 246, 247, 248, 249, 251, 253, 254, 259, 260, 261, 262, 263, 265, 266, 267, 270, 272, 309, 310, 314, 315, 318, 319, 321, 324, 327, 328, 329, 333, 334, 338, 339, 340
kidney failure, 6, 7, 36, 37, 38, 39, 44, 45, 78, 164, 324, 328
killer cells, 169
kinase activity, 163
kinetic model, 267, 268, 272, 277, 278, 279, 285, 286, 288
kinetics, 19, 20, 176, 191, 203, 279, 280, 319

L

labeling, 22, 23
laboratory studies, 25
laboratory tests, 68

laceration, 54
landscape, 3, 4, 7, 331
languages, 321, 326
L-arginine, 261
laws, 24, 339
laws and regulations, 24
LDL, 173, 186, 209, 310
leaching, 76
lead, xviii, 23, 38, 39, 45, 91, 115, 125, 126, 136, 137, 139, 142, 144, 158, 174, 175, 176, 180, 194, 200, 201, 202, 251, 252, 253, 254, 255, 256, 257, 258, 259, 260, 261, 262, 263, 264, 296, 299, 300, 301, 303, 310, 314, 316, 335, 339
leadership, 23, 27
leakage, 75
lean body mass, 139, 141, 176
learned helplessness, 70, 81
learning, 54, 81
left ventricle, xviii, 138, 311
legislation, 1, 14, 15, 16, 17, 25, 72, 123
legs, 328
leisure, 68
leptin, 213
lesions, 215, 216, 307
lethargy, 129
leucocyte, 184
leukemia, 165
liberalization, 68
life expectancy, 43, 45, 61, 311, 322
life quality, 181
lifetime, 38, 43, 179
ligand, 210, 217
light, 14, 19, 103, 116, 128, 286
Lion, 181
lipid metabolism, 259
lipid peroxidation, 255, 258, 261, 262, 263
lipoproteins, 173, 177
liver, 4, 26, 137, 194, 203, 205, 258, 259, 263, 287
liver disease, 26, 287
locus, 165, 178
logistics, 58
longitudinal study, 100, 260
loss of appetite, 176
low risk, 298
low-grade inflammation, 168, 170
lumen, 117
Luo, 217
lupus, 67
lying, 291
lymphocytes, 170, 171, 174, 177, 179, 187

M

macrophages, 167, 168, 169, 170, 171, 173, 174, 175, 183, 184, 185, 189

magnesium, 210, 216, 264, 288

magnetic resonance imaging, 144

magnitude, 89, 116, 137, 141, 274

majority, xviii, 25, 50, 74, 78, 106, 115, 139, 144, 152, 270, 288, 290, 296, 333, 334

malignancy, 60, 179

malignant hypertension, 6

malnutrition, 104, 108, 140, 148, 150, 151, 161, 164, 168, 176, 178, 189, 193, 194, 195, 196, 197, 200, 201, 202, 203, 204, 247, 251, 254, 255, 256, 257, 258, 261, 263, 310, 317, 318

man, 15, 49, 61, 136, 195, 203

management, 3, 6, 7, 17, 20, 21, 23, 24, 25, 30, 39, 41, 50, 81, 102, 110, 116, 123, 128, 129, 131, 138, 139, 141, 148, 214, 245, 247, 248, 249, 291, 306, 308, 311, 314, 315, 318, 319, 321, 326, 333, 334, 335, 337, 339, 340

manipulation, 117, 161, 181

manufacturing, 12, 18, 273

mapping, 296, 298, 304, 306

marital status, 14

marrow, 169, 248

Maryland, 13

mass, 20, 67, 107, 111, 115, 139, 140, 141, 144, 146, 147, 148, 150, 151, 154, 155, 158, 159, 160, 165, 174, 176, 177, 195, 197, 200, 201, 219, 244, 267, 268, 269, 272, 274, 275, 276, 277, 278, 280, 282, 284, 288, 289

mast cells, 169

materials, 5, 7, 12, 325

matrix, 173, 208, 209, 210, 216, 217

matter, 300

maturation process, 298

measurement(s), 11, 61, 142, 148, 150, 151, 200, 258, 267, 269, 273, 278, 279, 285, 286, 287, 288, 290, 302, 311, 322, 323, 325, 329, 330, 332, 334

mechanical ventilation, 132

media, 177, 207, 208, 209, 213

median, 17, 26, 61, 89, 93, 107, 323

mediastinitis, 315

mediation, 171

Medicaid, 14, 22, 33, 63, 64, 132, 305, 322, 325, 329, 332, 337, 338

medical, 4, 5, 14, 15, 18, 20, 24, 25, 36, 38, 39, 40, 42, 45, 49, 59, 60, 81, 104, 108, 109, 123, 124, 125, 127, 128, 130, 131, 185, 262, 296, 311, 312, 322, 326, 328, 333, 335, 337, 338

medical care, 328

medical history, 296

Medicare, 1, 14, 16, 17, 18, 22, 24, 25, 26, 29, 33, 38, 63, 64, 65, 72, 73, 78, 113, 124, 132, 201, 305, 321, 322, 325, 329, 332, 333, 334, 337, 338

medication, 75, 105, 147, 168, 335, 336

medication compliance, 336

medicine, 6, 7, 132, 243

melanoma, 159

mellitus, 189, 306, 310

membrane permeability, 266, 284, 287

membranes, xviii, 3, 4, 5, 12, 13, 117, 157, 158, 180, 182, 189, 191, 192, 271, 272, 280, 282, 285, 289

memory, 169, 187

menopause, 310

mental health, 128, 321, 323

mesothelium, 275, 276

meta-analysis, 182, 244, 245, 246, 248, 251, 252, 260, 301

Metabolic, 164

metabolic acidosis, 36, 151, 155, 156, 162, 195, 202, 203

metabolic pathways, 152

metabolic syndrome, 151, 213, 218

metabolism, 51, 104, 110, 137, 149, 150, 152, 160, 162, 174, 177, 181, 187, 189, 203, 205, 211, 212, 213, 214, 219, 246, 248, 259, 310, 321, 328, 335

metabolites, 194, 314

metabolized, 314

metals, 76, 194, 251, 252, 257, 259, 263

metastatic disease, 27

methodology, 25, 26

methylation, 314

metropolitan areas, 108

Mexico, 89, 97, 102, 199

Miami, 13

mice, 138, 158, 159, 160, 162, 165, 166, 182, 187, 188, 209, 210, 212, 213, 214, 215, 216, 217, 259, 263

microgravity, 166

micronutrients, 194

microorganisms, 99

migration, 170, 173, 213, 332

military, 9

mineralization, 24, 207, 210, 214

miniature, 9, 67

Minneapolis, 204

miscommunication, 46, 128

mitochondria, 152, 156

mixing, 66, 67, 76, 285

models, xviii, 10, 98, 153, 154, 155, 156, 158, 159, 176, 193, 194, 195, 210, 211, 213, 214, 246, 267, 274, 281, 331, 332, 338, 339

modifications, 12, 19, 76

molecular biology, 31

molecular weight, 189, 265, 272, 273, 276, 277, 280, 284, 286, 287, 314

molecules, 20, 91, 92, 93, 96, 100, 106, 109, 173, 175, 180, 188

monolayer, 209

morbidity, 20, 24, 30, 31, 32, 33, 51, 65, 78, 98, 100, 103, 104, 111, 115, 116, 132, 135, 136, 139, 150, 160, 167, 207, 208, 214, 243, 251, 258, 259, 263, 266, 305, 310, 311, 317, 318, 321, 322, 323, 329, 334, 335, 336, 339

mortality, xvii, 17, 19, 20, 21, 22, 24, 30, 31, 32, 33, 40, 49, 58, 80, 85, 86, 88, 89, 95, 96, 97, 100, 103, 104, 105, 106, 109, 110, 111, 114, 115, 116, 120, 126, 132, 135, 136, 139, 140, 144, 146, 150, 160, 161, 167, 168, 170, 177, 178, 182, 184, 189, 200, 202, 204, 205, 207, 208, 212, 214, 215, 218, 243, 245, 247, 249, 250, 251, 252, 254, 255, 256, 257, 258, 259, 260, 261, 262, 263, 271, 290, 304, 305, 310, 311, 315, 316, 317, 318, 321, 322, 323, 327, 329, 334, 335, 336, 340

mortality rate, 19, 24, 49, 87, 89, 96, 100, 104, 105, 106, 109, 167, 253, 256, 271, 311, 315, 323, 335

mortality risk, 80, 104

motivation, 41

mRNA(s), 153, 154, 155, 164, 165, 166, 179, 189, 194, 195, 203, 218

mucous membrane, 61

multidimensional, 321, 322

multiple factors, 309, 310

multiple regression analysis, 256, 257

multivariate analysis, 89, 90, 255, 315

murder, 57

muscle atrophy, 159, 160, 162, 163, 164, 165

muscle extract, 163

muscle mass, 151, 154, 155, 158, 159, 160, 165, 278, 280

muscle relaxant, 313

muscle stem cells, 165

muscles, 154, 155, 159, 160, 268, 285

muscular dystrophy, 155

mutation(s), 158, 165, 210, 212, 219

mycobacteria, 187

myocardial infarction, 311

myocardium, 140

myofibroblasts, 211

myosin, 152, 154, 163

N

Na^+, 136, 137, 140, 142, 143, 144

NaCl, 135, 136, 137, 138, 139, 143

nares, 178

National Institutes of Health, 69, 82, 98, 196, 261

natural killer cell, 169

nausea, 129, 142, 176

necrosis, 169, 183, 184, 188, 191, 258, 263, 310

neglect, 147

nephrectomy, 55, 58, 64, 160

nephritis, 3, 144

nephrologist, 14, 15, 26, 35, 36, 37, 38, 39, 40, 43, 44, 61, 71, 107, 129, 132, 303, 313, 314, 335, 338

nephron, 132

nephropathy, 165, 212, 218, 253, 260

nephrotic syndrome, 138

nephrotoxic drugs, 50

nervous system, 31, 137, 138

Netherlands, 5, 16, 89, 101, 198

neurohormonal, 177

neuropathic pain, 129

neuropathy, xvii, 129, 176, 296, 311

neutropenia, 191

neutrophils, 169, 171, 173, 180, 186

New England, 13, 315, 318

New Zealand, 80, 89, 98, 126, 299, 324

nickel, 257

nitric oxide, 137, 147, 169, 174, 181, 183, 186, 255

nitric oxide synthase, 169, 174, 183, 186

nitrogen, 16, 162, 173, 176, 203, 317, 319

Nobel Prize, 153

nodules, 209, 211

norepinephrine, 137

North America, 97, 102, 106, 340

NSAIDs, 314

nucleus, 152, 156

nurses, 37, 73, 78, 129, 132, 300, 301

nursing, 14, 42, 115, 116, 120, 300

nursing home, 42

nutrient,(s) 101, 150, 176, 194, 205

nutrition, xviii, 23, 24, 93, 130, 150, 161, 164, 181, 193, 194, 197, 200, 201, 202, 205, 317, 335, 336

nutritional assessment, 337

nutritional status, 103, 106, 110, 142, 150, 161, 176, 189, 193, 195, 197, 201, 202, 204

O

obesity, 51, 113, 163, 177, 193

obstacles, 46, 115
occlusion, 300
oedema, 204
Office of Management and Budget, 18
OH, 211, 213
operations, 54, 311
opioids, 129
opportunities, 26, 37, 334, 337
optimization, 49, 58, 312
organ(s), xviii, 3, 49, 50, 51, 52, 53, 54, 55, 56, 57, 58, 59, 60, 61, 63, 64, 138, 145, 152, 208, 216, 252, 258, 280, 312, 313, 316
organic compounds, 252
organism, 136, 173
osmosis, 10, 12, 13, 29
osmotic pressure, 12, 194
ossification, 208, 210
osteoarthritis, 154, 155
osteoclastogenesis, 217, 218
osteodystrophy, 24, 129, 208, 211, 212, 214, 215, 218, 220
osteomalacia, 212, 219
osteomyelitis, 129, 178
osteopathy, 104
osteoporosis, 210, 217
outpatients, 168
overlap, 296
overnutrition, 177
overproduction, 171, 256, 258
oversight, xvii, 1
oxalate, 248
oxidation, 161, 173, 186
oxidative stress, 168, 169, 170, 176, 178, 186, 189, 190, 256, 258, 262, 263, 310
oxygen, 169, 256, 258, 261

P

pain, 119, 123, 126, 129, 130, 131, 133, 296, 314, 322, 328, 332
pain management, 129
palate, 215
palliative, xviii, 26, 27, 123, 126, 128, 130, 131, 335
palpation, 300
paradigm shift, 124
parallel, 3, 11, 29, 188
parathyroid hormone, 162, 219, 248, 254, 256, 312, 328
parathyroidectomy, 328
parenchyma, 57
parents, 15, 59, 104, 108, 109
participants, 36, 46, 63, 97, 128, 257

pathogenesis, 178, 184, 207, 208, 209, 213, 214, 246, 256, 257, 258
pathogens, 170, 171, 174, 190
pathology, 204
pathophysiological, 162
pathophysiology, 138, 161, 196, 334
pathways, 136, 152, 164, 171, 180
patient care, 23, 24, 44, 194, 202, 321, 332
patient rights, 24
pattern recognition, 170
payment reform, 1, 20, 25, 124
payroll, 124
pedal, 145
peer influence, 39
peptide(s), 137, 142, 146, 153, 155, 160, 174, 250, 286
percentile, 53
perfusion, 54, 58, 64, 311, 315
pericarditis, 311
periodontal disease, 202
peripheral blood, 177, 179, 184, 185, 191
peripheral blood mononuclear cell (PBMC), 179, 184, 191
peripheral vascular disease, 26, 202
peritoneal cavity, 17, 75, 86
Peritoneal dialysis, 1, 17, 29, 77, 79, 100, 102, 113, 272
peritoneum, 75, 272
peritonitis, 76, 85, 90, 91, 93, 97, 98, 99, 101, 178
permeability, 12, 29, 137, 180, 191, 195, 197, 203, 266, 272, 284, 287, 290
permission, 57, 115, 196, 197, 199
permit, 54, 140
peroxidation, 255, 258, 261, 262, 263
peroxide, 179
personal communication, 15, 16
personal values, 41
personality test, 15
pH, 151, 157, 158
phagocyte, 190
phagocytosis, 168, 171, 173, 174, 179, 183, 187
pharmaceutical(s), xvii, 95, 130
pharmacokinetics, 129, 178, 246, 267, 313
pharmacology, 161, 263
pharmacotherapy, 56
phenotype(s), 158, 208, 209, 210, 212, 213, 214, 219
Philadelphia, 13, 27, 81, 123, 144, 145, 161, 243
Philippines, 69
phlebotomy, 38
phobia, 71

phosphate, 25, 91, 92, 93, 96, 103, 104, 106, 107, 108, 110, 111, 120, 121, 156, 162, 176, 207, 209, 210, 211, 212, 213, 214, 216, 219, 258, 265, 270, 271, 280, 282, 289, 290, 310, 312
phosphate-binders, 103
phosphorous, 208, 209, 212, 213, 214
phosphorus, 4, 24, 99, 100, 106, 107, 108, 109, 115, 119, 208, 212, 216, 219, 322, 323
phosphorylation, 156, 158, 174, 180, 208
physical activity, 310
physical environment, 24
physical exercise, 330
physical features, 138
physical health, 321, 322, 324
physical properties, 272
physical therapy, 130
physicians, 7, 15, 16, 23, 26, 27, 37, 69, 70, 71, 73, 78, 124, 128, 129, 130, 131, 132, 201, 299, 303, 332, 333, 338
Physiological, 246
physiology, 269
PI3K, 156, 164
pigs, 16, 118
pilot study, 121, 122, 148
placebo, 22, 189, 198, 200, 250, 253, 254, 328
plants, 256
plasma proteins, 274, 287
plastics, 5, 10, 12, 29
platelets, 182, 313
platform, 337
playing, 170, 176
pleasure, 42, 46, 143
pleural effusion, 316
pneumonia, 168, 181
Poland, 12
policy, 16, 17, 18, 51, 63, 64, 68, 300
polio, 295
pollution, 257, 262
polycystic kidney disease, 138
polymer(s), 7, 9, 12, 291
polymorphism(s), 54, 63, 158, 170
pools, 19
population, 2, 18, 19, 20, 36, 53, 70, 73, 96, 97, 98, 100, 113, 114, 115, 120, 121, 124, 129, 130, 143, 170, 177, 178, 179, 189, 193, 200, 202, 251, 252, 254, 255, 257, 258, 259, 260, 309, 310, 311, 312, 313, 315, 316, 317, 321, 322, 323, 329, 333, 334, 335, 336, 337, 339
porosity, 28
portability, 115
positive correlation, 257
post-transplant, 50, 51, 52

potassium, 11, 51, 104, 108, 115, 145, 270, 288, 313, 314, 323
potential benefits, 272
poverty, 121
precipitation, 207, 210, 211, 212
pregnancy, 262
preparation, xvii, 43, 53, 76, 77, 80, 144, 246, 296, 312, 333, 334, 335, 336
preparedness, 26
preservation, 28, 40, 93, 126
President, 132
pressure gradient, 117, 139
prevention, 91, 146, 189, 190, 214, 310, 314, 317
priming, 185
principles, 20, 124, 126, 130, 131, 267, 273, 338, 339
probability, 131
probe, 40, 142
professionalism, 126
professionals, 46, 83, 126, 130, 246, 340
profit, 14, 18, 66, 72
profitability, 18
prognosis, 2, 26, 31, 125, 127, 129, 151, 176, 181, 190, 309, 311
pro-inflammatory, 168, 170, 171, 173, 176, 180
project, 13, 22, 337
proliferation, 72, 77, 158, 159, 169, 171, 173, 175, 209, 215, 216, 219, 303, 307
promoter, 156, 169, 184, 218
prophylaxis, 75, 190
proposition, 334
prostaglandins, 137
protection, 54, 55, 169, 263
protein kinase C, 145
protein structure, 181
protein synthesis, 150, 154, 156, 160, 205
proteins, 108, 149, 152, 153, 154, 155, 158, 163, 169, 171, 173, 175, 185, 187, 207, 208, 209, 210, 211, 216, 274, 287
proteinuria, 51
proteolysis, 152, 154, 155, 157, 158, 160, 163, 164
prototype(s), 1, 5, 6, 7, 11, 16, 67, 76, 118, 261
psychologist, 70
psychosis, 325
psychosocial conditions, 103
psychosocial factors, 130, 131
psychosocial stress, 310
PTFE, 308
pulmonary edema, 147
pulmonary embolism, 4
pumps, 66, 117, 275
pure water, 10, 13, 76

purification, 4, 5, 13
purity, 76, 180, 192
pyrophosphate, 217

Q

quality assurance, 273
quality control, 24, 273
quality improvement, xviii, 26, 44, 338
quality of life, 1, 21, 23, 26, 31, 32, 58, 65, 69,
    74, 78, 81, 83, 85, 93, 94, 97, 98, 101, 103,
    104, 105, 107, 108, 110, 111, 114, 115, 119,
    120, 123, 124, 126, 127, 130, 131, 135, 244,
    265, 266, 290, 321, 322, 324, 325, 328, 329,
    330, 335, 337, 338
quantification, xvii
quartile, 257
Queensland, 85

R

race(ing), 158, 165, 208, 298, 299, 323
racing performance, 165
radicals, 157, 158, 170, 174
radius, 284
reactant, 212, 218
reactions, 75, 129, 153
reactive oxygen, 169, 255, 256, 258, 261
reactivity, 174, 186, 256
reality, 5, 14, 19, 50, 51, 54, 60, 121, 268
reasoning, 42, 116
recall, 98
receptors, 159, 170, 171, 173, 184, 185, 208
recognition, 129, 170, 171, 207, 331
recommendations, 15, 23, 25, 32, 35, 128, 298,
    312, 333
reconciliation, 337
reconstruction, 307
recovery, 57
recruiting, 89
recurrence, 129
red blood cells, 152, 249, 313
redistribution, 142
reform, 1, 20, 25, 124, 332, 337, 338
regenerated cellulose, 5
Registry(ies), 3, 19, 54, 64, 77, 89, 95, 97, 98,
    102
regression analysis, 92, 94, 255, 256, 257, 258
regression model, 323
regulations, 24, 30
regulatory oversight, 1
rehabilitation, xviii, 14, 28, 65, 69, 71, 79, 81,
    103, 104, 108, 135, 144, 203, 330

rehabilitation program, 330
reimburse, 17, 72
reinforcement, 71
rejection, 7, 32, 51, 54, 63
relevance, 63, 137
reliability, 141, 144, 324
relief, 42, 126
renal cell carcinoma, 60, 64, 262
renal dysfunction, 181, 257
renal failure, 3, 15, 16, 18, 28, 30, 31, 32, 49, 66,
    67, 70, 82, 104, 109, 122, 159, 162, 163, 179,
    181, 183, 186, 188, 189, 203, 204, 205, 218,
    246, 247, 248, 252, 259, 260, 263, 264, 298,
    312, 313, 314, 317, 319
renal osteodystrophy, 24, 129, 208, 211, 212,
    214, 215, 218, 220
renal replacement therapy, xvii, 33, 42, 104, 109,
    116, 121, 181, 195, 204, 252, 266, 296, 310,
    311, 318, 334, 335, 336
renin, 36, 137, 138, 141, 310
repair, 71, 256, 306
reparation, xvii, 53
replication, 178
requirements, 24, 44, 71, 115, 141, 178, 249, 314,
    339
research funding, 66
researchers, 322
resection, 60
reserves, 165
residues, 210
resistance, 67, 149, 154, 163, 176, 181, 185, 202,
    247, 248, 259, 275
resolution, 297
resources, 13, 18, 23, 26, 37, 58, 63, 64, 107,
    114, 115, 116
respiratory failure, 315
response, 18, 23, 26, 42, 56, 108, 137, 143, 149,
    154, 155, 156, 157, 158, 159, 160, 164, 168,
    169, 170, 171, 174, 175, 177, 178, 179, 180,
    182, 185, 192, 202, 203, 218, 219, 246, 248,
    297, 302, 313, 314, 323, 324, 326, 327
responsiveness, 156, 177, 247, 248
restless legs syndrome, 328
restoration, 54, 212
restrictions, 17, 78, 103, 104, 108
retardation, 108
reticulum, 152
retirement, 119
retirement age, 119
revenue, 124
rewards, 20
rickets, 212, 219
rights, 24

risk(s), 6, 21, 22, 23, 24, 26, 31, 39, 43, 45, 49, 51, 53, 57, 58, 59, 60, 61, 64, 68, 70, 75, 80, 83, 87, 90, 93, 94, 100, 101, 104, 117, 127, 129, 135, 139, 150, 160, 161, 167, 168, 177, 178, 179, 181, 182, 190, 201, 205, 208, 212, 214, 216, 220, 252, 253, 254, 255, 257, 259, 261, 262, 263, 266, 271, 289, 290, 298, 309, 310, 311, 312, 313, 314, 315, 317, 318, 319, 324, 325, 327, 328, 332, 333, 335, 336, 337, 338, 339, 340
risk factors, 21, 31, 167, 177, 179, 181, 190, 214, 253, 261, 262, 309, 310, 317, 319
RNA, 178
rodents, 156
root, 273, 276, 284
routes, 136
rubber, 12
rules, 301
rural areas, 109

S

sadness, 39
safety, 9, 24, 52, 70, 72, 76, 250, 258, 289, 302, 308, 331, 332, 333
salts, 142
sampling error, 52
sarcopenia, 151
saturated fatty acids, 173
saturation, 248
savings, 26, 108, 120, 332, 337, 339
scarcity, 15, 116
school, 15, 67, 71, 97, 98, 103, 104, 105, 108
science, xvii, xviii, 11, 49
scientific progress, 207
scientific publications, 201
sclerosis, 208
scope, 50, 136
second generation, 77
secretion, 137, 170, 173, 184, 194, 213, 259
selenium, 173, 263
self-awareness, 127
senescence, 180
sensation, 127
sensing, 145, 207
sensitivity, 62, 63, 111, 141, 252, 255, 257, 258
sensors, 117, 137
sepsis, 154, 155, 156, 164, 165, 178, 299, 315
septic arthritis, 178
sequencing, 44
serine, 156
serotonin, 313

serum, 6, 21, 24, 30, 78, 107, 140, 151, 155, 160, 162, 166, 168, 170, 171, 175, 176, 179, 180, 181, 182, 183, 184, 188, 193, 194, 195, 196, 197, 200, 201, 202, 203, 204, 205, 207, 208, 209, 211, 212, 213, 214, 216, 218, 248, 252, 253, 254, 257, 259, 271, 290, 313, 319, 322, 324, 325
serum albumin, 21, 78, 151, 162, 193, 194, 195, 196, 197, 200, 201, 202, 203, 204, 205, 252, 257, 322, 324, 325
serum bicarbonate, 155
serum cholinesterase, 319
serum ferritin, 248
service provider, 332
services, 1, 9, 13, 17, 18, 24, 25, 27, 38, 44, 71, 120, 124, 325, 332, 338
sex, 61, 94, 277, 323
sexual activity, 60, 324
sexuality, 321
SGOT, 323
shape, 6, 9
shear, 181, 191
sheep, 158, 246
shock, 169, 173, 177, 185, 187, 189
shortage, xvii, 51, 59
shortness of breath, 316, 327
showing, 66, 93, 176, 299
side effects, 176
signal transduction, 208
signaling pathway, 156, 158, 159
signals, 158, 163, 182, 250
signs, 75, 127, 129, 141, 181, 296
simulation(s), 19, 78, 82
Sinai, 6, 113
single pass system dialysis machine, 1
skeletal muscle, 152, 158, 162, 163, 164, 165, 177, 189
skeleton, 208, 213, 214
skin, 16, 60, 61, 75, 137, 174, 178, 186, 190, 297
skin cancer, 60
smoking, 214, 262, 263, 310
smooth muscle, 173, 208, 209, 210, 211, 216, 219
smooth muscle cells, 173, 209, 216
social consequences, 104
social environment, 105
social life, 105, 327
Social Security, 14, 16, 33, 132
Social Security Administration, 33, 132
social services, 325
social work interventions, 325
social workers, 37, 73, 324
socialization, 69

society, 114, 115, 119

sodium, 3, 10, 11, 85, 92, 93, 100, 115, 136, 140, 141, 143, 144, 145, 146, 147, 165, 209, 259, 285, 288, 314

software, 270, 326

solution, 3, 11, 54, 86, 115, 314, 327

space shuttle, 166

Spain, 90

specialists, 23, 37, 38, 298, 303

species, 169, 173, 255, 256, 258, 261, 277

specific gravity, 197

specifications, 24

spectroscopy, 142, 148

speech, 28

spending, 25, 124, 339

spirituality, 131

spleen, 258, 263

Spring, 245

stability, 5, 68, 189, 314

stabilization, 334, 336

staff members, 178

staffing, 121

stakeholders, 20, 25, 51, 59, 60, 61, 62, 63, 119

standard deviation, 327, 328

standardization, 4

starvation, 154, 160, 195, 197, 203

state(s), 19, 24, 39, 44, 51, 55, 56, 70, 126, 137, 138, 141, 144, 148, 151, 158, 162, 168, 176, 177, 192, 194, 203, 208, 209, 244, 247, 249, 267, 271, 278, 282, 290, 298, 313, 315, 325, 332, 334, 336

steel, 6, 66, 76

stem cells, 165

stenosis, 211, 296, 297, 299, 300, 301, 311, 313, 318

sterile, 54, 75, 76, 116, 120, 180, 192

steroids, 21

stimulus, 209

storage, 54, 64, 137, 177

stratification, 33

stress, 25, 68, 147, 168, 169, 170, 171, 173, 176, 177, 179, 181, 182, 186, 189, 190, 191, 194, 256, 258, 262, 263, 310, 311

stressful life events, 329

stretching, 276

stroke, 115, 120, 315, 316, 319

strontium, 264

structure, 1, 24, 25, 154, 181, 219, 332, 339

style, 43, 69, 115

subcutaneous injection, 61, 160

subgroups, 178

substitution, 108, 109, 139, 173

substrate(s), 149, 152, 153, 154, 155, 161, 162

Sudan, 69

Sun, 148, 164, 188

supervision, 71, 115

supplementation, 186, 187, 193, 201, 204, 205, 206, 248, 336

supplier, 72

suppression, 138, 160, 168, 169, 170, 173, 174, 178, 187

surface area, 30, 31, 179, 266, 267, 269, 272, 273, 275, 276, 277, 284, 290, 291

surgical intervention, 120, 311, 316

surgical technique, 53, 54, 302

surrogates, 130

surveillance, 61, 179, 190, 300, 304, 322

survival, xvii, 7, 19, 21, 26, 33, 39, 45, 46, 47, 51, 59, 61, 63, 64, 65, 69, 77, 78, 80, 81, 82, 83, 88, 89, 90, 92, 93, 96, 97, 98, 99, 101, 102, 105, 106, 109, 110, 111, 121, 126, 132, 135, 139, 141, 144, 147, 159, 160, 162, 168, 174, 176, 177, 178, 182, 183, 205, 255, 264, 266, 270, 271, 289, 290, 297, 304, 306, 308, 309, 316, 317, 329

survival rate, 64, 105

susceptibility, 170, 174, 177, 185, 189

sustainability, 336

Sweden, 11, 67

swelling, 296

Switzerland, 246

sympathetic nervous system, 138

symptoms, 16, 18, 31, 71, 75, 100, 103, 129, 130, 131, 140, 141, 142, 191, 244, 266, 271, 296, 311, 327, 328

syndrome, 138, 151, 176, 204, 208, 213, 218, 247, 261, 310, 328

synthesis, 46, 150, 152, 154, 156, 160, 162, 168, 173, 176, 179, 184, 191, 194, 195, 202, 203, 204, 205

systemic lupus erythematosus, 67

systolic blood pressure, 138, 323

T

T cell, 185, 186, 187, 188, 190

T lymphocytes, 187

tactics, 36

Taiwan, 90, 251, 257, 262

target, 21, 22, 32, 96, 138, 145, 209, 216, 219, 290, 299, 312, 336

taxes, 124

taxonomy, 151

TCR, 184

teachers, 105

team members, 25, 37, 61

teams, 26, 36, 38

technical support, 72

technician, 15, 24, 120

techniques, 4, 28, 55, 125, 141, 150, 266, 278, 290, 302, 303, 304, 314

technology(ies), xvii, xviii, 1, 3, 7, 8, 9, 10, 13, 21, 27, 43, 65, 71, 78, 148, 295, 302, 339

teens, 197

telephone, 71, 75, 326

temperature, 53, 54, 67, 76

terminal illness, 127

testing, 23, 69, 141, 253, 254, 289, 297

tetraflouroethylene, 9

textbook, xviii, 145

thalassemia, 248

therapeutic goal, 19

therapeutic interventions, 81

therapeutics, 136

therapy, xvii, 1, 3, 4, 6, 7, 9, 14, 15, 16, 17, 25, 26, 27, 33, 35, 36, 38, 39, 40, 41, 42, 43, 45, 47, 50, 83, 85, 86, 89, 94, 95, 99, 104, 107, 108, 109, 113, 114, 115, 116, 119, 120, 121, 123, 124, 125, 126, 127, 128, 129, 130, 131, 135, 136, 139, 144, 154, 161, 174, 175, 176, 177, 178, 181, 185, 187, 188, 195, 203, 204, 214, 218, 244, 246, 249, 251, 252, 253, 254, 260, 264, 266, 296, 302, 310, 311, 313, 315, 318, 334, 335, 336, 337, 338

thoughts, 39

threonine, 156

thrombosis, 54, 57, 297, 298, 299, 302

time constraints, 60

time frame, 52, 327

time periods, 91, 178

tissue, 7, 16, 53, 75, 138, 141, 158, 171, 177, 213, 251, 258, 263, 275, 278, 281, 285, 302, 306

TLR, 171, 173, 178, 190

TLR2, 171, 178

TLR4, 171, 173, 178, 190

TNF, 159, 160, 163, 170, 171, 173, 174, 175, 176, 178, 179, 183, 187, 310

TNF-alpha, 183

TNF-α, 160, 170, 171, 174, 175, 176, 178, 179

tobacco smoke, 257

tooth, 215

total cholesterol, 177

total energy, 194

toxic effect, 252, 256, 257, 258

toxic metals, 251, 252, 259

toxicity, xvii, 129, 169, 176, 178, 184, 252, 262, 263

toxin, 182, 272

trace elements, 251, 252, 259, 263

training, 6, 15, 42, 44, 68, 71, 72, 73, 75, 81, 86, 91, 129, 321, 328, 329, 330

training programs, 72

transcription, 152, 153, 156, 158, 159, 162, 163, 164, 174, 186, 203, 208, 209, 215, 216, 250

transcription factors, 152, 153, 156, 158, 162, 164, 174, 186, 208, 216, 250

transduction, 208

transferrin, 203, 248

transformation, 176, 255

transforming growth factor (TGF), 158, 208, 211, 218

transfusion, 5, 174, 179

transgene, 163

translation, 325

translocation, 177, 188

transmission, 49, 60, 61, 178

transparency, 62

transplant, 1, 7, 16, 23, 26, 32, 38, 39, 40, 41, 49, 50, 51, 52, 53, 54, 55, 56, 57, 58, 59, 60, 61, 62, 63, 64, 69, 72, 78, 80, 247, 302, 319, 324

transplantation, xviii, 6, 7, 16, 28, 35, 38, 39, 41, 50, 51, 52, 53, 54, 55, 56, 58, 59, 60, 62, 63, 64, 72, 76, 103, 104, 174, 181, 309, 310, 314, 333, 335

transport, 54, 86, 91, 92, 95, 96, 100, 176, 180, 192, 212

transportation, 45, 73, 115, 120, 252

trauma, 155, 164

treatment, 1, 3, 5, 15, 16, 17, 18, 20, 22, 25, 26, 28, 31, 32, 37, 38, 40, 41, 43, 46, 52, 65, 66, 67, 68, 69, 70, 71, 72, 73, 75, 76, 77, 78, 79, 80, 81, 82, 89, 91, 92, 95, 98, 104, 105, 110, 111, 114, 115, 116, 121, 124, 125, 128, 135, 136, 139, 140, 141, 142, 143, 144, 146, 150, 151, 159, 173, 175, 176, 178, 179, 180, 186, 188, 191, 200, 205, 211, 212, 213, 214, 218, 219, 243, 245, 246, 248, 249, 250, 262, 265, 266, 267, 270, 272, 280, 291, 301, 302, 303, 305, 307, 310, 312, 317, 321, 323, 329, 330, 333, 334, 336

treatment methods, 301

trial, 19, 21, 22, 31, 69, 81, 86, 89, 91, 94, 95, 96, 98, 99, 100, 107, 108, 109, 110, 111, 118, 124, 125, 128, 130, 144, 146, 147, 148, 150, 155, 181, 189, 200, 204, 205, 206, 243, 244, 245, 298, 306, 308, 327

tumor(s), 60, 159, 183, 184, 191, 212, 219, 258, 263

tumor necrosis factor, 183, 184, 191, 258, 263

Turkey, 90

turnover, 19, 149, 150, 152, 156, 162, 164, 174, 176, 211, 212, 213, 214, 218, 219
twins, 63
twist, 137
type 2 diabetes, 189, 244, 253, 306
tyrosine, 163, 250

U

ubiquitin-proteasome system, 149, 152, 162, 164
UK, 28, 69, 95, 101, 265
ultrasonography, 304, 305
ultrasound, 142, 287, 296, 297, 298
unacceptable risk, 117
underlying mechanisms, 190
undernutrition, 177
uniform, 20, 24, 300
Union Carbide, 12
United States (USA), xvii, 1, 6, 14, 15, 17, 19, 22, 28, 29, 31, 30, 32, 35, 49, 50, 64, 65, 70, 72, 73, 78, 81, 82, 86, 87, 89, 98, 106, 126, 129, 135, 149, 161, 164, 165, 179, 190, 193, 196, 198, 199, 254, 261, 295, 303, 304, 309, 317, 321, 331, 332, 333
universe, 185
updating, 278
urban, 108, 255
urban areas, 108
urea, 3, 5, 19, 20, 22, 30, 67, 91, 92, 96, 118, 119, 169, 176, 205, 265, 266, 267, 268, 269, 270, 271, 272, 274, 275, 276, 277, 278, 279, 281, 282, 283, 284, 285, 286, 287, 288, 314, 319
uric acid, 286
urinalysis, 51
urine, 3, 94, 96, 139, 143, 168, 195, 262, 270, 271, 288, 314, 333
urologist, 12
US Department of Health and Human Services, 331
UV, 286, 287

V

vaccinations, 336
vaccine, 185, 336
validation, 318
valuation, 41, 98, 248, 262
valve, 211, 217, 310, 311, 312, 315, 316, 317, 318
valvular heart disease, 316, 318
vanadium, 251, 252, 259, 264
variables, 30, 36, 69, 89, 98, 161, 255, 256, 282, 298, 305, 323

variations, 24, 30, 270, 297, 322
vascular surgeon, 302
vascular system, 104, 136
vascularization, 215
vasculature, 57, 211, 214, 296
vasoconstriction, 138
vasodilator, 291
vasopressin, 137
vasopressor, 56
vehicles, 252
vein, 55, 297, 298, 300, 302, 304, 306, 313
velocity, 215
venipuncture, 28
venography, 306
ventilation, 132
ventricle, xviii, 138, 311
ventricular arrhythmias, 138
vertebrates, 4
vertical integration, 18
vessels, 54, 57, 79, 209, 211, 297, 301, 302, 313
virus infection, 178, 190
viruses, 179
viscera, 56
viscosity, 275
vitamin C, 248
vitamin D, 25, 187, 211, 212, 217, 219
vitamins, 194
vomiting, 129, 176

W

war, 5
Washington, 7, 9, 11, 15, 16, 64, 65, 66, 67, 68, 69, 70, 74, 75, 76, 77, 80, 81, 132, 207, 339, 340
waste, 150, 332
wastewater, 257
water, xvii, 9, 10, 13, 24, 66, 71, 72, 73, 76, 108, 115, 116, 121, 136, 137, 139, 142, 143, 145, 194, 202, 252, 259, 266, 267, 268, 269, 270, 272, 273, 274, 275, 276, 277, 278, 279, 280, 282, 285, 287, 288, 290
water quality, 24
weakness, 115
wear, 116, 117
weight gain, 45, 104, 121, 135, 139, 140, 291
weight loss, 177, 310
weight reduction, 147
well-being, 31, 74, 78, 124, 202, 322, 328, 329
whales, 277
white blood cell count, 258
white blood cells, 323
wires, 7

Wisconsin, 321
withdrawal, 126, 127, 129
wood, 4, 9
workers, 35, 37, 39, 73, 139, 257, 262, 324, 327
workload, 328
workplace, 262
World War I, 7
worldwide, 76, 107, 113, 115, 129
wound healing, 167, 168, 181
wound infection, 168, 181, 315, 319

Y

yield, 4, 158, 278
young adults, 109, 215

Z

zinc, 215, 256, 264